SAGE LIBRARY OF SOCIAL RESEARCH

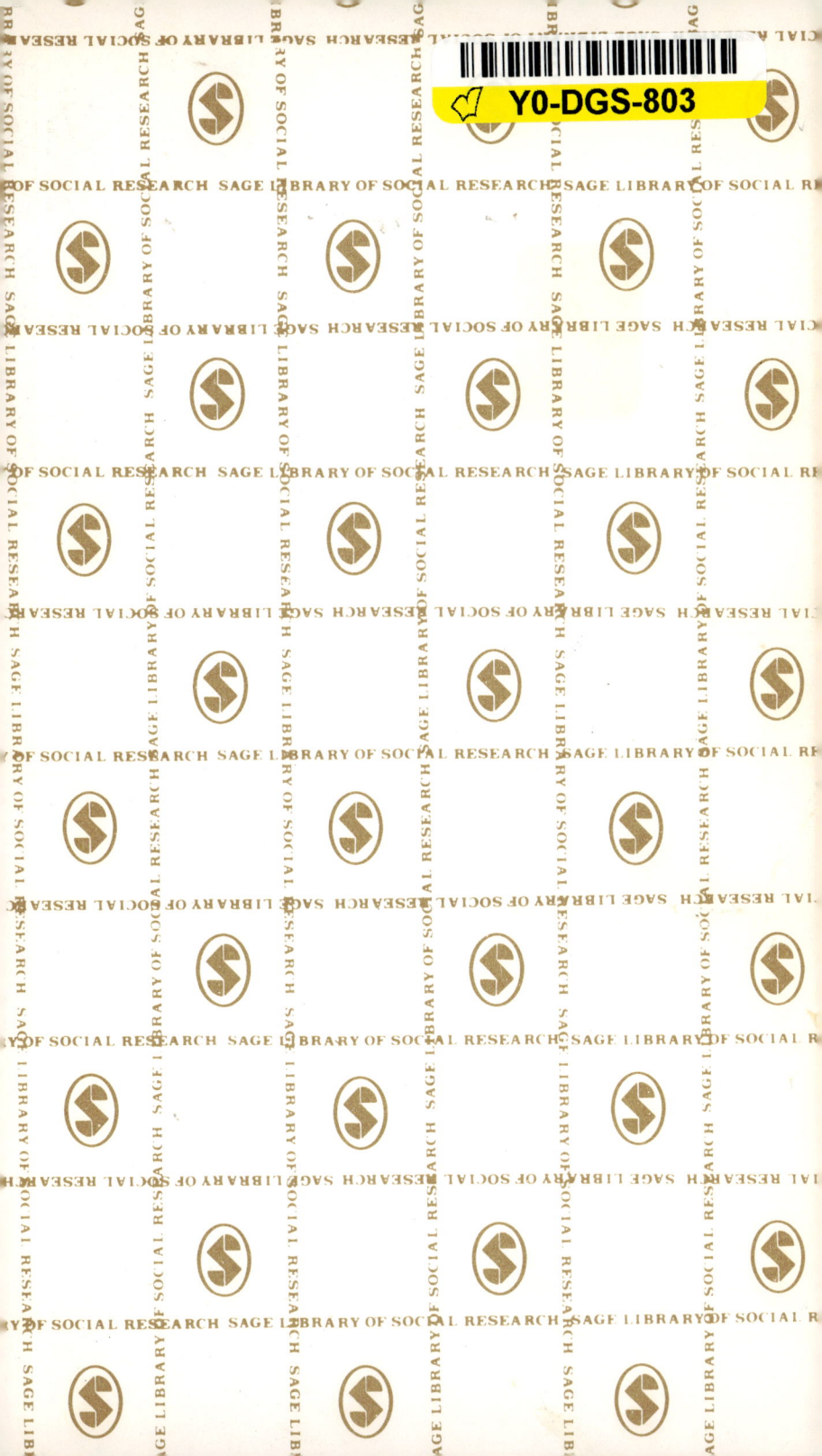

THE CANCER MISSION

Volume 103, Sage Library of Social Research

SAGE LIBRARY OF SOCIAL RESEARCH

1 Caplovitz **The Merchants of Harlem**
2 Rosenau **International Studies & the Social Sciences**
3 Ashford **Ideology & Participation**
4 McGowan/Shapiro **The Comparative Study of Foreign Policy**
5 Male **The Struggle for Power**
6 Tanter **Modelling & Managing International Conflicts**
7 Catanese **Planners & Local Politics**
8 Prescott **Economic Aspects of Public Housing**
9 Parkinson **Latin America, the Cold War, & the World Powers, 1945-1973**
10 Smith **Ad Hoc Governments**
11 Gallimore et al **Culture, Behavior & Education**
12 Hallman **Neighborhood Government in a Metropolitan Setting**
13 Gelles **The Violent Home**
14 Weaver **Conflict & Control in Health Care Administration**
15 Schweigler **National Consciousness in Divided Germany**
16 Carey **Sociology & Public Affairs**
17 Lehman **Coordinating Health Care**
18 Bell/Price **The First Term**
19 Alderfer/Brown **Learning from Changing**
20 Wells/Marwell **Self-Esteem**
21 Robins **Political Institutionalization & the Integration of Elites**
22 Schonfeld **Obedience & Revolt**
23 McCready/Greeley **The Ultimate Values of the**
24 Nye **Role Structure & Analysis of the Family**
25 Wehr/Washburn **Peace & World Order Systems**
26 Stewart **Children in Distress**
27 Dedring **Recent Advances in Peace & Conflict Research**
28 Czudnowski **Comparing Political Behavior**
29 Douglas **Investigative Social Research**
30 Stohl **War & Domestic Political Violence**
31 Williamson **Sons or Daughters**
32 Levi **Law & Politics in the International Society**
33 Altheide **Creating Reality**
34 Lerner **The Politics of Decision-Making**
35 Converse **The Dynamics of Party Support**
36 Newman/Price **Jails & Drug Treatment**
37 Abercrombie **The Military Chaplain**
38 Gottdiener **Planned Sprawl**
39 Lineberry **Equality & Urban Policy**
40 Morgan **Deterrence**
41 Lefebvre **The Structure of Awareness**
42 Fontana **The Last Frontier**
43 Kemper **Migration & Adaptation**
44 Caplovitz/Sherrow **The Religious Drop-Outs**
45 Nagel/Neef **The Legal Process: Modeling the System**
46 Bucher/Stelling **Becoming Professional**
47 Hiniker **Revolutionary Ideology & Chinese Reality**
48 Herman **Jewish Identity**
49 Marsh **Protest & Political Consciousness**
50 LaRossa **Conflict & Power in Marriage**
51 Abrahamsson **Bureaucracy or Participation**
52 Parkinson **The Philosophy of International Relations**
53 Lerup **Building the Unfinished**
54 Smith **Churchill's German Army**
55 Corden **Planned Cities**
56 Hallman **Small & Large Together**
57 Inciardi et al **Historical Approaches to Crime**
58 Levitan/Alderman **Warriors at Work**
59 Zurcher **The Mutable Self**
60 Teune/Mlinar **The Developmental Logic of Social Systems**
61 Garson **Group Theories of Politics**
62 Medcalf **Law & Identity**
63 Danziger **Making Budgets**
64 Damrell **Search for Identity**
65 Stotland et al **Empathy, Fantasy & Helping**
66 Aronson **Money & Power**
67 Wice **Criminal Lawyers**
68 Hoole **Evaluation Research & Development Activities**
69 Singelmann **From Agriculture to Services**
70 Seward **The American Family**
71 McCleary **Dangerous Men**
72 Nagel/Neef **Policy Analysis: In Social Science Research**
73 Rejai/Phillips **Leaders of Revolution**
74 Inbar **Routine Decision-Making**
75 Galaskiewicz **Exchange Networks & Community Politics**
76 Alkin/Daillak/White **Using Evaluations**
77 Sensat **Habermas & Marxism**
78 Matthews **The Social World of Old Women**
79 Swanson/Cohen/Swanson **Small Towns & Small Towners**
80 Latour/Woolgar **Laboratory Life**
81 Krieger **Hip Capitalism**
82 Megargee/Bohn **Classifying Criminal Offenders**
83 Cook **Who Should Be Helped?**
84 Gelles **Family Violence**
85 Katzner **Choice & the Quality of Life**
86 Caplovitz **Making Ends Meet**
87 Berk/Berk **Labor and Leisure at Home**
88 Darling **Families Against Society**
89 Altheide/Snow **Media Logic**
90 Roosens **Mental Patients in Town Life**
91 Savage **Founders, Heirs, & Managers**
92 Bromley/Shupe **"Moonies" in America**
93 Littrell **Bureaucratic Justice**
94 Murray/Cox **Beyond Probation**
95 Roberts **Afro-Arab Fraternity**
96 Rutman **Planning Useful Evaluations**
97 Shimanoff **Communication Rules**
98 Laguerre **Voodo Heritage**
99 Macarov **Work and Welfare**
100 Bolton **The Pregnant Adolescent**
101 Rothman **Using Research in Organizations**
102 Sellin **The Penalty of Death**
103 Studer/Chubin **The Cancer Mission**
104 Beardsley **Redefining Rigor**
105 Small **Was War Necessary?**
106 Sanders **Rape & Woman's Identity**
107 Watkins **The Practice of Urban Economics**

THE **CANCER** MISSION

Social Contexts of Biomedical Research

Kenneth E. Studer
and **Daryl E. Chubin**

Foreword by **Robert S. Morison**

Volume 103
SAGE LIBRARY OF
SOCIAL RESEARCH

SAGE PUBLICATIONS Beverly Hills London

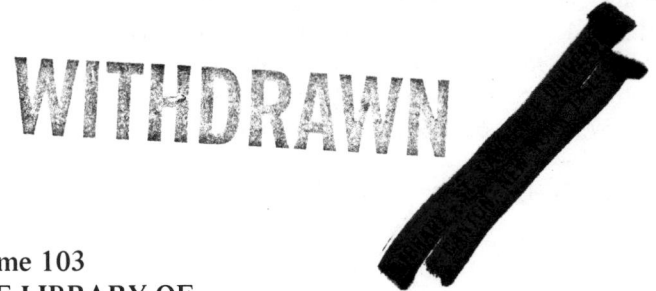

For information address:

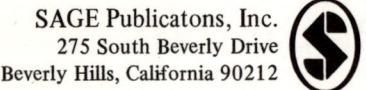

SAGE Publicatons, Inc.
275 South Beverly Drive
Beverly Hills, California 90212

SAGE Publications Ltd
28 Banner Street
London EC1Y 8QE, England

Printed in the United States of America

Library of Congress Cataloging in Publication Data

Studer Kenneth E.
Viruses and cancer.

(Sage library of social research ; v. 103)
Bibliography: p.
1. Viral carcinogenesis–Research–History.
I. Chubin, Daryl E., joint author. II. Title
[DNLM: 1. Cell transformation, Viral. 2. Neoplasms–Etiology. 3. Oncogenic viruses. 4. Reverse transcriptase. 5. Research. QZ202 S933v]
RC268.57.S8 616.99'4071 80-10312
ISBN 0-8039-1423-7
ISBN 0-8039-1424-5 pbk.

FIRST PRINTING

CONTENTS

To Elaine and Vicki

FOREWORD

There are a number of ways of reading this book—as a narrative account of a recent Nobel-worthy discovery, an exercise in the sociology of small group behavior, a critique of current theories of scientific creativity, an evaluation of the technique of citation analysis, or as an introduction to policy making in an era of Big Science. Indeed, it has something to contribute in all of these areas. But I suspect that what the authors want us to find in it most of all is an empirical approach to the epistemological problems of the life sciences. This possibility is all the more intriguing because I do not believe that this is what they had in mind when they began.

Through a series of the kinds of accidents that befall retired professors, I happened to find myself housed beside them when they started planning to exercise their recently acquired sociological tools on some segment of the scientific community. I had never seen anything like this effort before; and I watched with awe as data were assembled, cards punched, and programs debugged.

Having been trained as a biological investigator a half-century before, I suddenly discovered that in matters of history of philosophy, I had been something called an "internalist" for most of my life. Nevertheless, I had recently begun to notice that events outside science such as Mary Lasker's cocktail parties or Sydney Farber's Jimmy Fund had something to do with the setting of science policy. Still, it was difficult to get over my initial impression that the generation of new ideas and new methods by individual scientists had something to do with the progress of science. After a year or so of casual conversation about these matters, the three of us separated in search of more stable employment and I heard only rather faint and incomplete accounts of what was going on.

Suddenly, after nearly five years, the completed manuscript appeared. Obviously, the sheer labor of production has been prodigious. Furthermore, this effort has been actually, not only nominally, interdisciplinary. The authors have refined what they already knew about contemporary quantitative sociology and added to it a working knowledge of one of the most intriguing and rapidly advancing areas of modern biology. They make no pretense of qualifying as bench investigators, but they clearly know what is necessary to qualify them as "participant-observers." Their use of this ancient anthropological technique to check the hypotheses developed from the ultramodern computer readouts is particularly impressive. Indeed, it is their principal tool for forging a firm bond between externalist and internalist interpretations.

What really carries the reader through the massive accumulation of data and interpretation is the repeated discovery of bits and pieces derived from still a third discipline–speculative philosophy. In spite (or perhaps because) of the fact that neither author is a philosopher, it is the occasional finding of epistemological raisins in their sociological cake that is likely to cause the greatest discussion and may ultimately give the book its greatest value.

Of course, it is obvious to anyone with a nodding acquaintance with the philosophy of science that the field has been almost wholly preoccupied with physics and mathematics. There are many reasons for this. By and large, it is easy to dissect and isolate physical systems into subsystems consisting of very few variables. When this is successfully done, it turns out that the physical models have a seductive similarity to mathematical models derived by quite different means. Among other things, this similarity between certain aspects of the tangible world and the intangible logical world of mathematics has led philosophers from Pythagoras to Eddington to assert that God is a mathematician. Often there is even a hint that the reciprocal is equally true and that man can claim relationship to God through his exercise of right reason. But not even Aristotle with his atypical concern for the living world could assert that God is a biologist.

As Ian Hocking has recently reminded us in his essay on "The Emergence of Probability," even the social origins of biology are suspect. Historically, biologists were barber-surgeons, quacks, and magicians engaged at worst in a form of trade and at best in something he calls "low science." Low science customarily accepts its inability to capture the *Ding an sich* and remains primarily concerned with signs related to actual states or events only by greater or lesser degrees of probability. There is little or no pretense about knowing the world "as it really is" or might be thought to exist in the mind of God. The latter has been left to high science, which has continued to flirt with the notion that science is primarily a matter of deducing or demonstrating how things really are. Such notions as simplicity and elegance are often cited as confirmatory evidence of demonstrated truth.

True enough, nineteenth-century biology made its run for simplicity and elegance with its rediscovery of the thesis that all life comes from an egg, the formulation of cell theory by Schleiden and Schwann, and the efforts of Starling and Bayliss to explain such medical phenomena as heart failure and edema formation in simple physico-chemical terms. Somehow or other, the simple and elegant explanations never stayed put. Unlike the situation in the solar system, the perturbations often loom larger than the "systematic" variations. It is possible that God said "Let Watson be," and all was light–for a few years; but as the present manuscript points out, by 1970 information began flowing from RNA to DNA in opposition to Watson's interpretation of the central dogma. Even earlier, it became clear that information only flowed at all if permitted to do so by largely unknown but possibly protein repressors, and already there are voices referring to the horrid possibility that information might flow on occasion from proteins to nucleic acids.

This is not to say that biology is fundamentally different from physics and chemistry, much less to join the unfashionable vitalists in their flirtation with entelechy and final cause. It seems at least equally likely that the simplicity and elegance which for so long distinguished the physical from the life sciences may be something of an illusion based on the ease with which certain limited subsystems can be isolated for study. The relative inability of biology to isolate subsystems from their contexts for any length of time may explain why, as this book points out, it is difficult if not impossible to identify Kuhnian revolutions in this area. Since biologists can never be sure of anything, there are no rigid conceptual structures requiring the violence of revolution for change. An evolution is both preferable and adequate in such circumstances. Of course, indications are that the days of pseudocertainty in physics are already over and that instead of biology gradually acquiring the attributes of high science, physics is coming down off its pedestal to read the signs of probability. A quarter of a century ago, it was this uncomfortable vision of coming inelegance that prompted Enrico Fermi to observe that he would have gone into botany if he could have foreseen the mess of "particles" which would result from cutting up the uncuttable.

In the past, movements toward the unity of science have usually assumed that the ultimate union would take place under the unsullied banner of physics and mathematics. But a more complex federation may be in the making, somewhat earthier perhaps and certainly with less concern for a divine order. If so, this present eyewitness account and statistical analysis of what biologists actually do may help to guide the way.

To one who grew up in the sphere of influence of Percy Bridgman, it is interesting to follow our present authors' discussion of the close relation between methods and concepts. Though Bridgman himself was a physicist, his ideas seem to have found their readiest welcome and made their most indelible mark in behavioristic psychology. Although conventional biologists may also have been more receptive to "operationalism" over the years than the physicists, most of them would probably disagree with orthodox behaviorism when it forbids the investigator to go beyond inputs and outputs to look inside the black box. Similarly, one may predict a lively discussion of the pages in this book which imply that the methodology is the message. Some will certainly wonder if the authors are not carrying empiricism rather far when they use the evidence of maximal citation to stake a claim of conceptual equality between Lowry et al., Darwinian theory, and the discovery of DNA.

In summary, this is an exciting book because it opens discussion of new ideas and new variations on some very old ones. Most significant, perhaps, is the effort to bring empirical evidence to bear on topics which have had to rely mostly on speculation and intuition. Particularly impressive in this connection is the effort to bring internal and external observations of scientific behavior into some kind of congruence. It is clear that, although the book is concerned with methodological and theoretical matters, the authors have had practical objectives in mind from the beginning. For two decades post-Sputnik, science policy has in theory been largely the prerogative of experienced men and women of sound judgment. In practice, it has also involved a number of special interests and people with axes to grind. Analysis of alternative forms of organization and funding have been noticeably and embarrassingly lacking. Only in the last few years has one been able to observe a tentative groping for indicators of the "health of science" to guide the nation in its choice of policies. From other directions come cries for greater relevance, more accountability, and wider participation in decision making.

In the present state of the art, the authors have doubtless been well-advised to concentrate on what they themselves have learned from one very small segment of the scientific world. Their references to policy are limited to sidelong glances at the peculiar combination of aspiration, improvisation, and self-interest exhibited by the National Cancer Program. But there is at least a hint that the infant science of science may be growing rapidly enough to have something more generally useful to tell policy makers in the not-too-distant future.

Robert S. Morison

ACKNOWLEDGMENTS

This study was born late in 1974 when we were associated with the fledgling Research Program in Social Analyses of Science Systems at Cornell University. Under the liberal direction of Robert McGinnis, a generous contract (N01-OD-4-2175) from the Office of Program Planning and Evaluation of the National Institutes of Health (overseen by Helen Gee), and the sage counsel of Robert Morison, we undertook to evaluate (quite presumptuously) the research activities and products of biologists who had been funded by the National Institutes of Health. The result–five years later–is this book.

During our Cornell period, K.E.S. produced a dissertation (Studer, 1977b) which is the basis for the present work. From Cornell, he moved to the Sociology and Anthropology Department at Virginia Commonwealth University (1977). For D.E.C., next came the History and Sociology of Science Department at the University of Pennsylvania (1976-1977), then the Department of Social Sciences at the Georgia Institute of Technology (1977).

Although Cornell provided the context for our initial conceptualizations, a one-year National Science Foundation grant (SOC77-11593) from the Science Policy Research Program to D.E.C. was decisive for bringing the work to fruition (thank you, Ron Overmann). It permitted us to interview the patient and dedicated scientists who were more than indulgent by first interrupting their busy schedules and then taking an active interest in sharing their insights. The commitment of each to recapture in 90 conversational minutes the history they made created exciting and informative exchanges that no student of science should forego. This may be our story, but it is their science. So thank you Stuart Aaronson, John Bader, David Baltimore, Joseph Beard, Louis Carrese, Gary Gerard, Raymond Gilden, Maurice Green, Robert Huebner, Frank Rauscher, Jeffrey Schlom, Sol Spiegelman, Howard Temin, George Todaro, and Sue Yang.

There are many other colleagues to whom our gratitude is due. Proceeding chronologically, we thank Daniel Sullivan, Edward Barboni, and Hywel White—our "physics specialty" counterpart in SASS—who taught us, often on a daily basis, the meaning of competition. The assistance of Janice Jannett and Rita Spyker in document retrieval and data coding was indispensible, too, for our research. Today we know that those were indeed the "best and worst of times" for all of us.

In addition to all of the aforementioned, the following offered valuable critical commentary on various versions of the chapters that follow: Eugene Burns, Diana Crane, David Edge, Ron Johnston, Roger Krohn, Robert McGinnis, Michael Mulkay, Dorothy Nelkin, Richard Rettig, and Henry Small. Some confidants whose kind and critical words gave sustenance were Richard Boyd, Tom Carroll, Everett Mendelsohn, Ian Mitroff, Sal Restivo, Maurice Richter, Arnold Thackray, and Stephen Turner.

With no embarrassment, we also thank the editors of three journals who deemed two chapters contained herein as unfit for publication; their rejections convinced us that certain excerpts would not stand alone, but required more coherent, book-length treatment. However, two excerpts did emerge into the light of print (Chubin and Studer, 1978, 1979). For permission to incorporate those papers into Chapters 3, 5, and 6, we thank Elsevier-North Holland Publishing Company. We also acknowledge the University of Chicago Press for permission to reprint in Chapter 2 a figure from Diana Crane's *Invisible Colleges.*

The Department of Social Sciences at Georgia Tech has been the organizational home for the final copy of this manuscript. Without Iris Mitchell's remarkable transcription of 25 hours of recorded interviews into more than 600 pages of double-spaced text, the study would have lacked a vital dimension. Jane Holley Wilson and Valarie Carter rendered copy out of cut, pasted, and scrawled drafts. And never failing to provide sound advice to D.E.C. were Jim Camp, Patrick Kelly, Melvin Kranzberg, Morris Mitzner, Alan Porter, Fred Rossini, and Jay Weinstein. Jon Johnston was a constant source of encouragement as the final manuscript took shape.

Finally, we salute the support, understanding, and faith of our respective families throughout the years that this book evolved. One or two sentences are woefully insufficient recompense for our wives, Elaine and Vicki, and D.E.C.'s children, Rand and Jessica.

Richmond K.E.S.

Atlanta D.E.C.

PART I: THE CULTURAL CONTEXT

CHAPTER 1

BIOLOGICAL "PROBLEM DOMAINS":
The History of Cell Transformation Research

The inescapable fact is that biomedical science is a complex, interrelated, n-dimensional universe. One can wish it were not, but it is. True, there are within it some large confluences of great density, such as cancer, but even this is inseparable from other large islands such as aging, human development, etc., which in turn relate to atherosclerosis and stroke. To look at any isolated fragment, no matter how large, apart from its innumerable major and minor connections in the vast network of relationships, would be at best naive and at worst self-defeating. This reality animates the processes that the scientific community has institutionalized in the NIH, to view biomedical sciences, to the extent possible, holistically and to thereby assess opportunities not in isolation but in the context of the past state of the art and recent changes in contiguous domains of science.

Dr. James A. Shannon
(quoted in U.S. Senate, 1971a:99-100)
Former Director
National Institutes of Health

The immunologists, the molecular biochemists, and the new generation of investigators obsessed with the structure and function of cell membranes have all discovered that they are really working together along with the geneticists, on a common set of problems: how do cells and tissues become labeled for what they are, what are the forces that govern the orderly development and differentiation of tissues and organs, and how are errors in the process controlled?

Dr. Lewis Thomas (1977:167)
President, Sloan-Kettering Institute

Introduction

When one surveys the scientific terrain of the modern world, he is struck by one prominent feature: Science is big (Weinberg, 1961; Price, 1963) and appears to differ radically from the science of the pre-World War II era in its impressive formal and informal organizational arrangements. Because this feature of modern science is amenable to study by historical and sociological techniques, it can readily be understood why the sociology of science has embarked on the organizational studies which so dominate it. What this has meant, however, is that the cognitive content and structure of the disciplines under scrutiny have receded from the purview of analysis. Ideas are seen as "ghosts in the machine" of science, a phenomenon whose substratum, society, can be analyzed without need of other explanatory principles (see Whitley, 1972).

The question "Are ideas independent or dependent variables for the sociologist of science?" calls forth the problem at issue. One would think that science as a human activity devoted to the creation of a corpus of knowledge would serve as the sociologist's focus of analysis. But that has decidedly not been the case. For if ideas and knowledge are independent variables, then the sociologist must become familiar with the "technical" literature to an extent that has not been deemed feasible. Rather, this function is relegated to the (intellectual) historian of science (King, 1971) because the tacit assumption of the sociologist is that ideas are somehow ancillary to the *real* process. Such a position does not imply, however, that ideas *consequently* are dependent variables. For if ideas and knowledge are dependent variables, then the relativism of sociology which was earlier implied in the sociology of knowledge tradition (Mannheim, 1936) is called forth. This position (e.g., Phillips, 1974; Barnes, 1974), of course, has been resoundingly rejected by the dominant tradition within the sociology of science (Merton, 1949; Storer, 1966; Ben-David, 1971).

Because ideas, the cognitive content of science, are so problematic for the sociology of science, they are commonly ignored (for discussion, see Blume, 1977; Mendelsohn, 1977). No viable medium for their entrée has been found or sought beyond the occasional gesture of seeking the consultation of experts in research areas. But can consultation ameliorate the situation when one's explanatory framework has already banished ideas from its domain? We think not. Thus we adopt as a principal goal of this research to develop a framework that will allow scientific ideas to assume a vital role in the explanation and prediction of scientific development.

We shall argue that only when contact is maintained with the cognitive domain of science does the sociology of science become relevant to science policy research. While the traditional orientation to the support of science has been "What will science give us for our money?", such investment metaphors best apply to sciences that can be co-opted by technical-production sectors of the economy, for example, nuclear science. Indeed, most models seem to work better the "harder" the science (Storer, 1967) and thus hold sway by combining the high prestige of technology-laden fields, such as nuclear physics, with a high yield of observable results, such as atomic energy.

Due to the more diffuse dependency relationships of much of science, however, the investment-production metaphor of science is often inappropriate:

> Not only must science seek truth, it must seek *relatedness.* The value of chemistry as a field can hardly be decided by the chemists alone; they must ask the biologists who need the results of structural chemistry to elucidate the genetic mechanisms of the cell; or they must ask the physicists who cannot probe nuclear magnetic resonances unless they understand how the chemical environment affects the details of their NMR signals; or they must ask the reactor technologist who needs the chemistry or protactinium to design a continuous purification system in a thorium breeder. And so it is with the rest of science. The scientific merit of a field must be judged in large part by the contribution it makes, by the illumination it affords, and by the cohesion it produces in the neighboring fields [Weinberg, 1967: 116].

If this complex interrelatedness factor is at work in the sciences Weinberg mentioned, it would appear to be the sine qua non of biomedical science. To understand and correspondingly make intelligent policy decisions concerning such sciences will thus demand that their interrelatedness be unraveled, their dependencies discovered, and their intellectual advances circumscribed.

We can proceed with the task as follows: First, it is well known that the post-Crick and Watson era has generated much research interest in the cell-transforming propoerties of DNA and RNA.[1] It appears that this locus of biological interest could provide a point of departure for analysis of the intellectual and social structures of science. By tracing backward from this contemporary problem, the social and intellectual roots of cell transformation could be uncovered. It would be possible to see, for instance, just how dependent the area was on Weinberg's criteria of relatedness. What, in a word, were the historical prerequisites for progress in this area? And when some fields as divergent as Mendelian genetics and cytology converge to create classical genetics, what is it that mediates the convergence (see Ruse, 1971a; Wagner, 1968; Allen, 1975)?

Second, if disciplinary convergences stimulate the growth and specialization of science, then science policy and the sociology of science would benefit by focusing on a research site whose mediating situation is a pressing social problem. The threat to health posed by dread disease represents such a social problem. *The* dread cell-transforming disease, second only to heart disease in number of lives claimed annually, is cancer. Yet *social* studies of cancer were, until recently (see Rettig, 1977; van den Daele et al., 1977; Bud, 1978; Chubin and Studer, 1978, 1979; de Kervasdoue and Billion, 1978; Petersen and Markle, 1979), nonexistent.

Third, with the contemporary emphasis on revolutionary episodes in science, theories of science have shifted their focus a priori away from the *process* whereby scientific innovations are made and nurtured. Rather than adopting a crisis orientation to science, that is, as social discontinuities and intellectual upheavals, we seek to trace the continuities and cumulative nature of a biomedical science. Such an effort to overcome well-entrenched views (for commentary, see Laudan, 1977; Edge and Mulkay, 1976) requires a clarification of vocabulary *prior* to analysis.

Our approach to analyzing biomedical specialties is predicated on a "confluence theory" of scientific development.[2] In its simplest form this approach suggests that various "lines of inquiry" converge on a set of problems or theories which, because of the nature of biological "objects," researchers active in the field can anticipate. Against a backdrop of contemporary theorizing about scientific growth and development, this "intuition" concerning the nature of biological research appears to generate several insights. A confluence theory, therefore stipulates the following:

First, the major advances within biomedicine occur when techniques, theories, and so on from other fields of science (e.g., chemistry, physics) converge to form a biological problem domain.[3] The biological sciences appear to be organized so that such confluences of ideas and specialties come to facilitate medical practice and, in turn, alleviate health problems (see Williams et al., 1976; Thomas, 1977; Comroe, 1978).

Second, the convergence of ideas and manpower on a problem domain does not imply that a new discipline or field has been created. Sociologists enamored of traditional ideas concerning institutionalization and professional identity (e.g., Ben-David, 1971) are often at a loss to find these characteristics in biological specialties. In a sense, the most stable characteristic of professional organizational units becomes more and more distant from the actual social practice of workaday biological science. The idea structure of the units (i.e., specialties) composing the biomedical sciences (and blurring the distinction between biology and medicine) has militated against balkanization. Consequently, new conceptions of scientific identity will have to be developed to fit biomedical reality (see Bhaskar, 1975).

Finally, an analysis of one biomedical domain will reveal that most growth models of science have tacitly assumed a view of the scientific reasoning process that is foreign to biology. Judgment must be deferred as to how well these models fit physics and chemistry, but the possibility that various regions of science require *different* models of growth is a provocative notion to entertain. Ziman's assertion that "the expertise of the professional scientist is his ability to 'think physically' or 'chemically'–to transform every problem into the concepts and formulae of his discipline" (1968: 71)–should be taken seriously by the sociologist who seeks to characterize growth and specialization within biomedicine.

A History of Cell Transformation[4]

The case of cell transformation aptly summarizes many aspects of the problem outlined above:

> The revolution in the life sciences . . . [namely, the discoveries concerning DNA beginning in 1944] has produced almost as remarkable and as unexpected results as the revolution in the physical sciences which was initiated by the discovery of radioactivity. The formal lines between the several disciplines have disappeared in biology just as they were forced to break down in the physical sciences. *It is no more possible now to make a clear distinction among cytologists, geneticists, immunologists or virologists than it is among chemists, physical chemists and physicists. They attend each other's meetings, present papers on associated problems, utilize materials, techniques and instruments that, 10 years ago, either they were not interested in or had not heard of; but most importantly they have come to speak a common language, which makes it possible for them to understand one another* [Horsfall, 1960; 2; italics added].

Although Horsfall probably overstates biology as an analogue of physics (radioactivity was neither the result nor the cause of the confluence of specialties in physics), his comments nevertheless are instructive. How is it that such a confluence of fields occurred? In retrospect, how were the intellectual currents in the various fields "preparing" for this new orientation to biomedical research? What were the various intellectual traditions that were to come together and foster a new set of researchable problems? These are the questions that will be addressed in this section.

Various strands of thought regarding cell transformation must be unraveled. For the sake of convenience the strands to be discussed will be labeled the (1) viral, (2) bacterial, and (3) molecular biological traditions. As shall be seen, it is entirely incorrect to presume that these traditions are dominated, respectively, by virologists, bacteriologists, and molecular biologists. The fact, however, that information on these traditions was readily retrievable from historical and review articles, as well as their focus upon clearly delineated objects, methods, and theories, make their choice advantageous.[5] This is also not intended to suppress the fact that biomedical orientations have historically changed in all of these areas. The early researchers, whose training was in medical pathology, for instance, no doubt thought in terms of trauma, damage to cells, or inflammation, rather than of cell transformation.

THE VIRAL TRADITION

The viral tradition within cell transformation extends back into the early decades of the twentieth century. It has been known as early as 1908 that leukemia in chickens (Ellerman and Bang, 1908) was caused by viruses. Because leukemia at this early date was not as yet classified as a cancer, however, the congruity of this early finding with the tumor (oncogenic) tradition was not initially apparent (see Shope, 1966). The real impetus of the oncogenic virus tradition was the first discoveries of virus(?)-induced tumors of chickens by Rous (1911a, 1911b) in *1911* (for which he did not receive the Nobel Prize until *1966*) in the United States and virtually simultaneously by Fujinami and Inamoto in Japan.[6] Because the Rous sarcoma could be easily identified with a neoplasm, the virus tradition of cell transformation may be said to begin with Rous and Fujinami. Unfortunately, the scientific community was not ready for a viral etiology of tumors and even less for a virally induced cancer. In fact, up until the 1940s, researchers tended to refer to a "filterable agent" or a "cell free agent" rather than to a "viral induction of tumors." It is difficult to deduce much from this semantic fact, however. Probably more important for this usage was the popular operational bias of scientists during this period. Viruses were defined in terms of the methods used to isolate them; they were filterable. They were thought of as agents that could not grow by themselves and could not be seen under a microscope. Reluctance to use the term was probably further reinforced by the common association of viruses with contagious processes. This was indeed an ominous thought.

Although other discoveries of viruses (filterable agents) were periodically made over the next several decades–49 such discoveries, listed in Appendix A, were made from 1908 to 1966–they were either limited to avian viruses, which were thought not to affect mammals, or they were mammalian (human, cattle) wart viruses which were deemed uninteresting because they were not malignant. The path-finding of the 1930s, beginning with Shope's work on rabbit fibroma (Shope, 1932) and rabbit papilloma (Shope, 1933) and the work of Bittner (1936) was of critical importance in connecting viruses with malignant growths. For the first time it appeared that some "agent" in mammals, probably viral, stimulated a malignant neoplasm. The case of rabbit papilloma was to provide the mammalian analogue to the earlier discovered avian (Rous) sarcoma. It was malignant, transmittable, and progressed like any carcinoma. Moreover, the virus manifested interesting properties when taken from its natural host, the cottontail rabbit, and injected into domestic rabbits. Although the domestic rabbits developed the same malignancies as their cottontail counterparts, inoculants prepared from the domestic rabbit tumors did not induce tumors. In fact, immunity to rabbit papilloma had developed. Shope (1937) simply designated this as a process whereby the virus was "masked." But henceforth, the search for immunogenic cures for cancer became much more plausible. The path was at least cleared for more research in this direction.

Shope's discovery of rabbit fibroma also stimulated much interest in the 1930s. Rous and Beard (1934-1935) discovered that sometimes the rabbit papilloma was also capable of progressing to a cancerous stage. Although in its native hosts, again cottontail rabbits, the fibroma was not necessarily lethal, it *was* found (Duran-Reynals, 1940-1941) to be so in young domestic rabbits. And it is imperative to note the work done by Ahlström and Andrews (1938) which suggested that viruses interact with chemical carcinogens (in their case, carcinogenic tar) in producing a more virulent form of malignant fibroma in domestic rabbits. The facts that viruses react differently in their natural hosts from other hosts and that carcinogens interact with viruses were, in later years, to stimulate studies of the chemical triggering of latent viruses and the concern that viruses may be lethal to humans, though humans are not their natural hosts (e.g., simian virus 40).

Perhaps the most outstanding of all discoveries in viral research during the 1930s was that by Bittner of the mouse mammary carcinoma virus (hence the eponymy "Bittner virus") and its mode of transmission. Theories of genetic heritability of cancer had been part of the dismal cancer science for some time (Slye, 1931; see also Williams, 1960) and so the search for the transmission mechanism from generation to generation was not without its research precedent (see Gross, 1970, for an excellent review). What Bittner succeeded in demonstrating, by using a simple yet elegant experimental design, however, was that the mouse mammary carcinoma was transmitted through the mother's milk to the infant. By removing at birth the infants of high breast cancer strain of mice from their mothers and allowing them to nurse from a low breast cancer strain, he was able to disconfirm the inheritance theory and replace it with an "extra-chromosomal influence" theory of transmission (Bittner, 1936). Further experimentation quickly confirmed Bittner's results and research was extended to study the hormonal changes necessary for the triggering of this tumor agent in adult female mice. At last, not only had the virus etiology of a carcinoma been specified but also its means of transmission had been demonstrated and its interaction with another bodily system had been shown as well. It appeared that the stage was set for rapid growth of viral research on cancer.

But this was not the case at all. What occurred, as can be seen from the entries in Appendix A, was a great "slowdown" (from the 1930s to the 1950s) in new discoveries of oncogenic viruses. Although a convenient explanation for this fallow period (as for the earlier period following Rous's discovery) may be a world war, another cultural fact of equal and opposing significance for the conduct of virally induced neoplasm research in the United States was the founding of the National Cancer Institute (NCI) in 1937 (see Strickland, 1972).

The Surgeon General had appointed a committee to outline the type of research that should be carried out by the anticipated research institute. A key sentence in the report succinctly summarizes the committee's orientation to virus research:

> It considered established that mammalian cancer was not infectious, and grouped viruses with other micro-organisms as etiological agents that may be disregarded [Bayne-Jones et al., 1938: 2123].

In Table 1.1, which summarizes all of the early research grants awarded by the NCI in its first five years of existence, one project on the "properties of the papilloma virus protein" and Bittner's research are recorded. It is also remarkable to learn that, "In making the first appropriation of $400,000 for the institute, Congress provided that $200,000 of the amount should be used for the purchase of radium" (Marshino, 1944:

(text continued on p. 25)

TABLE 1.1 NCI Grants-in-Aid Certified for Payment from August 5, 1937, to June 30, 1943[a]

Grantee	Years Paid	No. of Grants[b]	Total Received[c]	Project Summaries
American College of Surgeons, Chicago	1938-42	4	$ 29,500	Clinical cancer service.
Barnard Free Skin and Cancer Hospital, St. Louis	1938-43	5	25,000	Experimental carcinogenesis.
Bittner, Dr. John J., Roscoe B. Jackson Memorial Lab., Bar Harbor, Maine	1938-39	3	14,360	Relation of nursing to breast cancer in mice.
California, U. of, Berekeley, CA	1938-42	6	93,250	Development of cyclotron for clinical research. Clinical investigations of cancer therapy with neutron ray. Testicular neoplasms. Effect of fast neutrons on cancer in humans.
Chicago Tumor Institute, Chicago	1941-42	2	27,500	Radiotherapy of radioresistant forms of cancer of the mouth, pharynx, and larynx.
Chicago, U. of, Chicago	1938-40	4	11,000	Purification of extracts of human gastric cancer. Relation of hormones to ovarian cysts. Tissue research on human-cancer etiology. Sex hormones and cancer.
Cincinnati, U. of Cincinnati	1938-43	7	27,508	Methods of diagnosis and treatment of cancer. Gastric carcinoma and chronic atrophic gastritis.

TABLE 1.1 NCI Grants-in-Aid Certified for Payment from August 5, 1937, to June 30, 1943[a] (continued)

Grantee	Years Paid	No. of Grants[b]	Total Received[c]	Project Summaries
Cornell U., New York City	1939-42	3	$ 16,400	Tissue metabolism fundamental to cancer. Quantitative study by in vitro methods of liver tumor in rats.
Duke U., Durham, N.C.	1938-40	2	3,625	Papilloma virus protein and related materials.
Harvard U., Cambridge, Mass.	1938	1	27,550	Synthesis of carcinogenic compounds.
Institute of Cancer Research, Columbia U., New York City	1938	1	8,500	Literature review to assist laboratory research workers and clinicians.
Roscoe B. Jackson Memorial Laboratory, Bar Harbor, Maine	1938-43	5	66,900	Research in genetics of cancer.
Louisiana State U., Baton Rouge, LA	1940	1	500	Photographic and art work in cancer research.
Martland, Dr. Harrison, chief medical examiner, Essex County, City Hosp., Newark, N.J.	1938	1	1,425	Osteogenic sarcomas in radioactive persons (dial painters).
Meharry Medical College, Nashville, Tenn.	1938-43	5	5,825	Establishment of record-keeping system for scientific and statistical studies.
Memorial Hospital, New York City	1940-43	3	13,300	Experimental study of tumor response to radiation. Metabolic studies on patients with gastric cancer.

TABLE 1.1 NCI Grants-in-Aid Certified for Payment from August 5, 1937, to June 30, 1943[a] (continued)

Grantee	Years Paid	No. of Grants[b]	Total Received[c]	Project Summaries
Michael Reese Hospital, Chicago	1940-42	2	$ 6,000	Significant factors in induced and spontaneous tumors. Caloric level of food intake and incidence of tumor formation.
Michigan, U. of, Ann Arbor, Mich.	1938	1	1,800	Biologic comparison of X-rays and neutrons.
National Research Council, Washington, D.C.	1938-41	3	7,000	Cooperation with American Registry of Pathology to collect and study tumors.
Nebel, B.R., New York State Agricultural Experiment Station, Geneva, N.Y.	1938	1	1,000	Cytology and physiology of non-green plant-tissue cultures.
Rochester, U. of, Rochester, N.Y.	1942	1	4,900	Metabolism in gastrointestinal cancer.
Society of the New York State Hospital, New York City	1939-42	2	11,000	Early diagnosis of gastric cancer and clinical methods.
Wallace, Dr. Edward, U. of, Cincinnati, Cincinnati	1938-40	2	5,850	Relation of pituitary gland to cancer. Climatic temperature and cancer in experimental animals.
Washington U., St. Louis	1940	1	16,000	Application of the cyclotron to treatment and study of cancer.

[a]Source: Adapted from Marshino (1944:433-435).

[b]Total number of grants 1937-43 = 66

[c]Total payment made 1937-43 = $425,693

432). It would appear that the NCI had a deeper commitment to theories of treatment than it had to discovering the etiology of cancer. But its founders also knew what they did not like—viruses—and this no doubt influenced, through funding of research at major universities, the energy expended on the discovery of new oncogenic viruses.

It is misleading to think, however, that the NCI was acting in a prejudicial manner toward the virus hunters. There is a real sense in which their discoveries were all premature. Stent has argued that "A discovery is premature if its implications cannot be connected by a series of simple logical steps to canonical, or generally accepted, knowledge" (1972: 84). But the crux of the matter is that precisely because the viral studies were embedded in "a series of simple logical steps to canonical, or generally accepted knowledge"—contrary to Stent—they were premature (see Glass, 1974). In the case of oncogenic viruses, the connections that were present within the literature on microbiology, immunology, genetics, cytology, and so on did not allow the theoretical "feedback" that would lead to mutual advancement of these disciplines.[7] It was not that connections were missing; rather, the connections that *were* made were analytically deficient and thus deceptive. Only with difficulty were the filterable agents called viruses, since techniques were lacking for analyzing such small microbiological units. Immunology had clarified the relationship to alien proteins, and thus the protein capsid portion of the virus was the focal point of interest, *not* the nucleic acid (RNA and DNA) component. A known propensity for family lines to manifest certain cancers made it easy to assume, in line with classic genetic theory, that transmission was direct and one of propensity or deficiency, rather than by an exogenous cause (see Slye, 1931). Who had ever "caught" cancer? Besides, chemical induction was already well known. And one cannot help but suspect that tumors themselves were thought of as quasi-inflammatory responses and not as the reshapers of cytological structure; in other words, cell transformation was not yet born.

In sum, at the cutting edge of research during the 1930s resided a body of information about oncogenic viruses that *was* readily integrated into the contemporary corpus of biological knowledge. Indeed, its integration was so thorough that the NCI and numerous other scientists could not envision it as the most fruitful line of research to follow. But virus research was no more premature than any of the other biological problem areas surrounding cancer research, and to say that all of a science of an era is premature robs prematurity of its meaning (see Wyatt, 1972, 1975; Lederberg, 1972; Olby, 1972).

THE BACTERIAL TRADITION

A better way to envision the growth of a research tradition which we have called viral cell transformation is to search for those historical points of intersection with other problem domains. The emerging confluence of viruses with an area that had concentrated on bacterial transformation provided one of the contexts for advancement. As Northrop has argued:

> If the transforming principle had been discovered and isolated before the discovery of the viruses, the latter would have been classified with the transforming principle, and it is doubtful if the parasite theory would have been accepted at any time [1962: 7].

But history does not unfold according to the dictates of an idealized analytical logic. The logic of the discovery process surrounding the transformation principle itself shows the circuitous route that discovery often takes.

When Griffith (1928) discovered pneumococcal type changes and for the first time labelled this process a "transformation," he was definitely not in some "teleological" fashion beginning a research tradition. The concern of his research was epidemiology and not molecular biology.

> Griffith's abiding interest, and his life's work, was the epidemiology of infectious disease and he believed that the proper understanding of epidemiological problems lay in more detailed and discriminating knowledge of infectious bacterial species and of the nature of bacterial variation. For him, therefore, as for nearly all medical bacteriologists of his time and for many years thereafter, the importance of transformation of pneumococcal types rested on the light it might throw on such problems as the evolution of bacterial virulence, the rise and fall of epidemics, and variations in the incidence of type infections. By any yardstick, the demonstration that such dramatic and specifically directed transmutations of both type and virulence might occur with considerable frequency, in epidemiologically well defined types of bacteria, was a startling enough revelation [Hayes, 1966: 12].

Given Griffith's concern for epidemiological problems, the modern molecular biological research tradition can still count him as a precursor, though it deals with an unanticipated consequence of his work. And its consequences probably would not have been so great except for the fact that "by 1928 it had been well established by particular work of Avery's laboratory [at Rockefeller Institute] that pneumococci fall into true-breeding immunologically specific types and their routes of infection can be traced by means of their polysaccharide capsules" (Hotchkiss, 1965: 4). In short, Griffith's work challenged the findings of one of America's most prestigious microbiological research groups located at the Rockefeller Institute: Act I had been witnessed, but the drama was not over. Avery's group replicated Griffith's work (Dawson, 1930) and then concentrated their efforts for the next 16 years on discovering the substance that was responsible for the transformation. In this fashion, a thought that was ostensibly easy to conceive in the context of epidemiology provided the crucial nexus for the development of another tradition (Olby, 1974a).

By tracing the important events from 1928 to 1961 in the genetic transformation of bacteria (see Appendix B) one notices that research was sluggish in the period after Griffith's discovery. Such an hiatus in a historical chronology provides a temptation once more for theorizing about the prematurity of the discovery (Stent, 1972) or the need for an anomaly, crisis, and revolution (Kuhn, 1962) before "progress"[8] could occur. But the shift in scientific focus elicited by the Griffith article was immediately significant, as can be seen from the review of the literature in the Avery et al. (1944) groundbreaking article (see Table 1.2). The very fact that the four replications of Griffith's experiments, which are cited in the Avery et al. review of the literature, occurred between 1928 and 1932, suggests the impact of the discovery. The subsequent multiple replication is one indication that the problem was well worth considering. Dawson and Alloway were even working in the same laboratory as Avery so that the continuity of the chain of transformation experiments was perhaps publicly underplayed by the "in-house" nature of the progress. In any case, this period of suspended belief in the era following Griffith's work—when old facts no longer seemed relevant—had the salutary effect of stimulating a typical, especially for biology, search strategy. The result was a looking outward from a problem nexus for relevant auxiliary information.

Avery's group was well aware, for instance, that experiments analogous to bacterial transformation had been carried out with viral transformation (Berry and Dedrick, 1936, and others in Table 1.2). A feature of their research, to be sure, was the complementarity of bacterial research by viral research which, at the same time, was altering the foundation of the former. The search for relevant information also threw into question old theories about the nature of the genetic material, but this time the questions—recurring ones at that (see Glass, 1965)—were weighed in a more propitious scientific and political climate.

(text continued on p. 31)

TABLE 1.2 Foundational Research in Cell Transformation as Seen by Avery et al.[a]

Year	Researcher	Reference	Location	Avery's Quote
1928	Griffith, F.	The significance of pneumococcal types. J. Hygiene 27:113	Ministry of Health Pathology Laboratory Great Britain	first described bacterial transformation in pneumococcus
1928	Neufeld, F., and Levinthal, W.	Beitrage zur variabilitat der Pneumokokken. Z. Immunitatforsch. 55:324	Institut Robert Koch, Berlin	confirmed original observations of Griffith
1930	Dawson, M.H.	The transformation of pneumococcal types. II. The interconvergence of type specific S pneumococci. J. Exp. Med. 51:123	Rockefeller Institute for Med. Res.	confirmed original observations of Griffith
1931	Dawson, M.H., and Sia, R.H.P.	In Vitro transformation of pneumococcal types. I. A technique for inducing transformation of pneumococcal types in Vitro. J. Exp. Med. 54:681	Dept. Med., Presbyterian Hospital, and the College of Physicians and Surgeons, Columbia, N.Y. *Sia on leave from Peiping Union Med. College, Peiping, China	confirmed original observations of Griffith
1932	Baurhenn, W.	Experimentelle Untersuchungen zur Variabilitat und zur analyse der R S-Umwandlung von Pneumokokken, mit besondern Berucksichtigung der Grunpe X. Centr. Bakt., 1. Abt., Orig., 126:68	Hygienischen Institute der Universitat Heidelberg	confirmed original observations of Griffith

TABLE 1.2 Foundational Research in Cell Transformation as Seen by Avery et al.[a] (continued)

Year	Researcher	Reference	Location	Avery's Quote
1932	Alloway, J.L.	The transformation in vitro of R pneumococci into S forms of different specific types by the use of filtered pneumococcus extracts. J. Exp. Med. 55:91	Hospital of the Rockefeller Institute for Med. Res.	"...showed that crude extracts containing active transforming material in soluble form are as effective in inducing specific transformation as are the intact cells from which the extracts were prepared."
1936	Berry, G.P., and Dedrick, H.M.	A method of changing the virus of rabbit fibroma (Shope) into that of infectious myxomatosis (Sanarelli). J. Bact. 31:50	Univ. Rochester, School of Med. and Dent.	"...succeeded in changing the virus of rabbit fibroma (Shope) into that of infectious myxoma (Sanarelli)."
1937	Berry, G.P.	Transformation of the virus of rabbit fibroma (Shope) into that of infectious myxomatosis (Sanarelli). Arch. Path. 24:533	Dept. Bacteriol. Univ. Rochester, Rochester, N.Y.	"...was successful in inducing the same Berry and Dedrick transformation using a heat-inactivated suspension of washed elementary bodies of myxoma virus. In the case of these viruses the methods employed were similar in principle to those used by Griffith in the transformation of pneumococcal types."
1937	Hurst, E.W.	Myxoma and the Shope fibroma III. Miscellaneous observations bearing on the relationship between myxoma, neuromyxoma and fibroma viruses. Brit. J. Exp. Path. 18:23	Bacteriology Dept., Lister Institute London	confirmed Berry and Dedrick and Berry's observations

TABLE 1.2 Foundational Research in Cell Transformation as Seen by Avery et al.[a] (continued)

Year	Researcher	Reference	Location	Avery's Quote
1941	Hoffstadt, R.E., and Pilcher, K.S.	A study of the 1A and OA strains of the Shope fibroma virus with special reference to the Berry transformation. J. Infect. Dis. 68:67	Dept. Bacteriology Univ. Washington, Seattle	confirmed Berry and Dedrick and Berry's observations
1942	Gardner, R.E., and Hyde, R.R.	Transformation of rabbit fibroma viruses (Shope) into infectious myxomatosis (Sanarelli). J. Infect. Dis. 71:47	Dept. Immun. and Filterable Viruses, School of Hygiene and Public Health, Johns Hopkins Univ., Baltimore	confirmed Berry and Dedrick and Berry's observations
1942	Houlihan, R.B.	Transformation of virus rabbit fibroma (Shope) into that of infectious myxomatosis (Sanarelli). Proc. Soc. Exp. Biol. Med. 51:259	Dept. Prev. Med., Univ. Virginia, School of Med., Charlottesville, Va.	confirmed Berry and Dedrick and Berry's observations

[a]Compiled from the citations in Avery, MacLeod, and McCarty (1944) and from information contained in the original articles.

Before we begin to follow the path that was to lead to the discovery of the DNA-RNA structure, we note that the "post-Avery" bacterial tradition (see Appendix B) shifted to the bacterial resistance to drugs and the analysis of transformation in human disease bacteria. In short, the field maintains close contact with epidemiology and the biomedical tradition that bore it. That this tradition articulates with immediate practical medical research should not go unnoticed.[9] Some of the developments in molecular biology which are about to be reviewed illustrate that potential paths of confluence in the biomedical sciences elude conventional classification (e.g., "theoretical" or "experimental") of some disciplines (e.g., elementary particle physics, see Sullivan et al., 1977a).

THE MOLECULAR BIOLOGICAL TRADITION

In the early decades of the twentieth century the most widely held view of genetic material was the "nucleoprotein theory of the gene" (Olby, 1974a). Some eminent biologists, however, toyed with the idea that nucleic acid was the fundamental genetic unit. Indeed, as early as 1869, Miescher had called attention to the importance of DNA (see Glass, 1965). But for numerous reasons, perhaps chief among them the inability to develop appropriate methods for assaying DNA, the protein theory gained acceptance. Hindsight tells us that the astonishing simplicity of the genetic code went unrecognized. Besides, proteins were much better understood and science was seeking answers in an area that already was sufficiently illuminated to make the search meaningful. This tactic might seem ludicrous, ex post facto, after advancements in other areas provided the researcher with a different set of intellectual guidelines. But at the time, the protein theory probably loomed as the only viable search strategy to follow. The noted American cytologist Edmund B. Wilson made this clear in 1925:

> It is an interesting fact, which has been emphasized by biochemists, that apart from the characteristic differences between animals and plants . . . the nucleic acids of the nucleus are on the whole remarkably uniform, showing with present methods of analysis no differences in any degree commensurate with those from the various species of cells from which they are derived. In this respect they show a remarkable contrast to the proteins, which, whether simple or compound, seem to be of inexhaustible variety. It has been suggested, accordingly, that the differences between different "chromatins" depend upon their basic or protein components and not upon their nucleic acids [quoted in Glass, 1965: 229].

Fisher in Germany (see Watson, 1970; Edsall, 1962) and others early in the twentieth century had already uncovered the basic structure of proteins. Much was known about the amino acids and the peptide bonding that went into the impressive "inexhaustible variety" of proteins. Nucleic acids, on the other hand, were extremely difficult to study largely because the methods available often destroyed (depolymerized, denatured) the very DNA or RNA that was being studied (Glass, 1965; Watson, 1970). This methodological blindness together with the relatively advanced state of protein chemistry made the protein theory very plausible, if not the only alternative worthy of exploitation. In short, protein was the most rational choice—the "sure bet"—for the biochemist of the time.

The odds of the biochemical wager shifted, however, as biochemistry developed. More was being learned about the functions of genes; notably the "one gene, one protein" hypothesis was developed by Beadle (1963; also see Olby, 1974a). The parameters of a better circumscribed domain of research began to emerge. The old theoretical barriers that did remain, such as the tetranucleotide hypothesis which oversimplified the nucleic acid and made it uninteresting to study, were to fall before the new analytical methods being developed in the 1940s.

For example, new methods were derived from the development of physical chemistry. The techniques of the organic chemists were, as earlier noted, destructive of the very molecules that were of growing interest to the biochemist:

> the protein chemist, before he could even start worrying about the detailed structure of a protein, needed to work very hard to be sure his protein was both chemically pure and biologically active. He had to devise gentle techniques for isolation, which avoided the usual strong acids and alkalines of organic analysis. Then he needed techniques to reveal whether his product was homogeneous, and hopefully, also to provide data on molecular size. For this sort of answer, the help of physical chemists was indispensible, and there developed a well-recognized new line of research investigating the physical-chemical properties of macro-molecules in solution [Watson, 1970: 61].

The pressure for the development of these new methods, as is intimated in this quote, came from an unflagging interest in proteins. Thus it is somewhat ironic that it was precisely these methods that eventually were to dethrone the nucleoprotein theory of inheritance and replace it with the DNA-RNA model.

In marked contrast to our presentation of the key events in the development of oncogenic virus research, research into the biochemistry of the transformation process is replete with references to new methodologies. The virus research which has been described could be called the Waring Blender-Berkefeld Filter tradition, but developments in cell transformation are virtually synonymous with the introduction of new methods in physical chemistry. A sentence from Avery et al. attests to the importance of the confluence of the rapidly developing physical chemistry methodology and this seminal research in cell transformation:

> The data obtained by chemical, enzymatic, and serological analysis together with the results of preliminary studies by electrophoresis, ultracentrifugation, and ultraviolet spectroscopy indicate that, within the limits of the methods, the active fraction contains no demonstrable protein, unbound lipid, or serologically reactive polysaccharide and consists principally, if not solely, of a highly polymerized, viscous form of desoxyribonucleic acid [1944: 156].

Electrophoresis had been developed in the late 1930s by Tiselius, ultracentrifugation had been developed by Svedberg in the 1920s, and ultraviolet spectroscopy came into its own in the 1930s (Sawyer, 1963; Edsall, 1962). It is not hyperbole to say that the work being done at the Rockefeller Institute by Avery's group depended on such advances in physical chemistry technique. When they added the caveat "within the limits of the methods," they were no doubt aware that many would say that there was protein contamination of their "transforming principle." But their careful methodological triangulation, using numerous techniques to confirm their hypothesis, revealed the state of the art of the physical chemist's tools and the need for improvement of such instruments before the science of molecular genetics could progress.

And indeed, when advances are recorded, new techniques also invariably seem to surface. When Chargaff (1947) overthew the tetranucleotide theory that had rendered DNA uninteresting, he did so by means of paper chromatography. He separated the components of DNA and discovered that the proportions of nucleotides did not support the conventional theories. And when Hershey and Chase (1952) were able to demonstrate that viruses inject DNA into the bacterial cell, their demonstration depended on the use of radioactive tracers. Building on the knowledge that protein contains sulphur but no phosphorous while DNA contains phosphorous but no sulphur, Hershey and Chase were able to utilize radioactive tracers to aid their research. By growing a bacteria culture in a medium containing radioactive sulphur, viruses that attack these bacteria will subsequently possess radioactive protein capsids. When these viruses in turn attack normal bacteria the question was, Did they leave their protein coats outside the bacteria or inject them into the bacteria? Hershey and Chase ascertained that the radioactive protein remained outside the cell. In one well-conceived experiment they confirmed the findings of Avery et al. (1944) and showed that DNA was the main information-bearing constituent of viruses.

If one considers the famous Crick and Watson conceptual "invention" of a double helical structure in 1953, one finds a physical chemistry technique at their side—X-ray crystallography. Although this method had been around since 1912 (see Law, 1973; Astbury, 1952), it was not until Bragg's student Bernal (1939) became deeply interested in discovering the structure of proteins that the technique became applicable to the macromolecule problem. When Crick and Watson were making the run for their discovery (Watson, 1968; Olby, 1970), they were running against another X-ray crystallographer, Linus Pauling, not to mention other Bragg students, such as Wilkins at King's College. The technique needed was clear to these men; the only questions were (1) who had the requisite skills to harness the method and (2) who had the requisite theoretical intuition to grasp the structure—*first*? Clearly, there is little room to doubt that the discovery of the double helical structure of DNA was largely dependent upon the development of X-ray crystallography.

From this cursory review of the molecular biology of the genetic substratum we observe a somewhat different set of people from that found in the bacterial transformation table (Appendix B). Although Avery's work intersects the bacterial transformation tradition, it is also at the critical nexus of the development of modern molecular biology. Likewise, it is not difficult to find others in Appendix B whose research interests intersect in intriguing and complicated ways with that of bacterial transformation. Ephrussi-Taylor (1951), for instance, is well known for refining the genetic theory of "crossing over"; others come to the field with interests in embryology or molecular biology. Hershey and Chase have been discussed among the molecular biologists, but if an analogous table to the bacterial transformation one based on researchers in bacteriophage were constructed, Hershey and Chase would definitely be included there, too. In the case of Avery, McLeod, and McCarty, they were quite aware of the viral research on transformation and saw it as paralleling their own research. More typically than not these pioneer researchers stood at the hub of numerous traditions.

Summary

The decision to include certain traditions of research in the above discussion was somewhat arbitrary, that is, "biased" by our knowledge of the history of the DNA-RNA revolution and an overarching interest in cancer research. Selection of other traditions, we hypothesize, would have yielded the same conclusion: Biology is organized such that the streams of thought necessarily intersect. Within this intellectual topography, streams can flow together for a while and then branch off again. This is more than a metaphor, however, since problem areas *do* come and go, created and antedated by discoveries and new knowledge claims. Yet the channels formed by the historical developments of biological specialties seem to remain as intellectual remnants for future reference. Once the short-lived "problem domain" discharges its centripetal forces into the formation of institutionalized disciplines and their specialties, the possibilities for future connectedness—as we shall see—often endure.

It is this distinctive rationality that seems to govern the biological sciences and helps to delimit the intellectual context for studying biomedical specialization. A sorting of intellectual traditions must precede attempts to understand any chronology of discovery and its social consequences within a domain. No such chronology, we would argue, can be established through manipulations emanating from a methodology that is uninformed by the research content and interests of those scientists being studied. Like a prism that scatters light, such a methodology may produce configurations which are interesting to behold but, without knowledge of its rationality, defy interpretation.

Without a model of how rationality advances in biology, and in view of the research traditions in cell transformation, the imposition of categories such as "methodological" and "conceptual" onto biological fields can only serve to mask the very structures sociologists need to perceive. It is exactly this imposition of a priori criteria that results in the "identification" of scientific specialties. What is identified for study, as we suggest in the next chapter, is nothing more than a social construction that is insensitive to the internal logic, or perhaps the confluence, of many traditions which create a problem domain. Ours, then, is an initial attempt to trace the ways of reason to, and in, these domains. For without this knowledge, there can be little understanding.

Many questions, of course, arise from our introductory discussion. Is the case of cell transformation generalizable to all of biomedicine? Has not the increased research specialization within biomedicine created a move ment toward esoterica (e.g., a chemical or molecular reductionism) which has rendered traditional confluence patterns obsolete? In Part II the analysis of the development of reverse transcriptase research will help answer some of these questions. Then the progress of the research arguments begun in the work of Ellerman and Bang, Bittner, Watson, and others will be placed in perspective.[10] It is the interplay of these traditions that will be seen from the perspective of reverse transcriptase research. In Chapter 2, however, the focus shifts to operational problems of definition and measurement, marking a transition from cell transformation in toto to one of its major traditions, research on viral transformation. As we gradually narrow the focus–from cell transformation to viral transformation to reverse transcriptase–the various dimensions of the research process, including its political context and laboratory structure, will emerge.

NOTES

1. Another consideration is, of course, the availability of numerous historical and philosophical discussions of recent developments in molecular biology. Of particular interest is the philosophical debate concerning reductionism in biology (see Hull, 1974; Ruse, 1971b, 1973; Schaffner, 1969, 1974, 1976; Smart, 1963). Schaffner's treatment of the *possibility* and yet the *peripherality* of reductionism in molecular biology is a particularly important consideration. Any hastily constructed *typologies* of the growth of biological science or the uncritical assumption that the *narrative* of a historical treatment of biology must follow the logic of reductionism seems to be totally unwarranted. The possibility that sociology might be able to contribute to this debate, we concede, was also an attraction for studying this area of biomedical science.

2. That biologists and management experts chose to call a plan for the reorganization of leukemia research (Special Virus Leukemia Program) the "convergence technique" (Baker et al., 1966; Carrese and Baker, 1967) denotes recognition of the structure of innovation within biomedicine. It describes how science should grow; what the sociologist can do is show *how* biomedicine *has grown.*

3. The concept of a research or problem "domain" which pervades the present work was developed without knowledge of Dudley Shapere's (1974) careful analysis of "scientific theories and their domains." Anyone familiar with Shapere's research will recognize, however, a great deal of resemblance between our basic interests and concerns. Shapere (1966, 1969a, 1969b) has consistently argued that the positivist distinction between observational and theoretical terms necessarily ends in a philosophical and analytical cul-de-sac. He proposes in its place the concept of scientific domains. The concept as Shapere developed it does not artificially separate the

analysis of science into the observational world as opposed to the theoretical world or into the distinction between the context of discovery and the context of justification. The views which Shapere ably criticizes can best be termed the Kuhnian tradition. Whether or not Kuhn (1962) still maintains or ever maintained the positions which sociologists ascribed to him is not as important as the recognition that many similar positions are part of the received wisdom of sociology. Thus Shapere's discussion of domains can be taken, *mutatis mutandis,* as a criticism of many positions espoused within the sociology of science.

4. This section makes no pretense of being an exhaustive treatment of the historical development of cell transformation research. The schematic nature of this treatment should not, however, deceive the reader into thinking that what is recounted is merely incidental to the argument of the following chapters. First, elaborating on what was said above, we agree with King that the "division between the history of scientific ideas and the sociology of scientific conduct, between the study of science as 'a particular sort of knowledge' and as 'a particular sort of behavior' has met with the ready consent of historians and sociologists alike. One can see why such a division of labor should appear so attractive to both sides—whatever its intellectual justification. *It saves intellectual historians from the indignity of being told that the 'real' causes of scientific growth lie beyond their professional comprehension; and it relieves sociologists of the necessity of understanding scientific ideas*" (1971: 4; italics added). This problem concerns the relationship of both sociology and history to the development of scientific ideas—one part of the old "internalist-externalist" debate (see Johnston, 1976; MacLeod, 1977; Spiegel-Roesing, 1977). The externalist part is addressed in Chapter 3.

Second, the internalist problem does not, of course, imply that previous historical analysis is of little value. Numerous histories and reviews have been consulted for the development of a history of cell transformation research. The histories of nucleic acid research included in Levene and Bass (1931), Chargaff (1947, 1955), and Davidson and Chargaff (1955) provide an interesting temporal perspective from which to view the beginnings of cell transformation research. Glass (1974), Stent (1972), Wyatt (1972, 1975), Olby (1972), and Lederberg (1972) all address the problem of "prematurity" in biological discoveries, in particular, the case of Avery. The development of the influential Rockefeller Institute, where Avery made his important discoveries, is ably chronicled by Corner (1964; see also Fruton, 1966). Hess (1970) and Waddington (1969) express views on the origin of molecular biology; Stent (1969) and Cairns et al. (1966) supplemented by Mullins (1972) provide a schematic view of the development of phage research. Carlson (1966), Glass (1965), Beadle (1963), and Wagner (1968) outline the history of modern genetics research which contributes to cell transformation research. The work on virus research is recorded in Shope (1966), the introductions to chapters in Gross's (1970) masterpiece on "oncogenic viruses," and a popular treatment by Williams (1960). For an approach to cell transformation from cancer research, other reviews and surveys can be found. Shimkin's (1974) reading list provides a survey of the literature. Reviews of the cancer literature, such as those found in Furth (1959) and Potter (1964), demonstrate better than most discussions of scientific development the scientist's ability to "use history" in anticipation of meaningful future research. This section on the history of cell transformation research is a *critical distillation* of information found in such reviews and histories (others are cited in the text) together with a reading of selected portions of the research literature.

5. We learned that the availability of review articles in various research traditions was more than a "convenience" for the historian or sociologist of science. Review articles represent ways which scientists orient themselves to "lines of inquiry"; they represent "streams" which separate meaningful evidential and substantive problem areas. The tables in this chapter and Appendices A and B, compiled from review articles, reflect the identification of scientists in terms of their contribution to "lines of inquiry."

6. The eponymous labeling of viruses after their discoverers, e.g., Rous sarcoma virus, can deflect interest from other research of immense importance. By reading contemporary American reviews of the origins of viral cell transformation research, one soon discovers that the research of Fujinami and Inamoto is seldom mentioned. It would appear from a cursory survey of reviews that reviewers with a European background are much more inclined to recognize the importance of this early Japanese research (see Gross, 1970; Maisin, 1949).

7. The power of the nonviral lines of research can be clearly seen in Little's (1941) review of the genetics of spontaneous tumor incidence. Of particular interest in Little's review is the manner in which he is capable of integrating Bittner's research and genetics. The influence and difficulties of Slye's (1931) genetic interpretation of leukemia can also be seen in the research of Cole and Furth (1941). For the record, however, the first textbook on virology did not appear until 1928 and it dwelled on how viruses and bacteria (supposedly) differed.

8. Recall that Kuhn (1970, 1974) claims that a paradigm shift does not represent progress toward truth in any absolute sense, a notion that his critics (notably Lakatos, 1971) have lambasted as irrevocably relativistic (also see Laudan, 1977).

9. For another excellent example of the intertwining of epidemiology, bacteriology, virology, and molecular biology within the biomedical research tradition, see Wood's (1961) discussion of the history of diphtheria research. The discovery that the virulence and toxigenicity of the diphtheria bacilli depended upon their being infected with bacteriophage provided a point of confluence for the various research traditions.

10. It must be emphasized again that when one is interested in studying the growth and development of knowledge (i.e., science) that the structure of argumentation, in short, rationality, must be properly introduced into the analysis. This has been made explicit in this chapter and underlies our entire analysis. As Boehme succinctly states, "In contrast to most other types of communication, scientific communication . . . is argumentation; the coherence of communication here is the coherence of an argumentative context. This thesis may seem trivial, but that it is not so is shown by the fact that scientific communication is frequently understood to be an exchange of information" (1975: 206; see also Hagstrom, 1965; Scherhorn, 1968).

CHAPTER 2

PHAEDRUS' KNIFE AND VIRAL CELL TRANSFORMATION

> Phaedrus was a master with this knife, and used it with dexterity and a sense of power. With a single stroke of analytic thought he split the whole world into parts of his own choosing, split the parts and split the fragments of the parts, finer and finer until he had reduced it to what he wanted it to be.
>
> You get the illusion that all those parts are just there and are being named as they exist. But they can be named quite differently and organized quite differently depending on how the knife moves [Pirsig, 1974: 72].

> A new catchphrase is "promoting the *diffusion* of scientific knowledge." Lord help us if we can't do better than let it *diffuse*. . . . Diffusion is an intermingling of molecules resulting from the random movement of each. It works rapidly over short distances such as micrometers, but takes forever over long distances. Can't we pinpoint where special new knowledge should go and get it there by special delivery [Comroe, 1978: 934]?

Introduction

The possibilities for dissecting the scientific world are well known to the sociologist of science. Conceptual knives can be wielded to slice science into cohorts, specialties, schools of thought—and justified according to various theoretical and methodological criteria. The sociologist is virtually assured that no one will ever replicate his work using precisely the same specifications because the probability of carving the same slice of science is minute.[1]

What is perhaps more vexing is the ease with which the sociologist assumes that all the specialties that can be named actually do somehow "exist." The initial criteria for circumscribing a specialty assure some unity–whether social, conceptual, or methodological–and are thus reassuring that one is on to something. And because there is an a priori base unity against which findings can be compared, the descriptive process can proceed unhampered.

Momentary reflection cautions, however, that if a specialty is a slice of the scientific world, it would behoove us to know if we were cutting through a cone (and getting conic sections) or through an amoeba (and getting fragments of unique shape and composition). Traditionally, historians and sociologists assumed that science was a linear phenomenon and that specialties were in essence part of a line segment. Others with distinctive views of science, such as Comte, might have seen a specialty as a vertical cross-section of a pyramid of learning which had sociology as its capstone. The point is this: One needs to know how to slice science into meaningful units; such choices must necessarily be made prior to empirical investigation (although they will be refined by such research) and they will have to be made in conformity with criteria that sociologists have until now neglected, namely, the ideas and "rationality" in the chosen specialty.

Rationality here refers to the peculiar "conduct of inquiry" (Kaplan, 1964), the "structure of argumentation" (Boehme, 1975), and the "ways of knowing," which embody "cognitive and technical norms" (Mulkay, 1972) and its equally esoteric "tacit knowledge" (Polanyi, 1966; Collins, 1974). When viewing science, the sociologist is witnessing the ongoing synthesis of the "context of discovery" and the "context of justification" through the scientist's own "logic-in-use" (see Kaplan, 1964). From the scientist's perspective this rationality tells one where to look for new evidence and how to support one's ideas; from the perspective of a specialty or research problem it defines what is "relevant" and thus specifies the confluence patterns of the "problem domain." In the preceding exploration of cell transformation, it was shown how research traditions give rise to problem domains in biology which are too short-lived to be called "specialties." Domains seem to form when ideas (experimental evidence, theories, and techniques) converge through "conceptual migration" (Mulkay, 1974b) on a new site. This new site, then, has its own rationality and derivative social structure.

In so *defining* problem domains (see Woolgar, 1976a) one still wields a methodological knife to isolate slices of biomedical science. Because these slices are "intellectually" generated, however, a coherent understanding of the slice can be attained which is complementary to the scientist's own understanding of the research process. Indeed, one can now strive for an interpretive context that is informed by more than operational or definitional fiat. With this understanding of the problems confronting the student of scientific specialties, it is incumbent upon us to outline the reasoning process which has led to the circumscription of problem domains within the specialty of viral cell transformation.

Operationalizing Problem Domains

Contemporary science demands that the social analyst develop new methodological tools. Visible responses to this demand represent variants on the traditional analysis of bibliographic distributions, the study of networks of scientific organizations (formal and informal), and the study of information flows by means of citation analysis (e.g., Price, 1965; Small and Griffith, 1974; Mullins et al., 1977; Breiger, 1976). All of these techniques are attempts to develop indicators for monitoring or reconstructing the state of science in an era in which traditional techniques have been found wanting. In the following we posit that new analytical tools *are* needed and attempt to define units of biological science which could benefit from such analysis.

In a review of quantitative studies of science, Gilbert and Woolgar argue that there are two fundamentally different approaches to the analysis of specialties:

> The first method starts with the available data and then arbitrarily chooses a description (usually in the form of a mathematical function) to fit the data. Predictions about future growth can then be made by extrapolation. The second method begins by making an hypothesis about a social process in science, based on either sociological investigation or on intuition [1974: 279].

These different orientations to research are called, respectively, the "description-prediction" approach and the "hypothesis-testing" approach. Our approach approximates the latter orientation. Yet strong reservations about the ability of sociologists to implement this approach must be entertained because of widespread unwillingness to take seriously the logic-in-use, the knowledge content, of the specialties studied. In Gilbert and Woolgar's terminology, our "intuition" is that the sociology of science cannot progress until the methods and goals of knowledge production (and not simply in terms of dichotomies, e.g., hard-soft and basic-applied) are made explicit. Furthermore, we contend that the proper definition of units for analysis is fundamentally a problem which is resolved by understanding the "ways of knowing" within a domain. To us this means immersion in the primary literature of "the science" of the domain.

By contrasting this approach with Crane's (1972) analysis of scientific specialty communities, which Gilbert and Woolgar take as indicative of the "hypothesis-testing" approach, the force of the present argument can be seen. In Figure 2.1, Crane (1972) summarizes the four stages of paradigm development based on *cumulative* literature growth, which she calls the "characteristics of scientific knowledge and of scientific communities at different stages of the logistic curve." This abstract formal typification is based on assumptions concerning the underlying diffusion and contagion processes that for Crane are seemingly the necessary and sufficient conditions of exponential/logistic growth. Her research design is clear:

> In order to test the hypothesis that science grows as a result of diffusion of ideas that are transmitted in part by means of personal influence, the growth rate of research areas in which scientists were known to have been interacting with each other and with scientists who had not previously published in the area was compared with the growth rate of research areas in which they were known not to have been interacting in this manner [Crane, 1972: 24].

The focus of Crane's research is on the attributes of communication networks–this is not the same as the structure of argumentation[2]–which determine the growth of disciplines.[3]

The question that overwhelms Crane's approach, or extensions of it, concerns the cognitive demands of a specialty on the interaction process. Without consideration of the way knowledge advances within a particular science, the sociologist shrinks from the crucial question, "How does thought advance within the social milieu?", and settles for answers to other questions, for example, "How do communities of scientists develop?" This latter question does not allow progress beyond the "description-prediction" approach, even if it is formulated in terms of a "hypothesis-testing" methodology. Indeed, in the practical application of the description-prediction approach, one is often forced to import in some ad hoc fashion elements of the intellectual tradition of a specialty to explain the various distributions. In the hypothesis-testing situation the questions can be formulated, and usually are, so as to firmly entrench them in traditional sociological perspectives (Gilbert and Woolgar, 1974). The intellectual structure can thus conceivably be dismissed as irrelevant and removed from the purview of the sociologist. Because the sociologist of science comes out of a tradition in which ideas can easily be considered epi-

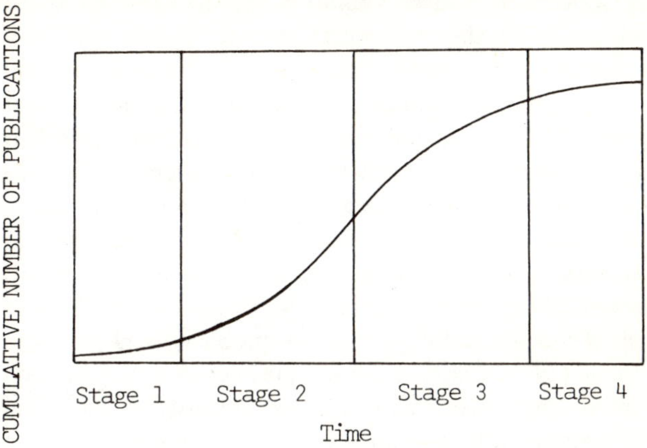

	Stage 1	Stage 2	Stage 3	Stage 4
CHARACTERISTICS OF KNOWLEDGE	Paradigm appears	Normal science	Solution of Major Problems	Exhaustion
			Anomalies appear	Crisis
CHARACTERISTICS OF SCIENTIFIC COMMUNITIES	Little or no social organization	Groups of Collaborators and an Invisible College	Increasing Specialization	Decline in Membership
			Increasing Controversy	Decline in membership

FIGURE 2.1 Characteristics of Scientific Knowledge and of Scientific Communities at Different Stages of the Logistic Curve[a]

[a]Reproduced from Crane (1972:172) by permission of The University of Chicago Press.

phenomena, or ideology (Barnes, 1977), and not, therefore, to be taken seriously, Gilbert and Woolgar's solution appears to be no solution at all.

The difficulty in the biomedical sciences is that confluences onto problem domains can cause very rapid changes of intellectual needs within an area. The intellectual unities that circumscribe problem domains have differing formative criteria and maintain the multidimensional connectedness with the larger field through the research interests of those scientists who work in them. It would appear that the duration of problem domains also varies greatly; answers are found, problems become irrelevant, scientists lose interest, hope, funding, and so on. Seldom, if ever, can these unities be said to represent the appearance of a paradigm, the development of normal science, the solution of major problems, and paradigm exhaustion, as Crane (1972) insists. They are much less pretentious, less organizationally interesting, or less visible to the sociologist, but their numbers and transience seem to create an overall complexity that must be grasped if the approaches of the Cranes and the Gilberts and Woolgars are to be reconciled and empirically explored.

It would appear that if one wants to study the growth and development of biomedical science, then the research site should be the problem domain. This is our choice for reconciliation; its exploration follows.

A BIBLIOGRAPHIC CHARACTERIZATION OF PROBLEM DOMAINS IN MEDICINE

There are numerous criteria that come to mind in trying to isolate problem domain formation.[4] Our criteria utilize bibliographic collection techniques that were developed to aid biomedical researchers, namely, those embodied in *Index Medicus.* We reason that the category system developed for this purpose reflects the rational structuring of this broad field. It is important to stress here that this index probably reflects the structure of biomedical fields all too well; the category system used in *Index Medicus* search modes is continually under revision and expansion to meet the needs of shifting research domains.[5] Although this complicates matters considerably, it derives from the complication of the biomedical world, which is precisely what our analysis is designed to capture.

Our hesitance to code the references found in the review articles we unearthed prompted us to consider the search capabilities of *Index Medicus.* This source, available on computer tape from 1964 to the present, contains the identical reference information found in hard-copy *Index Medicus* except it is in more accessible form. Likewise, the mode of access is through keywords which are attached to the articles after a reading of each article. The keywords are assigned to either the "IM"–a central part of the research–or "NIM"–mentioned in, but not central to, the research–pool. The accessing procedure is simply a matching of keywords to retrieve articles. The keywording structure is hierarchical which permits selection of terms at various levels of generality (National Library of Medicine, 1974), but it also forces one to utilize the most specific terms because if a specific term is present, the more general category is omitted. The search mode utilizing these terms is set-theoretic, that is, the intersections, unions, and complements of various sets can be defined. Thus, with knowledge of these tools, the terminal can become the site of a precisely controlled fishing expedition.

Convinced that in viral cell transformation, species of viruses are more identifiable and meaningful "fish" than the genus cell transformation, a search was carried out accordingly. Prior experimentation with the keyword structure also recommended this strategy: Search terms are added annually, rendering a tracing of certain broad keyword lineages difficult at best. First, all the keywords that described viruses were distinguished. Some would be searched exclusively under the most specific terms, others would be aggregated via "union" statements and then intersected with transformation terms. Four such terms were adopted: oncogenic/viruses, sarcoma/experimental, neoplasms/experimental, and cell-transformation/neoplastic. This latter term is a refined version of neoplasms/experimental introduced in 1968. Second, a series of searches for the total literature corresponding to the viruses were programmed; the frequencies of various characteristics of the IM keywords are described below. These two procedures yield a set of references which, when distributed over time, give us a chronological picture of a research topic. Thus, the methodology augments the expertise of *Index Medicus* editors with an agenda of search statements to produce various literature curves.[6]

The task is to find segments of research traditions which represent problem domains within the cell-transformation literature. These units should be particularly amenable to further, more rigorous, less aggregated analysis. Initially, we sought to study all of the cell-transformation literature; then the more modest goal of collecting data on *experimental* cell transformation was attempted, only to realize that even this effort posed an impossible task of data collection. We would have to choose between chemical transformation and viral transformation as a frame of reference. It became obvious that if *Index Medicus* was to be our research tool, then viral transformation was our choice. The appeal of the *Index Medicus* keyword system and the hopes of exploiting the content analysis which it afforded were highly attractive. We were also advised that research linking viruses to cancer seemed more robust than the chemical carcinogenesis literature.[7] It was through these considerations that the process of selection favored viral transformation as the initial research site.

By using the *MEDLARS* system, we retrieved a body of literature on viral transformation published for the 10-year span, 1963-1972 (Figure 2.2). It can readily be seen that the literature produced during this period was growing at a rapid rate. It thus manifests those characteristics of growth which have often assured students of contemporary science that they are studying a viable, "hot" area of research. The author distributions (Figure 2.3) also suggest that the area was recruiting new researchers at a rate indicative of a tremendous growth potential. When the percentage per year of new authors in the specialty begins to stabilize in 1967-1968,[8] it stabilizes around the 65% level. This means that 65% of the authors in any one year are completely "new faces," but this does not give any indication of how many of these new authors remain active and survive in the area. By eliminating authors who publish only one or two articles in the entire viral cell transformation set and graphing the distribution of those authors who publish each year (Figure 2.3), it can be seen that the growth is fairly constant. Constant linear growth in the number of highly published authors publishing per year suggests that a solid core of researchers in viral cell transformation is forming, but with its membership limited to a small fraction of the total publishing author set. If the number of authors with two or fewer articles is a fairly constant proportion of the highly published author set, then the rate of increase of the slope of the curve would also increase proportionally. By combining a fairly stable linear development of the number of authors publishing three or more times within the specialty with a recruitment structure (inferring that most low publishers are graduate or postdoctoral students), one could "explain" much of the rapid rate of growth in authors in viral cell transformation.

If, in addition to this inference, one would apply a theory concerning the increased combinatorial possibilities of individuals and ideas within the ever-expanding laboratories (see Shockley, 1957), a theory of the exponential growth of the literature of viral cell transformation could be developed: The more individuals within a laboratory structure, the more potential for the combination of ideas. One can only relate to a limited number of individuals, and the locations of viable laboratories is institutionally and financially finite. Perhaps, too, the seeming exponential-logistic growth of the biological sciences could be attributed to basic manpower (see McGinnis, 1972) and to intellectual processes as have been enumerated above. If

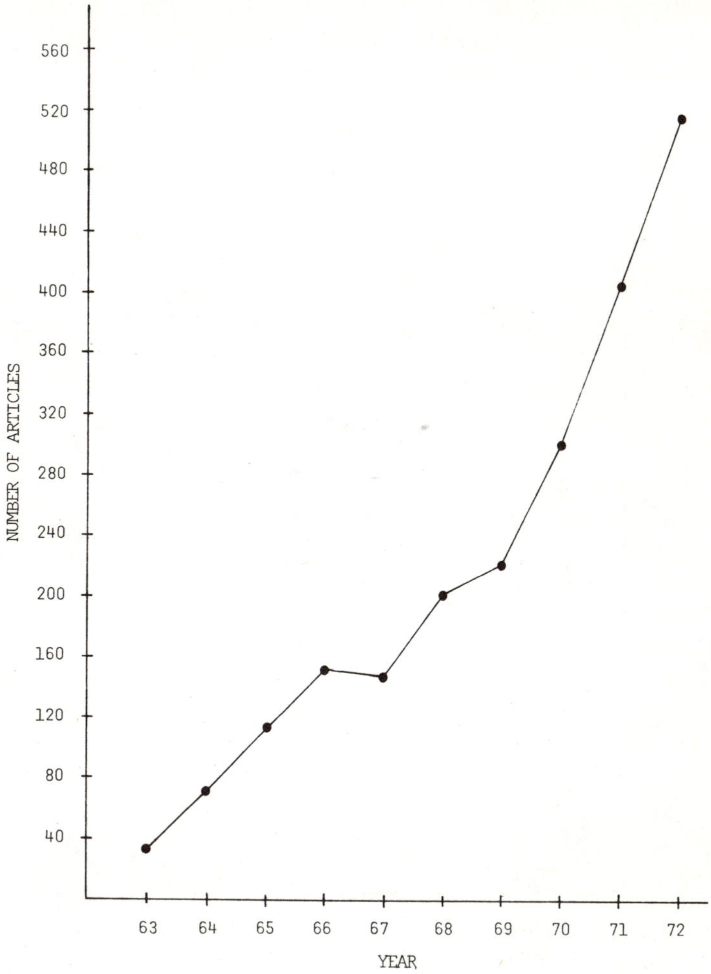

FIGURE 2.2 Number of Cell Transformation Articles per Year

such would prove to be the case, then it would be of great interest because the generator of the growth curve would be attributed to apprenticeship, an intellectual process which is too often overlooked (Zuckerman, 1977).

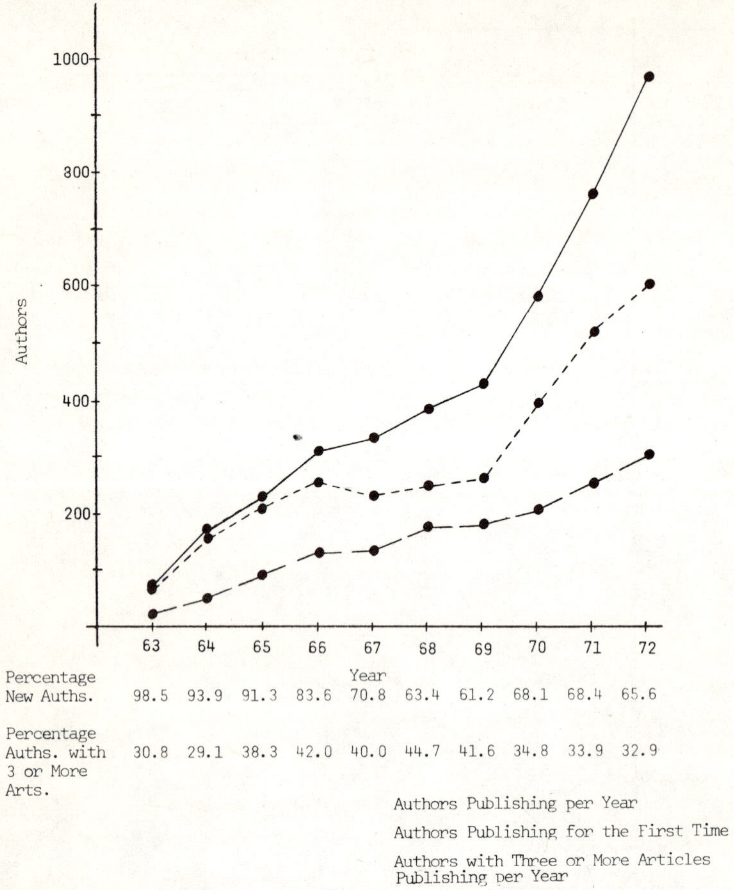

FIGURE 2.3 Number of Cell Transformation Authors, Number of First-Time Authors, and Number of Authors with Three or More Articles, 1963-1972

Because the theory of a binary diffusion process (see Hamblin et al., 1973) underlies the logistic process, it is often assumed that the "contagion" model must be creating the exponential growth of science:

> the exponential growth of scientific knowledge can be interpreted as a "contagion" process in which early adopters influence later adopters, which in turn creates an exponential increase in the numbers of

> publications and the numbers of new authors entering the area. The rate of expansion will vary depending upon the number of people with whom each scientist has personal contact [Crane, 1972: 23].

Couched in these terms, the explanation of growth loses sight of the process of scientific argumentation. An alternative explanation would allow that some "combinatorial" properties of ideas are enhanced by, for instance, the expansion of laboratory size (Pelz and Andrews, 1976). Then the theory would not depend solely on a diffusion process but on the stimulation of research capabilities. If the contagion process concentrates on the analogue of a general social information process (which works for diseases, population expansion, product diffusion, and so on), the alternative modeling approach would ask what is the structure of rationality within a problem domain? How does this process under "normal" conditions develop an exponential growth pattern? Eventually, it could ask, how would one intervene in the developmental process to stimulate the mechanisms of knowledge production?

Put another way, one can never know a priori from the shape of a distribution what generated it. Until one gains knowledge of the construction or programs of research on less aggregated levels within the specialty (see Studer, 1977a), one will never know what lurks behind literature curves. Thus, the methods utilized to decompose the growth curves of a specialty must apply knowledge of technical content as a criterion in isolating specialties for study, rather than impose as an explanation of specialty growth a social mechanism that is alien—or at least related in unknown ways—to this content.

To overcome such a priori model building, it is necessary to investigate a technique that will efficiently isolate research domains within specialties. In this spirit, we explore the MEDLARS technique. Recognizing that it has its difficulties, we are sensitive to the danger of overinterpreting the data received from MEDLARS.[9] But there is no better way to test data of the type needed for specialty studies than to utilize novel techniques and note their inherent limitations. In the following, as the large viral cell-transformation literature is decomposed into smaller problem domain units, the strengths and weaknesses of MEDLARS will be exposed.

The results of various literature searches through *Index Medicus* are graphed in six figures. The graphs are broken down into *total* distributions—the total number of articles retrieved from the file by an appropriate keyword(s)—and *major component* distributions—keyword(s) defining the primary research orientation of the article. In addition, the subset of each literature set which had a more direct bearing on virally induced cancer was retrieved (using the keywords "neoplasms/experimental," "oncogenic/viruses," and others) and has been labeled the *oncogenic component.* One anomaly on two of the graphs requires clarification: The subset "oncogenic component" appears to be larger than the total number of articles for the year. This occurs because the oncogenic component curve represents publication years whereas the total distribution is based on indexing years.[10]

By inspecting Figures 2.4 to 2.7 in succession, it can be seen that the literature curves for adenovirus (DNA), herpes virus (DNA), Friend virus (RNA), and avian leukosis virus (RNA) exhibit markedly different distributions. It is also quite clear that the two RNA virus literatures seem to have a much greater proportion of their research devoted to oncogenesis that that on the DNA viruses. But those with the higher percentage, it should be noted, also represent smaller bodies of literature. It would appear that the nononcogenic portion of all the curves is growing more rapidly than that specifically classified in *Index Medicus* as relevant to cancer research. Because such distinctions within the literature could conceivably signal a fractionation of intellectual interests within a specialty, this should inform its selection for analysis. If one wants to study a particular confluence of ideas within a biological specialty, then criteria *other* than apparent growth must be considered.

Such consideration is further illustrated by the adenoviruses (Figure 2.6) and the herpes viruses (Figure 2.7). Both of these viruses were intensively studied in the late 1950s due to their link with cold sores, respiratory infections, and afflictions of the central nervous system. In the 1960s, however, there was renewed interest in these viruses as possible causes of cervical cancer. It is conceivable, and quite likely, that the growth and decline in the literature production for these viruses are very closely associated with the immediate clinical interest in disease treatment. The relative complexity of these viruses, however, makes them less attractive as "model viruses" for the cancer researcher than other DNA viruses such as simian virus 40 (Dulbecco, 1974). Thus, although research on these viruses would no doubt be interesting to study if one wanted to demonstrate the relationship of clinical and nonclinical research, other choices would be preferable if one sought a domain representing how research central to the fight against cancer is structured.

In contrast, Friend virus is more central to cancer research (it is a murine leukemia virus) and also presents us with an intriguing picture of its bibliographic development (Figure 2.6). Gross's characterization of the

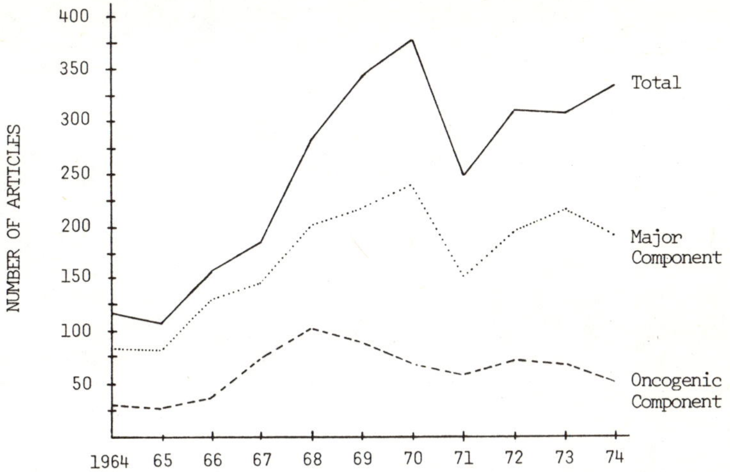

FIGURE 2.4 Growth of Literature on Adenovirus (DNA)

origins of research on the Friend virus greatly aids the understanding of its literature distributions:

> This curious syndrome seems to be a true "laboratory disease" and appears to be exceedingly rare under natural life conditions, if it occurs spontaneously induced in the laboratory by inoculating susceptible mice with a virus which was isolated originally from a Swiss mouse by Dr. Charlotte Friend (1956) at the Sloan-Kettering Institute in New York City [1970: 533].

This intimate connection with the research laboratory withdraws research on Friend virus from the pragmatics of epidemiology and treatment that often disperse the research interests attending other viruses. But a laboratory disease, we thought, might not be the best place to begin research into problem domain formation. Any conclusions that one might reach on the basis of the structure of the problems within this area might be treated as far removed from the mainstream of biomedicine. Nevertheless, other considerations favor its selection: The research did deal with mouse leukemia and therefore had a large oncogenic component; the research began in the recent past and therefore one could easily capture its entire history; it did manifest growth spurts coupled with interesting declines and plateaus reminiscent of post-Cancer Act acceleration; and above all, Friend

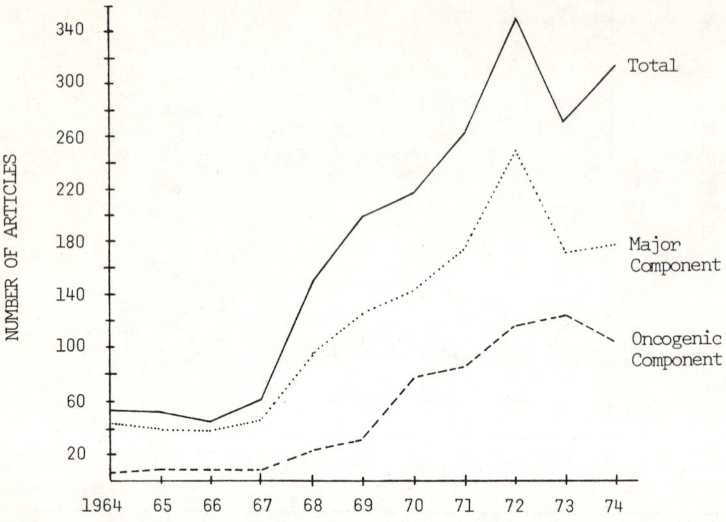

FIGURE 2.5 Growth of Literature on Herpesvirus (DNA)

virus in an RNA virus and RNA viruses have become more important for biologists as their oncogenic potential has been confirmed. Even though Friend virus is only one of several known murine leukemia viruses, as a "model virus" for leukemia research, it had something to offer that neither adenovirus or herpes virus possessed, namely, its unambiguous relationship to the war on cancer. With no major breakthroughs in Friend virus research, one would be able to develop a clear view of the policy impact of increased funding on a relatively stable area of research. Finally, it would be researchable because the body of literature on Friend virus in relatively small, but we continued to look elsewhere (Hackett, 1979, did not).

The two important papova viruses–simian virus 40 (SV40; Figure 2.8) and polyoma virus (Figure 2.9)–have relatively short histories: Polyoma was discovered by Gross in 1965 and SV40 was discovered by Pay and also by Sweet and Hilleman in the process of safety testing poliomyelitis vaccines in 1959-1960. Their importance to contemporary cancer research has been succinctly described:

> The reason that SV40 and polyoma virus have received ever-increasing attention during the past few years is that they provide a model system in which at least some of the events that lead to tumor formation in animals can be duplicated *in vitro*. The central phe-

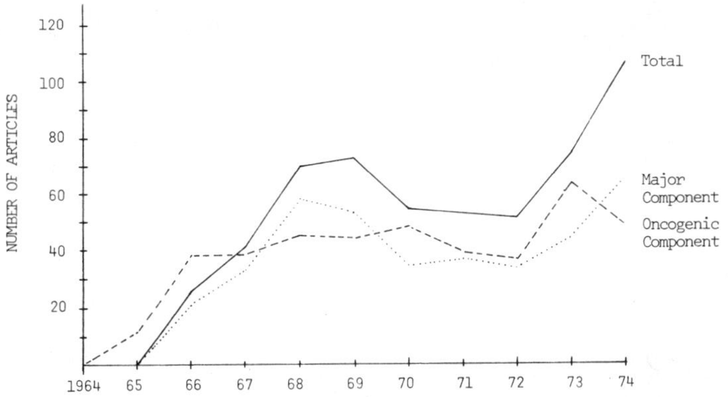

FIGURE 2.6 Growth of Literature on Friend Virus (RNA)

> nomenon of the model system is transformation. When cultures of cells are infected, a fraction of them assumes a net set of stable properties which closely resemble the properties of cells derived directly from virus-induced tumors. The model system is useful because it enables us to study in a quantitative way the interaction of the viruses with genetically homogeneous populations of cells free of interference from the host immune system, and it allows us to use the techniques of molecular biology to investigate aspects of the virus-cell interaction that are inaccessible in whole animals [Sambrook, 1972: 142].

And again,

> A number of attributes have encouraged the selection of SV40 as the viral agent for so many studies: it can be readily propagated and accurately assayed in tissue culture; it can transform cells *in vitro* as well as induce tumors *in vivo*; it has a limited content of genetic information; and its nucleic acid can be isolated in an infectious form [Butel et al., 1972: 2].

SV40 enjoys great popularity among cancer researchers because of its ability to transform cells in the laboratory situation. Unlike Friend virus, however, SV40 is often found as a "latent" virus (Gross, 1970) in monkey kidney cell cultures. Because such viruses are sometimes oncogenic in their nonnatural hosts, it was cause for concern when a virus with oncogenic potential was found in poliomyelitis vaccines. The question "Could SV40

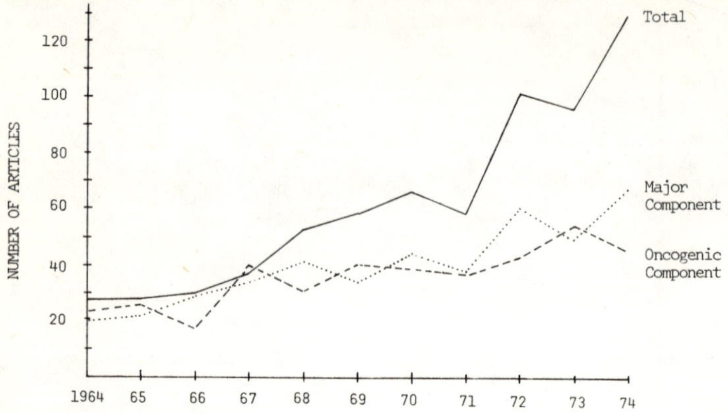

FIGURE 2.7 Growth of Literature on Avian Leukosis Virus (RNA)

transform human cells?" was therefore a question of real concern when it was discovered in the monkey kidney cells that were used to produce vaccines. Research on SV40 was thus doubly stimulated, first by its potential threat to humans and second because it proved to be a model DNA virus suited for laboratory experimentation. It was, after all, a primate virus with oncogenic potential and this fact alone was enough to bring it toward center stage in the war against cancer.

Thus of the three papova viruses, papilloma virus (or human wart virus, not discussed because of its tangential relationship to cancer research) and polyoma virus seem to be relatively isolated from the mainstream of cancer research. But in the case of SV40, one can see the take-off of interest in using this virus to induce sarcomas. In Figure 2.8 the oncogenic portion of the SV40 literature is decomposed into the three segments that are usually labeled "oncogenic component" on the graphs. The choice of keywords which indicate an interest in viral oncology is consistent with the growth of the experimental sarcoma classification that virtually parallels the growth of SV40 research. Is the source of the drop in 1973 in the experimental sarcoma category a shift in the literature or is it due to changes in the keyword system?

For an initial analysis of problem domain formation, then, what are the drawbacks to studying the viruses discussed above? First, the body of literature of all of them except Friend virus seems to be larger than is necessary for our purposes. Second, the research on all of these viruses

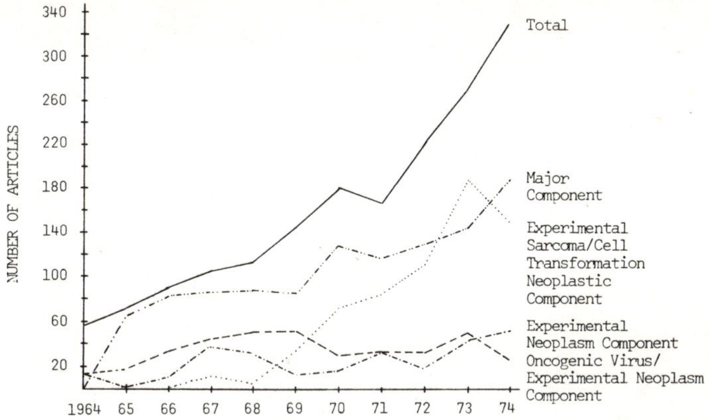

FIGURE 2.8 Growth of Literature on SV 40 Virus (DNA)

seems to be dominated by what is commonly, and pejoratively, called "normal science" (Kuhn, 1962). This makes the areas relatively unattractive because the confluence patterns would most likely be distributed over a longer duration, somewhat analogous to the historical development of cell transformation in toto, and hence would not encompass the drama of a domain created by an important discovery and sustained by a noticeable influx of ideas, researchers, and money. Eventually one would want to compare the seemingly slow accretion of knowledge in areas such as Friend virus with the rapid confluence of ideas in the form of dramatic discoveries.

If one could find a discovery that seemingly revolutionized a specialty or one of its component problems, and if its argumentation structure could be discerned, then perhaps a basis could be found for studying the continuities of the process of scientific growth. Contrary to our initial impression, therefore, it may be necessary to demonstrate the continuous process of confluence of ideas onto problem domains within a context in which one might suspect that a radical break with, or quantum leap from, the past had occurred. In short, there seems to exist in the contemporary virus literature discussed above no dramatic event to test the most crucial aspects of a confluence theory of scientific progress.

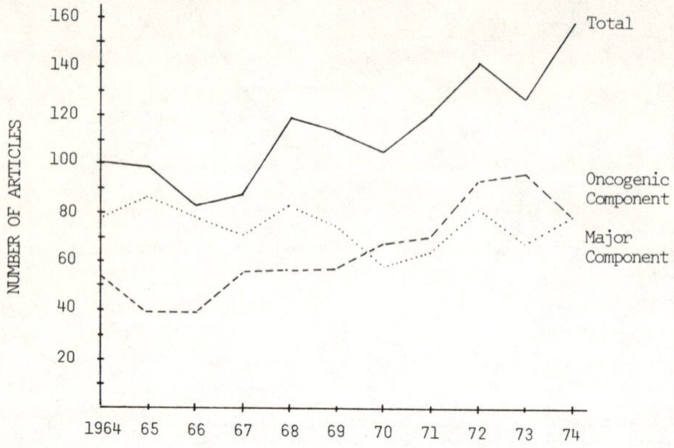

FIGURE 2.9 Growth of Literature on Polyoma Virus (DNA)

REVERSE TRANSCRIPTASE: A SALVAGED RESEARCH SITE

The case of avian leukosis virus, another seemingly uninteresting virus, supplies the missing event. Avian leukosis virus is notable as the earliest (Ellermann and Bang, 1908) group of oncogenic viruses discovered. From Figure 2.5 it can be seen that it was a relatively modest area of research until the 1970s. Then the literature growth rate increases much the same as it did for SV40 and Friend virus. A plausible explanation of this take-off is the increased governmental spending on cancer during this period; this may have been the reason why the SV40 and Friend virus literature accelerated at that time. In the case of avian leukosis virus, however, an intellectual event of great promise for cancer research coincided with increased federal funding. There was some experimental evidence concerning the means by which a class of oncogenic RNA viruses replicates:

> These results demonstrate that there is a new polymerase inside the virions of RNA tumour viruses. It is not present in supernatants of normal cells but is present in virions of avian sarcoma and leukemia RNA tumour viruses. The polymerase seems to catalyse the incorporation of deoxyribonucleotide triphosphates into DNA from an RNA template. . . . If the present results and Baltimore's results with Rauscher leukaemia virus are upheld, they will constitute strong evidence that the DNA provirus hypothesis is correct and that RNA tumour viruses have a DNA genome when they are in cells and an

> RNA genome when they are in virions. This result would have strong implications for theories of viral carcinogenesis and, possibly, for theories of information transfer in other biological systems [Temin and Mizutani, 1970: 1213].

The avian leukosis (myeloblastosis) virus had become the site of research in viral enzymology. It had certain laboratory characteristics that made it particularly amenable for study:

> The new availability of DNA copies of oncogenic viral RNA genomes appears to have particular importance due to the potential usefulness of these products in searchers for viral genomes and viral genome expression by hybridization techniques. The demonstration by Spiegelman et al. that purified polymerase from avian myeloblastosis virus, which *appears safe to handle and is available in large quantities,* can transcribe the RNA of other viruses to specific DNA products is particularly gratifying [O'Connor, 1973: 1177; italics added].

The large quantities of the virus came from the laboratory of Joseph and Dorothy Beard at Duke[11] which was supported by NCI's Special Virus Cancer Program to supply this virus to the world research community. With the discovery of the DNA-polymerase of avian leukosis virus and its appealing laboratory properties, plus its availability in large quantities, the stage was set for a research and literature explosion.

Of course, other viruses as well were used in this enzyme research, for example, Rauscher mouse leukemia virus and Rous sarcoma virus. Searches through *Index Medicus* revealed that these literatures were prohibitively large. Thus, a means of incorporating these other viruses into the problem domain was to redefine the problem as the replication of viruses which use a DNA intermediary. The study of RNA-directed DNA-polymerase, more popularly known as "reverse transcriptase," seemed to possess the crucial characteristics we sought: small enough in size to allow intensive research, yet potentially the site of discoveries of tremendous import for cancer control and, therefore, of policy relevance.

Indeed, the experimental discovery of reverse transcriptase (Baltimore, 1970; Temin and Mizutani, 1970) would put to rest the "Central Dogma" of DNA transcription. In the same year that Watson reiterated that "RNA never acts as a template for DNA" (1970: 331), it was decisively shown that this was not the case. Some molecular biologists were even declaring the "end of progress" arguing that if the Central Dogma did not essentially say it all, then what remained to be said was trivial (see Stent, 1969). For

Stent (1969), "success has dulled the sensibilities," and the "latter-day achievements" suggested to him that there are few surprises left.[12]

The "surprise" of reverse transcription is therefore of interest to the social analyst of science as an example of the process of scientific argumentation and refutation. Because it appears to have triggered a major change in both theory on and experimentation with RNA viruses, it allows one to compare how ideas are formulated and pursued through the pre- and postdiscovery periods of a biomedical domain. In Figure 2.10, the explosive exponential growth of reverse transcriptase research is seen to differ markedly from the Friend virus curve. By simply comparing the growth curves, it is tempting to ascribe great excitement and even importance to the discovery and elucidation of the reverse transcription process. Certainly if the distributions were reversed one would have to rethink the roles played by the respective problem domains within biomedicine. But precisely because it is *always* possible to "rethink" the significance of a research area *after* one has seen its literature distributions, it is difficult to ascribe a necessary relationship between the cognitive and the quantitative state of a domain. Thus, the sociologist who points to interesting "bumps" on literature curves and suggests that they indicate key intellectual events, will find any quantitative distribution of the literature ex post facto "interpretable." What must be specified a fortiori are the processes which underlie logistic growth, for example, those responsible for the reverse transcriptase literature curve in Figure 2.10.

The "salvaging" of reverse transcriptase as the research site for domain study is also significant since much of the biomedical community thought that the Virus Cancer Program of the National Cancer Institute was spending an inordinate amount of money on RNA virus research and not enough on the DNA viruses. The Zinder Committee (discussed in the next chapter) suggested that the funding of research was too one-sided and that it indeed would be embarrassing if papova (DNA) viruses would prove to be of key importance in the conquest of cancer. Due to National Cancer Institute research priorities, however, research on *RNA* viruses thrived. And because the discovery of reverse transcriptase allowed the development of new assay techniques for RNA viruses, research on reverse transcriptase has also experienced tremendous growth and specialization. While it may not be representative of biomedical domains, reverse transcriptase has certainly been the site of much pomp and controversy in the contemporary saga of viruses and cancer.

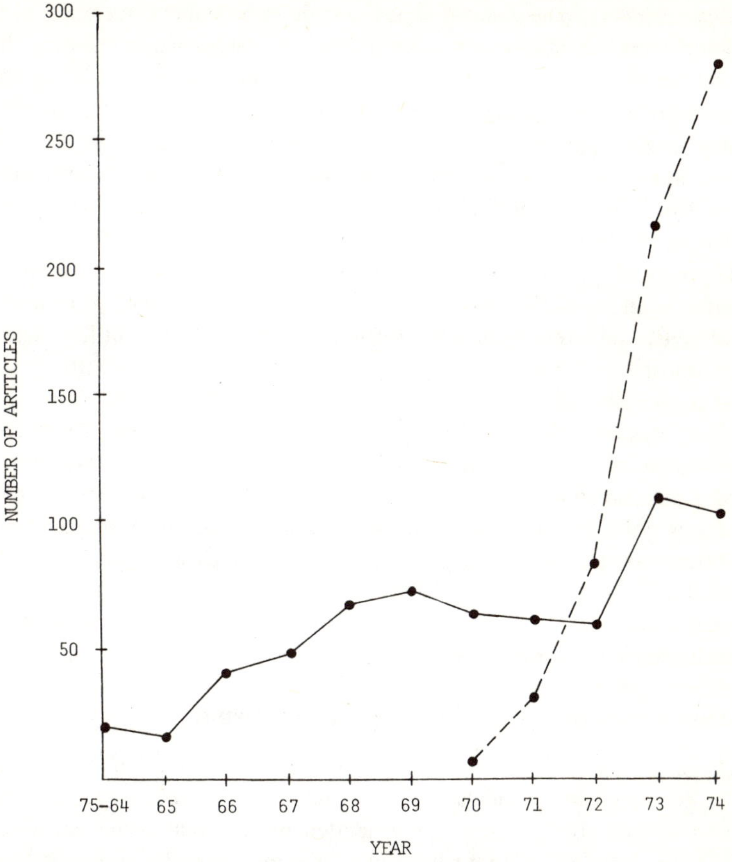

FIGURE 2.10 Frequency Distribution of Articles over Time on Reverse Transcriptase and Friend Virus

The Interviews

The foregoing chronicle might prompt one to ask (again?) would it not have been better to go directly to experts in viral cell transformation and inquire of them which areas should be studied? Would we not have arrived at the same conclusions with much less effort? The answer is, not surprisingly that, if at all possible, one should obtain expert guidance in choosing specialities for analysis. But the "insiders" of a field often perceive it so selectively as to enforce a certain theory of scientific development (see Mulkay, 1974a). The fishing expedition described above specifies what type of "fish" our research is attempting to catch. While enlisting the assistance of expert insiders, the sociologist must be cognizant of the position of such individuals within a research area and should critically review their opinions. Historians, of course, are accustomed to such evaluations of experts' testimony; the sociologist must learn to be equally critical of the views of their expert informants. We tried to do so while soliciting the testimony of specialists in reverse transcriptase. But we were able to challenge their views only because of our knowledge of technical content, that is, of *their* research. The rich commentary they provided us (featured in subsequent chapters) further attests to the force of knowledge that boosts problem domains into the consciousness of scientists and science analysts alike.

Our reasons for interviewing reverse transcriptase researchers and administrators were to identify and then speak to individuals who occupied *particular* positions in various networks. But the sampling of networks is quite unlike conventional designs which seek to optimize representativeness, and therefore generalizability, through a random selection procedure (see Granovetter, 1976). What follows, then, is a methodological statement about our interviews as one source of data among many on the reverse transcriptase domain.

THE METHODOLOGY OF STRUCTURAL INTERVIEWING

Because any social network is a structural representation of relationships generated by particular behavior, for example, authorship, one can derive any number of networks generated by different behaviors which relate the *same* set of individuals in numerous ways. To compound the sampling problem, any behavior and relation formed by it can be disaggregated over time. Such disaggregation lends a dynamic dimension to the static structural representation. Disaggregation also multiplies the number of network structures, each of which can be thought of as a sampling frame. The choice then becomes whether to sample *each* frame, say, by year and generating relation, or somehow to juxtapose the frames to reveal patterns of variance and invariance in positions across networks. Structurally, the individual whose position in a network changes by year and relation may be as "interesting" or valuable for interviewing purposes (if not more so) as one who is "strongly tied" in every network. This is the crux of Granovetter's (1973) perceptive argument that sociometrically there is strength in "weak ties."

How, then, does one "preserve" the social processes underlying structural representations by sampling (i.e., "operationalizing") the network? For sure, one must sample purposively, not randomly, and in the absence of sociometric data, rely on visual inspection of the structures themselves: What are the configurations? Which dyads and triads appear repeatedly? Is their position (or physical location) on the network "map" relatively stable? Do they disappear in some years and on some relations and then reappear? These questions disclose the nature of the task. After studying pictures[13] of structured relations (see Chapter 5) and noting some of the patterns implied in the above queries, we began to perceive certain individuals and laboratories as important targets for further examination. Combined with our knowledge of intellectual events and principal characters in the narrative history of reverse transcriptase, these structural data offered another perspective (or set of perspectives) on visible researchers and organizational sectors, namely, those emerging from various bibliographic generators of networks, for example, coauthorship and cocitation.

Structural sampling must utilize this abundance of information: It must draw on the array of available empirical information to determine who should be selected for interviewing.[14] Targets may be selected, therefore, for their consistency of position in different networks, their centrality in some, their peripherality in others, their organizational setting, and their links to others in the relevant research populations. The rationale for sampling according to multiple criteria is that structural positions and relations are assumed to condition one's perceptions of the phenomena in question. What structural sampling seeks to tap is the divergence of perspective that participation in a social system, for example, a formal communication network, entails. Interviewing the designated targets of a structural sample will presumably develop insights about not only one's participation in the network but also one's perspective on whether the network really exists, how it has evolved, and why.

Structural interviewing thus operationalizes the notion of "triangulation" (Webb et al., 1966). The ability to approach one's subject in a myriad of ways (i.e., through multiple indicators) should indeed seem to be vital for faithful reconstruction of a problem domain. There is always sufficient measurement error in any kind of social data to lend doubt to the researcher's findings and interpretations. Rather than belabor or bemoan this point, social scientists should *assume* its veracity and adopt a skeptical, but constructive measurement posture: Treat data as a tentative baseline, as an approximation to refine and on which to build with the collection and analysis of *other* data.

Structural interviewing does this in two ways: It builds on structure (i.e., generated networks) and recognizes the credibility of one's perspective on the structure, his/her role in creating it, sustaining it, and so on *without* attributing credence to views based on structural position alone, for example, centrality. Credence stems from the collection of views, the assimilation of perspectives from different vantage points in the network(s). In short, structural interviewing is a "convergence technique" (Carrese and Baker, 1967). Indeed, such structural interviewing allows the "outsider" to glimpse through "insider's" eyes without becoming either blinded by insider's vision or resolutely myopic as outsiders (particularly social scientists studying natural scientists) tend to be.

To recapitulate, structural interviewing is an approach to scientific "objects" that begins with a known subject matter and is a proxy for nothing except the clearly unfeasible alternative of interviewing a population. It derives from multiple networks or clusters and, as a small sample technique, it requires the findings of such analyses, for example, of cocitations,[15] to inform both the actual sampling, and the interviewing itself.

Our sampled reverse transcriptase (RT) targets and their respective organizational sites are summarized in Table 2.1. Again, the interviews were intended to elicit recollections and subjective perceptions to compare with other observations which, we claim, endow the process of reconstructing a domain with evolutionary and integrating perspectives. What follows is a test of our claim: a description of how (1) the targets were contacted, (2) the interview sessions were conducted, and (3) the methodology of structural interviewing can be used to reconstruct an oral history of a problem domain through a composite of protagonists' accounts.

INITIAL CONTACT

Each interview target (or "subject") was sent a personalized letter in January or February of 1978. This letter described the purpose of the research and carried an admission that, after collecting and analyzing substantial bibliographic and biographic data, we as "outsiders" lacked the insights that only researchers working in a problem area can provide. Two or three sentences describing our perception of the subject's contribution to RT research followed, plus an invitation to share his/her perspective with us in a 30-minute "conversation." A self-addressed, stamped postcard accompanied the letter asking the subject to indicate specific dates within the month (the bulk of the interviews occurred in February and March 1978) which were most convenient. The subject was instructed that soon

TABLE 2.1 Initial Structural Sample of Local Organizational Sites for Targeted Interviewing of RT Researchers

Local Organizational Site	Interview Targets: Primary	Interview Targets: Secondary
Government:		
Laboratory of Tumor Cell Biology, NCI	Gallo, Robert C. Smith, R. Graham	-
Viral Carcinogenesis Branch, NCI	Parks, Wade P.	Huebner, Robert J.
Viral Leukemia and Lymphoma Branch, NCI	Aaronson, Stuart A. Scolnick, Edward M. Todaro, George J.	Ross, Jeffrey
Primate/Quasi-goverment:		
Bionetics Research Lab (Litton)	Reitz, Marvin S.	Ting, Robert C.Y. Wu, Alan M. Yang, Stringner S.
Flow Lab	Gilden, Raymond V.	-
Medical School:		
Institute of Cancer Research, College of Physicians and Surgeons, Columbia University	Spiegelman, Sol Schlom, Jeffrey	Axel, Richard Baxt, W. Gulati, Subhash C. Hehlmann, R.
Institute for Molecular Virology, St. Louis University School of Medicine	Green, Maurice	Gerard, Gary F. Grandgenett, Duane P.
Academic Departments:		
Department of Biology, Massachusetts Institute of Technology	Baltimore, David Verma, Inder M.	Huang, Alice S. Temple, Gary F.
McArdle Lab, University of Wisconsin	Temin, Howard M.	-

after receiving this card, we would be in contact by phone to confirm a date and time for our meeting.

Table 2.2 contains the names of the interview targets with whom we spoke and their respective institutional/organizational sector, which helped to frame their selection. A comparison of Tables 2.1 and 2.2 reveals that our targets, regardless of sector, were most receptive to our invitation to talk. This receptivity was reflected in their candor, sincerity, and genuine interest in our work. We also succeeded in speaking with almost everyone we had hoped to see. The responsiveness of all far exceeded our expectations.

Based on our reading of *Science* reports and hearing colleagues' predictions about the unwillingness of NCI researchers to discuss the cancer war, we decided to contact NCI people *before* we ventured into academic labs, particularly the ones where the discovery of the enzyme had been made. Fortunately, our concern was unfounded. So long as we were "neither from the Washington *Post* nor named Dan Greenberg," as one of our subjects put it, the meeting was a welcome opportunity; for some it was a veritable catharsis to discuss highly visible and controversial, in-house projects (a theme elaborated below).

TABLE 2.2 RT Interview Subjects, by Organizational Sites

Sites	Interview Subjects
Government	Aaronson, Stuart
	Bader, John[a]
	Carrese, Louis[b]
	Huebner, Robert
	Rauscher, Frank[c]
	Todaro, George
Private	Beard, Joseph
	Gilden, Raymond[e]
	Yang, Stringner[f]
Medical School	Gerard, Gary
	Green, Maurice
	Schlom, Jeffrey[g]
	Spiegelman, Sol
Academic Department	Baltimore, David
	Temin, Howard

[a]Head, Cell Growth Regulation Section, Chemistry Branch, NCI; interviewed on recommendation of early subjects.

[b]Associate Director for Program Planning and Analysis, Office of the Director, NCI, interviewed on recommendation.

[c]Former director, NCI; currently, Executive Vice-President, American Cancer Society; interviewed on recommendation.

[d]Sole supplier (on NCI contract) of Avian Myeloblastosis Virus and purified reverse transcriptase; interviewed as most acknowledged in RT literature; Emeritus Professor of Surgery at Duke University; currently President, Life Sciences Research Labs, St. Petersburg, FL.

[e]Currently at Federick Cancer Center, Frederick, MD (managed by Litton-Bionetics).

[f]Currently at Laboratory of Cell Biology, NCI.

[g]Currently Head, Breast Cancer Section, Laboratory of Viral Oncogenesis, NCI.

Two NCI luminaries whom we were unable to see were Robert Gallo and John Moloney.[16] Partly due to our disappointment over missing these targets (although only Gallo was originally targeted)–and partly based on our realization that NCI program heads and lab researchers regard NCI administrators, planners, and policy implementers with a mixture of perplexity and suspicion–we agreed that the subjects of such ambivalence deserve close attention. Our choices, though not necessarily representative, were Frank Rauscher, former NCI Director, and Louis Carrese, Associate Director for Program Planning and Analysis. Carrese was particularly receptive to our questions and spoke in animated fashion for two and a half hours about the incredulity harbored by NCI researchers about his office.[17] Rauscher, now an Executive Vice President of the American Cancer Society and unanimously respected by the NCI researchers we interviewed, was the epitome of public relations.[18]

THE INTERVIEW SESSIONS

The interviews took place in the office or lab of the subject.[19] With one exception, the subject was engaged in a three-way conversation with both of us. Each session was recorded with the permission of the subject, who was informed that he or she would be sent for review a copy of material containing quoted excerpts from the interview. In this way, both the accuracy and the context of quoted statements would be preserved.[20]

In all cases, one of us spent five to seven minutes recounting the origin of the study, its guiding questions, and progress to date. As we became more adept at tailoring our introductory remarks to the role of the subject's work in the RT saga, we succeeded in establishing rapport earlier in the conversation. The one element contributing to the rapport, however, was intellectual—our conversance with the *science* of the subject's research. Our ability to discuss experimental and theoretical issues, for example, the provirus hypothesis and the unreliability of inhibitor data, made us credible, curious social scientists who had taken our subject matter and its creators very seriously. This ability to enter the biologist's world of discourse requires ample preparation—especially an awareness of historically significant events (not just discoveries, but conferences and less official public exchanges) and a knowledge of researchers' whereabouts, collaborators, and programs at various times. Without this reservoir of pertinent facts, one simply cannot ask pertinent questions[21] (see Mulkay, 1974a).

This is one critical difference between social networking and structural interviewing. Structural interviewing surmounts, or at least erodes, the intellectual barrier between the natural scientists and his social scientist-interrogator. Our subjects sensed our effort to surmount this barrier. After opening with queries about whether the subject was surprised by the discovery of RT, what his or her research focus was at the time, and whether this focus changed soon after the discovery, we eased into discussion of the subject's organizational setting (e.g., the structure of his lab, division of labor within it). The conversation then gravitated to the question of antagonism between NCI and academic labs. This was our typical point of departure into the policy area (e.g., effects of the war on cancer on one's research and lab structure, and the reaction to the Zinder Committee report criticizing in general the contract mechanism at NCI and particularly the Special Virus Cancer Program).[22] This is not to say that the interviews were so structured that topics were not addressed in other sequences; they were. With a one-page schedule of topics before us, in no case was a topic untouched for lack of time. And as anticipated, we found the interviews to be quite intense. The advantage of our both being present at each interview was clear inasmuch as one of us would pursue a line of questioning, allowing the other to formulate and phrase questions privately; the other would then enter the dialogue anew. The mental concentration required to process answers and prepare related questions was exhausting. In most cases, both we and the subject were drained after 90 minutes.

Near the end of the interviews, the subjects were asked to suggest the names of colleagues whose insights they valued and who they thought would be willing to speak to us. It was overlap in these "snowballed" names that led us to NCI administrators, but confirmed that our selection of the literature-based structural sample was well-founded.[23] We close this chapter with some observations on the use of interview data for reconstructing the history of a problem domain.

THE USE OF PROTAGONISTS' RETROSPECTIVE ACCOUNTS IN THE PRESENT STUDY

Foremost among the precedents for the interviewing we did are Edge and Mulkay's (1976) analysis of the development of radio astronomy in Britain and Zuckerman's (1977) study of American Nobel laureates. Each of these researchers has reflected on methodology, particularly on the interaction between interviewer and scientist-interviewee (Mulkay, 1974a; Zuckerman, 1972, 1977: Appendix A). Now we reflect on our experience as a guide to interpreting the excerpts presented (in subsequent chapters) to augment other kinds of evidence.

Underlying our concern for reflection is not merely the reactivity of the interview as a data source. Of course, the interview is a social act and sociologists are wont to make it a self-fulfilling prophecy. But interviewing scientists, whether or not they qualify as "ultra elites" (to use Zuckerman's designation of the laureates) presupposes a theory of data. Our theory coincides putatively with that articulated by Mulkay (1974a): Interviewing re-creates, within the bounds of recollection and self-justification, the chronology of actions and reactions which are rarely registered in even the most introspective scientific writing.[24] Interviewing helps, in short, to demythologize—to distinguish historical accuracy from scientific accuracy, "great men" from great acts.

Perhaps the best example of the interview as a demythologizing tool involves the triad of reverse transcriptase codiscoverers, the Nobel laureates Temin and Baltimore plus the unsung NCI microbiologist John Bader. Bader refused to stake a claim in 1969 based on his inhibitor data—data which prompted Green to postulate the existence of an RNA-directed DNA polymerase[25] (Green and Gerard, 1974). To rely solely on written accounts of the events culminating in the discovery (as we shall see in Chapter 4), one would credit Temin with bold hypothesizing in 1964 and dogged determination in conducting six more years of experiments before demonstrating the plausibility of the hypothesis. Baltimore, while a newcomer to the research site, would share the credit for executing the crucial experiment, too. Bader today remains an obscure footnote in the history of the discovery. That his work paralleled Temin's is suggested once in the latter's Nobel address (Temin, 1976).

From our interviews, however, it would seem more than justified that the uncited, unfeted Bader share some of the recognition allotted Temin and Baltimore. Baltimore confesses that he "jumped the fence" for two days to do the experiment. The virus used was obtained by a phone call to his old friend and NCI project monitor George Todaro. Ironically, around this same time, Bader's request for virus from the Viral Oncology Program was declined because he was not a contractor doing research in that area.[26]

Thus, the Temin-Baltimore triumph is a far more intriguing story when told orally than when pieced together from documents. It is more than a story of one man being anticipated (Bader), another moving patiently and inexorably toward the discovery (Temin), and a third independently duplicating the discovery, almost on a lark (Baltimore). The discovery of reverse transcriptase took at least six years and many personalities to unfold. The retelling took—and yielded—much more.

Structural interviewing thus adds a dimension to the fathoming of fact from perception by socially (re)constructing reality in the most basic sense. Although far from definitive, such interviewing can play an integral part in clarifying the precise interplay between the cognitive and the social in science.

Conclusions

In Chapter 1 confluence patterns in biomedicine were viewed within the history of cell-transformation research. The gradual convergence of research traditions was not difficult to perceive when the developments in question were separated by years of careful research. Today the same history of biology is being "compacted" by the sheer amount of effort of an expanding body of biologists. What once took place in "slow motion" has now been accelerated. It is therefore incumbent on the social analyst of science to develop new techniques for illuminating the changing structures of biology. While the temptation is great to insulate ourselves from the immense complexity of the large biomedical research enterprise and to postulate that certain social structures found in other groups and in other sciences are also present within biomedical science, this chapter has counseled another course. To wit:

> Virologists have begun to recognize that the problem is substantially more complex than they had originally anticipated. Although some still argue that a tangible oncogenic human virus will eventually be isolated, a growing number of investigators have concluded that this approach may be futile and have thus begun to reconsider the fundamental concepts of the nature of viruses and their role in animal biochemistry.
>
> If viruses do play a causative role in human malignancies, these scientists suggest, it is most likely that the active agent is an incomplete or defective portion of one virus—or perhaps of several viruses—whose normal function is beneficial to the host. Research on oncogenic animal viruses, as a consequence, has been somewhat de-emphasized as investigators have pressed the search for virus fragments or information in human tumors [Maugh, 1974b: 1181].

Indeed, as this shift occurs, new keywords will develop describing the types of particles under analysis, for example, A-, B-, C-type particles (see Bernhard, 1958, 1960). The keyword method described above endows one with the capability to distinguish an area such as reverse transcriptase and capture its literature soon thereafter. Upon characterizing this literature, strategically located researchers can be identified and interviewed to gain insiders' perspectives on the unfolding domain. Dissecting such literature-based shifts in the foci of biomedical research thus becomes the work of latter-day Phaedruses.

If the development of science resides in more than organizational innovation, then it is a disservice to biomedicine to analyze its structures without reference to the research problems involved, the intellectual innovations, and the innovators themselves. Why this can be a disservice to biomedicine is the focus of the following chapter. Viewing the politics of cancer, biologists have often argued that their research requires a certain funding structure. Consequently, the dominant social positions of both individuals and government laboratories, as induced by the new funding structure, are often singled out for criticism. We shall see in Part II how such criticism impinged upon the reverse transcriptase domain. But first we must examine how the United States' war on cancer set the stage for biomedical research policy and criticism.

NOTES

1. As stated, this reads like a blanket criticism of case studies; it is not. Comparative studies, because they are typically defined along methodological dimensions, are equally vulnerable to the criticism.

2. Structure of argumentation, logic-in-use, discovery process, and rationality will be used interchangeably throughout this chapter and those to come.

3. Theoretically, once the research is completed and the hypothesis confirmed, one could reverse the order (Crane does not, although it is implicit in her functionalism) and say something about the state of a science based on the structure of its communication network. The implication in this reversal would be that policy decisions could be made on the basis of the "ripeness" or "take-off potential" of a specialty. If its communication network manifests a certain structure, then the growth rate of the specialty could possibly be further stimulated by enhancing the social prerequisites of growth.

4. The most common criteria usually are consistent with Law's (1973) tripartite specialty classification; predictably, "look and ye shall find" specialties "organized" around these principles. Law's three types, technique- or methods-based, theory-based, and subject matter specialties, may fit the rationality of the physical sciences (see Sullivan et al., 1977a), but seem inappropriate for biology. Griffith et al. (1974), as reviewed in the previous chapter, commit the same albeit methodological misjudgment in naming cocitation clusters. The organizing principle or dynamic differs in each cluster; one can neither assume nor declare them to be identical for all sciences.

5. The conventional approach to the study of specialties is through the literature. Variations on this approach include exhaustive bibliographies, review articles, and the selection of representative journals by specialists themselves. For cell transformation, as for biological specialties in general, none of these variations, if used alone, would yield a set of publications that could be analyzed as the outcome of specialty activity. The use of these variations in combination, though desirable, is unfeasible for cell transformation: there are no exhaustive bibliographies (review articles retrieve manageable samples of articles but with unknown biases), and a selection of journals typically generates a visible, and therefore unrepresentative, subset of literature. Information scientists have, of course, grappled with these problems for some time. For an overview, see Brittain and Line (1973); for a recent assessment of the retrieval capability of various existing indexing services, see Jones and van Rybergen (1976). Most relevant to our present concern, however, are information services in biomedicine (see Heumann, 1974). An early survey of *Biological Abstracts* is reported by Glass (1955), while Lancaster (1968), Virgo (1970), and Day (1974) have evaluated *Index Medicus* and *MEDLARS* (Medical Literature Analysis and Retrieval System, the "on-line" computer version of *Index Medicus*). For a full description of *MEDLARS*, see National Institutes of Health (1975).

6. However, we by no means abandoned use of other search modes. The clinical/medical orientation to literature indexing of *Index Medicus* continued to be monitored for biases (especially of exclusion) by checking subject entries in *Biological Abstracts* and articles which emerge due to high citation counts. In fact, the basic article set for reverse transcriptase analyzed in Part II represents the union of a search

of *Index Medicus, Biological Abstracts,* and the *Source Index* of the *Science Citation Index.* It would seem that the best strategy is to intersect as many sources as possible. Such comparisons must continue if an accurate time series is to be maintained. Because indexing services tend to change their journal sets and coverage within journals, and because the drift of a substantive problem may alter its definition and the location of the relevant literature, one must always keep abreast of how this will affect the retrieval properties of the literature. Without a sensitivity to "retrieval effects," growth and decline of a specialty literature may be more artifact than fact.

7. Dr. Robert S. Morison was instrumental in sensitizing us to the urgency within the biomedical community of understanding the role of viruses in human neoplastic disease. Why our choice was altogether fortuitous only became apparent later.

8. It is obvious that in the first year, 1963, the number of new authors must equal total number of authors. Stabilization occurs when the supply of previously published authors and the recruitment process for new authors achieve a relative equilibrium.

9. One must entertain the possibility that the growth of the literature in cell transformation is simply an artifact of the retrieval system. Could not the growth of the literature be confounded by the increased funding of *MEDLARS* during this period which in turn expanded their collection and indexing capabilities? Could not the increased emphasis on cancer in the cancer war era have influenced not only the actual research effort in viral cell transformation but also raised the awareness of content analysts who append keywords to the articles? Is it not possible that the growth of the literature retrieved is simply the result of a semantic shift (see Rose, 1967) and what was actually relevant to the domain in the past is overlooked because of our "Whiggish" contemporary orientation to word usage? The fact of the matter is that such arguments persist unless and until research is actually done using bibliographic data and then one observes their limitations. Our approach assumes that no one approach to the data is sufficient to warrant complete trust. Data must be allowed to criticize themselves, as it were, by means of approach from different perspectives.

10. The total counts are based on information supplied by the *Index Medicus* system, the other distributions have been *computed* from computer printouts provided by the *Index Medicus* system for each of the viruses.

11. The Beards, now "retired," head Life Sciences Research Labs in St. Petersburg where AMV is grown in chicks, purified into reverse transcriptase, then packaged and shipped free of charge to NCI contractors. Such renewable "sole source" contracts for the production and delivery of virus and/or enzyme is most economical. Yet none has succeeded like the Beard contract which was first established as a subcontract of a Sol Spiegelman research contract. Dr. Spiegelman of the College of Physicians and Surgeons, Columbia University, has been a primary consumer of AMV and an acknowledged leader in viral oncology research.

12. Such overstatements often accompany a major discovery. It is for this reason, among others, that the passion of the moment must be viewed with a cooler detachment that accrues over time. Hence, we interviewed in the winter of 1978 many of the principal researchers in reverse transcriptase (see Chapter 4).

13. The "pictures" were produced by a multidimensional scaling routine which translated frequencies (or strengths) of pair-wise relationships into distances within a network of points (i.e., people) depicted in two dimensions (for details, see Appendix C).

14. Structural sampling is somewhat akin to "dimensional sampling" (Arnold, 1970), a framework for drawing a small purposive sample representative of a population on n specified dimensions. The dimensions framing a structural sample are network positions and organizational ties, that is, lab sites where authors perform, collaborate, complete, and cite (for a recent university-framed sample, see Friedkin, 1978).

15. Recall that cocitation analysis establishes linkages between pairs of documents listed in the bibliographies of articles in some citing literature. The resulting set of cited documents represents a "map of science" never before visible in the research literature (see Small, 1973; Small and Griffith, 1974; Griffith et al., 1974). These retrieved documents cluster in various subject areas of science and allegedly reveal the structure which connects subjects as well as those documents which dominate in a certain area.

16. The latter was contacted less than two months after he had been rather unceremoniously removed as head of the Special Virus Cancer Program, the NCI program which, upon review in 1973 by the Zinder Committee, came to be perceived as embodying all the vices of big contract research and few of the virtues. The meaning of Moloney's "promotion" to Assistant Director of the NCI at the request of Arthur Upton was clear to our subjects. They advised we "leave Moloney alone," while Moloney's secretary suggested we talk to his "acting" successor, John Sibal. For various reasons, we declined this option.

The failure to see Gallo was of a different sort. His travel schedule simply did not permit our meeting. A chance to interview a long-time associate of his was discouraged by one or two of our NCI subjects who said our persistence to see Gallo would be rewarded ("Gallo is a dynamic guy"; he is also a staunch advocate of contract research and channeling "unlimited" sums to cancer research).

17. There was a vindicating, yet compassionate tone to this interview. In fact, Carrese said that he would encourage an assessment of the planning and policy which has emanated from his office for the last 15 years; it would reduce much misunderstanding about his "systems" approach as well as his mediating role vis-à-vis Congress and NCI researchers.

18. However, he was anything but evasive; he was circumspect and demanded that we discuss the ultimate purposes of our study *before* he allowed us to switch on the cassette recorder. Once satisfied, he produced a fluid 90 minutes of information and pledged to assist us in securing some important documents which had eluded us for months.

19. Within three weeks of each interview, we sent a note of thanks to each subject for his/her cooperation and with an assurance that we would keep them apprised of, and indeed enlist their skills to evaluate, our findings.

20. None of the subjects balked at our recording procedure, though several used the apparatus to differentiate "on-the-record" from "off-the-record" commentary. On occasion, we were asked to "switch off" in preparation for an especially candid, and sometimes ugly, remark. Naturally, we complied with such requests. Sometimes we were surprised when sensitive remarks warranted such a request, but none was made.

21. Also, a "learning effect" takes place when successive interviews are conducted during a period of only a few weeks. This effect surely polishes the syntax, phrasing, and delivery of questions, but it also heightens the interviewers' anticipa-

tion of replies to those questions. When one gains facility with one's research instrument, there is a need to compensate for inflections and facial expressions which may inadvertently cue the subject that "I'm curious as hell about your response, but I think I know what you're going to say," or "I've asked this delicate question of all the previous subjects; now how forthright are you going to be?". The way we compensated for such stirrings was to preface the question with a naive remark such as, "Because we are not formally trained as biologists . . . ," or "We realize now that the Cancer Institute is so vulnerable; it is constantly in the public eye, yet it seems to have unduly attracted much bad press . . . ," or stronger yet, "We were frankly critical of the NCI and hence deliberately chose to interview NCI personnel before visiting the academic researchers. . . ." Whether we were convincing is unknown, but we suspect that the subject, upon hearing such an admission, was more inclined to share a confidence that he ordinarily would not. This is pivotal in the interviewing of scientists: One must give a little to get a little. One must strike a balance between credible and informed interviewer, on the one hand, and confidant and respectful seeker of valuable new information, on the other. Above all, one must doggedly pursue the subject who, in the same interview, can adopt the posture of public relations man, intellectual, healer, bureaucrat, visionary, friend, and adversary. As interviewers, we became sensitive to such changes in character; we tried to adapt accordingly. Refusal to answer a question was rare; a smokescreen was more frequent, but with two interviewers and 90 minutes or more of conversation, questions can be reworded, digressions can be stymied, rapport can be built. In very few instances did we feel our control over the situation slipping. Even those few subjects who sought to set the boundaries for the discussion at the outset of the interview became less defensive, their answers more fluent. They carried the discussion; we merely clued them into the problems and issues we wished to discuss.

22. In only one case did the subject continuously evade our policy queries by deflecting them into rambling technical expositions. Upon terminating this interview, we vowed, out of our dissatisfaction, to elicit more direct answers and to develop in subsequent interviews other subjects' perceptions of this remarkable man whose professional style, as we later learned, tended toward long-winded but perceptive and optimistic statements about cancer prevention programs.

23. Still, researchers in foreign countries and on the West Coast of the United States (particularly the Bishop group located at the University of California Medical School in San Francisco) had to be omitted from consideration due to time and budget constraints. *Curricula vitae* were requested from these 26 scientists, as they were from the subjects we did interview. Chapter 5 presents a career analysis of our interview subjects and mail respondents.

24. Woolgar (1976b) has found, for example, that "discovery accounts," as developed in a series of interviews over two- to three-year periods, tend to be unreliable, that is, subjects juxtapose, delete, and generally scramble events. "The facts" assume a status that is less stable and authoritative than the historical record shows.

25. Bader, the prototypical textbook scientist, confessed "no regrets" for his behavior: "I've always had the feeling that ideas were a dime a dozen. And for anybody to go around making conjectures and hypotheses, it may be interesting, but, really, that's blowing in the wind." Our impression is that he might have been more assertive, but the "unimpressive" label hung on him by a few of our subjects seemed little more than ignorance of the man.

26. Bader (1978) also pointed out that the first article on the requirement for DNA synthesis in reproduction of RNA tumor viruses is his 1964 one, published five to six months *prior* to Temin's statement of the provirus hypothesis. Written history attributes to Bader a *1965* article (appearing in the same journal as the 1964 one, *Virology*) that builds on Temin's hypothesis. As for the criticism that data produced by inhibitor research is of questionable validity, Bader suggests without rancor that this is not a problem for a careful experimenter, but that Temin's experiments were sloppy. This may have accounted, in part (as other of our subjects conjectured), for Temin's departure from the California Institute of Technology and the hubris attributed to him by his postdoctoral supervisor there, Harry Rubin. Rubin remained skeptical about the discovery of reverse transcriptase, even after the enzyme activity was observed in a wide array of viruses (Spiegelman et al., 1970). The existence of the DNA provirus was finally confirmed to the satisfaction of virologists by Hill and Hillova's (1972) demonstration of infectious DNA for Rous sarcoma virus (Temin, 1976).

CHAPTER 3

THE POLITICS OF CANCER:
Funding the Mission

> Cancer is not simply an island waiting in isolation for a crash program to wipe it out. It is in no way comparable to a moonshot—to a Gemini or an Apollo program—which requires mainly the mobilization of money, men and facilities to put together in one imposing package the scientific knowledge we already possess.
>
> Instead, the problem of cancer—or rather the problem of the various cancers—represents a complex, multi-faceted challenge at least as perplexing as the problem of the various infectious diseases. . . . We have barely begun to perceive the fantastic array of causative factors involved in cancer, the methods by which they work, and the agencies by which they may be controlled. We are not yet ready to start a countdown for an anti-cancer blast-off, no matter what emotional appeal such an approach may have to the public.

Philip R. Lee (in U.S. Senate, 1971a: 140-141)
Chancellor,
University of California

> Internal NCI affairs are very complex, and outsiders comment on them at their peril because there are so many political issues involved.

Howard M. Temin (quoted in Wade, 1976: 531)
Nobel Laureate

Introduction

The evolution of a U.S. cancer research policy, established in 1937 with the creation of the National Cancer Institute,[1] was interrupted by the passage of the National Cancer Act in 1971.[2] Even the prospect of a National Cancer Authority, envisioned in Senate Bill S.34 as separate from the National Institutes of Health (NIH) and possibly administratively independent of NCI, had generated scientific, organizational, and political cross-currents that were seldom found in earlier, small-scale biological research. As some (notably, Weinberg, 1965) had predicted, the time had come for Big Biology: In the past Big Physics met with success, so now the national funding focus must shift to the biological sciences. There was to be a "war on cancer" waged with the influx of moneys into cancer-related research (Kalberer, 1975 and Figure 3.1).

Elsewhere (Chubin and Studer, 1978), we have discussed in broad strokes how the evolutionary course of basic cell transformation research was profoundly altered.[3] In this chapter, we seek to augment this critical discussion with detailed observations (some of the first-person variety) on the early stages of the cancer war, its programmatic priorities, and outcomes.

DECLARING WAR ON CANCER

The major impetus for expanding cancer research was heralded by former President Nixon's second State of the Union Message which included "an appropriation of an extra $100 million to launch an intensive campaign to find a cure for cancer" (U.S. Senate, 1971a: 74). This request elicited an overwhelmingly positive response. Cancer as a symbolic threat was seemingly capable of unifying both Congress and the electorate (as Vietnam had not). In turn, it was difficult for scientists to find fault with this increased subsidy of biological science, given the broader context of slackening governmental support of science (Strickland, 1972). As Rettig, in his thoroughly insightful *Cancer Crusade: The Story of the National Cancer Act of 1971,* states:

> In political terms, the Act is of interest because it indicates how a small but powerful elite composed of private citizens mobilized sufficient political resources to secure passage of legislation opposed by the National Institutes of Health and by most of the biomedical scientific community. In policy terms, the Act captures much of the current conflict between the public and its elected representatives eager to see life-saving and life-prolonging results flow from biomedical research and, on the other hand, a scientific community acutely conscious of the long time and great uncertainty characteristic of the process by which medical research is translated into clinically useful results [Rettig, 1977: xiii].

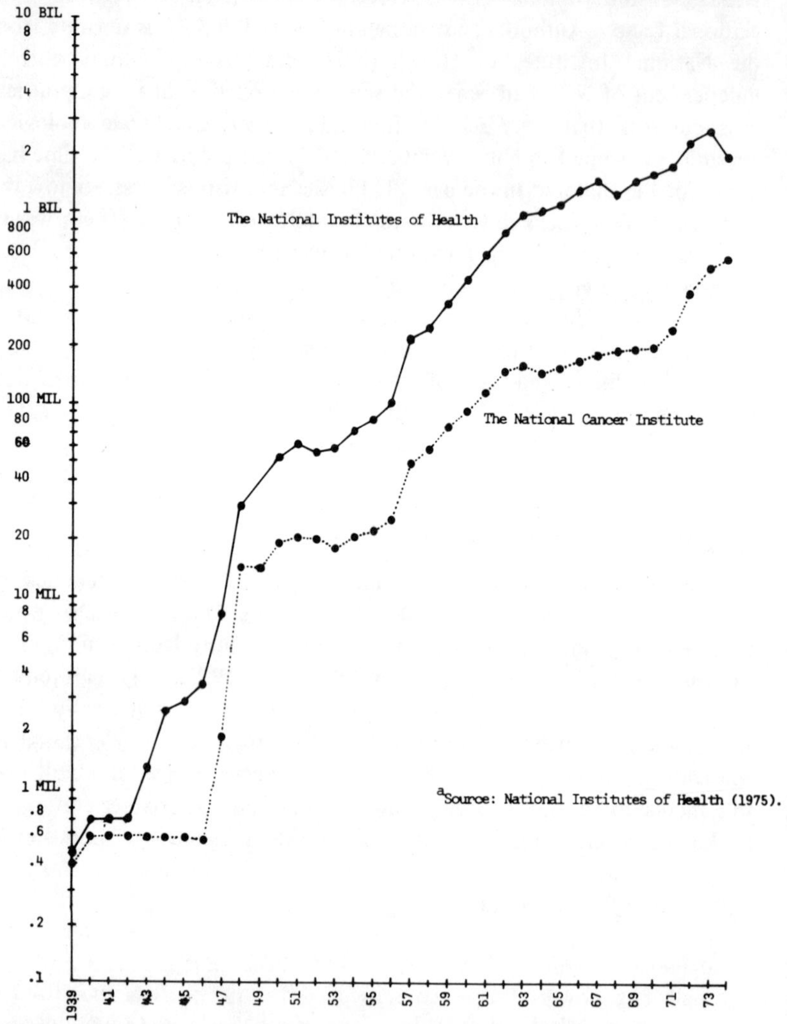

FIGURE 3.1 Amount (in Logarithms) of Appropriations to the National Institutes of Health and to the National Cancer Institute, 1939-1974[a]

Predictably, some reservations about the funding of cancer research were expressed. Dr. Campbell Moses, medical director of the American Heart Association, noted before the Senate Subcommittee on Health,

> that if the state of research in cancer makes reasonable such a comprehensible effort to the control of cancer today, an exactly parallel effort is even more appropriate in the field of heart disease. In the cardiovascular field, we know that the expansion of our research effort, and the comprehensive full-scale application of the fruits of already available research and technology, would save lives now [U.S. Senate, 1971a: 231].

That the cardiovascular field (which studies the number one killer, heart disease) was ripe for research, riper in fact than cancer, was of little *political* significance, however. As Senator Edward Kennedy remarked at the close of Moses's testimony, "There are those who say if you can't get a raise yourself, the best thing that can happen is for the fellow next to you to get a raise" (U.S. Senate, 1971a: 232).[4]

But how would the Cancer Act be administered? Whether it be administered autonomously as a NASA-type special project or as part of the existing NIH organization was an issue of research styles and reasoning processes within biomedicine. Taken at face value, at least provisionally, the scientists' expressed concern was for how biomedicine should interface with the existing organization.[5] Aside from the inevitable charges of favoritism and the abuse of power, the scientists' rhetoric centered on impediments to the advancement of knowledge inherent in the "mission mentality." What is at issue was the cognitive orientation toward research mobilization which the biomedical scientists shared and which accounts for their critical posture toward new funding mechanisms.

The biomedical researcher in the 1960s had already witnessed the pressures toward bigness and the scientific difficulties with mission-oriented research. As Health, Education and Welfare Secretary John Gardner cautioned:

> We must not imagine that dollars and large-scale organization are an adequate substitute for ideas and a sound scientific base. Where the ideas and the scientific base do not exist, it is possible to waste vast amounts of money under the banner of practicality [1966: 1602].

This caveat was echoed with even greater intensity by former (1955-1968) NIH Director Shannon in whose view, according to Strickland,

> Targeted research, research aimed at finding cures for particular health problems, was . . . not only the most expensive but certainly the most wasteful kind. The waste was not limited to dollars, but included use of scientific energies, for research efforts narrowly aimed at single targets could restrict the beneficial effects of the internal dynamics of science. Moreover, for NIH to place too much emphasis on directed research would be to retard the development of science in another way: it could artificially skew the production of new medical scientists [1972: 189].

Nevertheless, by early 1971 it was clear that the NCI was destined to be reorganized in accordance with a new mission-oriented mandate. When Congress established the Special Virus Leukemia Program in 1965 with an appropriation of $10 million, it became obvious what Congress had in mind. It wanted results. And to get results this program engaged in more contract research than had been the custom of any NIH agency (see Kalberer, 1975: 475f). Such contract research reflected a new type of planning premised on the operations research strategies that had worked for other areas of science.

Director Carl G. Baker, Frank Rauscher, the newly appointed Chairman of the Special Virus Leukemia Program, and Louis M. Carrese, a systems management specialist, set out to develop a "rational" basis for mission-oriented (therefore, contract-oriented) cancer research (Baker et al., 1966; Carrese and Baker, 1967; see Culliton, 1973). Although recognizing the limits of organizational theory when applied to biomedical research programs, they nevertheless assumed that at least one virus is an indispensible element for the initiation (directly or indirectly) of at least one kind of human leukemia (including lymphoma) and that the virus persists in the diseased individual (Baker et al., 1966). The emphasis on the viral etiology of cancer, in particular the importance of RNA viruses, had been organizationally blessed.[6] Contract research on the viral hypothesis would be a "programmatic" weapon in the cancer war arsenal. Still, medical researchers demurred. Some, like John A. D. Cooper, president of the Association of American Medical Colleges,[7] were disdainful (in testimony before the health subcommittee) of the nonscientists' view of how scientific "answers" materialize:

> An unfortunate misconception apparently is developing that the mere injection of additional federal cancer research funds will produce somehow an instant cure for cancer. Its equally misleading corollary is that the key to the conquest of cancer . . . lies in the managerial efficiency and the capacity of the medical-industrial complex [U.S. Senate, 1971a: 391].

A stark contrast to this view is provided by Benno Schmidt, who chairs the National Panel of Consultants on the Conquest of Cancer, forerunner of the existing President's Cancer Panel:[8]

> The valid analogy is not the scientific analogy but the organizational analogy. The cancer program, in order to succeed, needs the same independence in management, planning, budget presentation and assessment of program that those programs [splitting the atom or the space program] needed [U.S. Senate, 1971a: 196].

Rauscher (1978), recalling the passion of the debate, moderates Schmidt's tone:

> I think so long as the plan is reflective of the state of the art and doesn't try to force the state of the art, and that was the big fear of course, that the bull's eye was going to be used to tell "John" what he was going to do, and what he couldn't do, for that matter. It never was intended that way. I was a scientist, still am, and I would have rebelled myself at that. Carrese understands this very well, but many people don't understand that he understands it.

Finally, as Nobel laureate and NCI critic James Watson asserts:

> High-quality cancer research is likely to be much more difficult to pull off than most other forms of biology. . . . We may not have even one really hot clinical lead that has a good chance to lead somewhere soon with a major cancer. So we must be much more careful than we have in the past as to what we allow our lobbyist friends to claim for us. . . . We should do the science we are trained for and not hold the carrot too close. . . . But if we respond to the fear of less cancer money for next year by flashing out even shakier new leads, say, in tumor immunology, to mask the fact that we still have not made the big breakthrough, we have nowhere to go but down [quoted in Hixson, 1976: 178].

So on the one hand, the biomedical community was(is) under great pressure to effect a cancer cure. Witness a question recently posed to the President's Biomedical Research Panel: "Why don't you people in the NIH and the medical schools spend less time 'understanding' disease and more time preventing or curing it?" (Culliton, 1976: 33). On the other hand, Watson's statement reflects the peculiar nature of biomedical progress, namely, it is difficult to predict where a "breakthrough" will occur.[9] In the "uneasy partnership" (Lyons, 1969) between government and science, the "fear of less cancer money for next year" elicits a public relations response from the scientist; this response *must* be that progress is being made.[10]

The separation of imposed social structures from the structure of biomedical progress seems to be the source of the scientists' concern. By being a visible symbol of malaise as well as a research problem, cancer is particularly vulnerable to political abuse. The growth in the number of cancer victims, the shift in the age structure of the voting population and its possible partisan manipulation, and the need for conspicuous investments in science in the face of its dwindling public image (see Morison, 1969; Shils, 1972a; Toulmin, 1972), all capture something of the political tensions pervading cancer research. Cancer epitomizes a need for political mobilization exceeded perhaps only by issues of national defense. As Cooper concedes:

> In an ideal world, the association would say there is no need for new legislation to carry out a new scientific offensive against cancer. But the situation being what it is, there clearly is going to be some legislation [U.S. Senate, 1971a: 393].

That "situation" was charged with political overtones, forces with which scientists were ill at ease. To compound the situation, House Bill H.R. 10681 was introduced. The role of the author of this bill, Representative Paul G. Rogers (D-Florida), in effecting the compromise that the National Cancer Act of 1971 represented has been underplayed. Rogers paraded before his subcommittee member after member of the biomedical community who

> went on record in opposition to an autonomous cancer agency . . . [supplying] . . . a refutation of the Senate [Kennedy] bill and justification for this [Rogers's] own. . . . The net effect was to suggest that the Panel of Consultants [led by Schmidt] supported only by the American Cancer Society [and Richard Nixon, as it

> were], was isolated from the mainstream of biomedical thinking [Rettig, 1977: 233].

It was also a Rogers-called witness who drew attention to the discovery of reverse transcriptase by Temin and by Baltimore, noting (1) that this advance offered promise of determining whether viruses cause cancer in humans and (2) that David Baltimore's work had been supported mainly by the National Institute of Allergy and Infectious Diseases. To Rogers, and undoubtedly his subcommittee, this basic scientist, who had unexpectedly contributed to cancer research from unrelated work, was an outstanding illustration of why the existing NIH should be preserved (Rettig, 1977).[11]

Although Congress was ultimately convinced of the necessity for continuing the new cancer program *within* the structure of NIH (in the form of a compromise of S.34 cum S.1828 and its House counterpart H.R. 10681), the *internal* politics of cancer remained tense. On December 23, 1971 as an invited guest described, the President

> came to sign the Cancer Act of 1971. Cancer research had entered the political arena. The Congressmen and Senators who guided the law into being smiled broadly as the cameras focused on them. Most of the scientists in the audience did not smile; many were worried. The hoopla surrounding the Cancer Act implied the conquest on cancer in the near future because a couple of hundred million dollars a year more were to be channeled into cancer research. Those of us there who knew the "state of the art" had cause to worry [quoted in Rettig, 1977: 277].

The Postact Mission and Cancer Research Organization

The demands of science, organization, and politics were and remain intimately intertwined in the campaign to conquer cancer. And the effectiveness of any evaluation of a program such as this demands that the various ingredients receive their due portion of credit and blame. As one might expect after more than eight years of the program, a lot of credit and blame is available. Daniel Greenberg (1975) has leveled severe criticism at the optimistic claims of finding a cancer cure that emanate from the National Cancer Institute, seeing such claims as politically motivated and statistically suspect.

Not surprisingly, there is a body of opinion, if not evidence, to counter Greenberg's charge. Many *cognoscenti* point proudly to the Virus Cancer (nee Special Virus Leukemia) Program. From our interviewees we learned:

> You can't mount a national effort when Dick Rauscher and John Moloney are sitting in their labs dispensing their own virus just to certain scientists. Great big technical problem. Can you produce viruses, virus preparations, of high potency, high infectivity, high purity, in vat quantities so that lots of people can work on them? Sure. That [Virus Cancer] Program did that.

> I think the NCI did a couple of things, and had to do some things, unlike the other institutes. First of all, we had a number of line items in our budget which were, in effect, a mandate from the Congress to do so much at such a level in a particular field, not in a project now, but in groups of projects. Cancer control is a good example. Not only is there a separate appropriation for that part of the program, but an authorization as well coming out of the Kennedy-Rogers committees. So part of what we did was in effect built in or locked in because of the mandates. We strove, and I think successfully, to maintain the emphasis and integrity of our basic laboratory structure within the institute, but we did one thing different; and I still believe strongly that this is the way to go. We relied—we made a conscious decision to rely on—our good bench people in-house to help us manage outside programming. Management, scientific-wise, Carrese-wise, in my judgment was as important as doing good science.

> There was one key feature of the [program] for which Rauscher and Moloney must take a lot of the credit. They foresaw, when the thing was going to expand, that there would be logistical problems in supply and demand. They knew there would be a requirement for viruses on a large scale, cell culture on a large scale, for animals, etc. So from the very beginning, they created a resource logistic mechanism which would solve that problem so that by the time that guys like me came into the field, and I said, "Now, look," I told them, for example, that I would isolate and purify reverse transcriptase for them within one year if they would give me enough virus, and I told them how much virus I needed. In fact, Joe Beard got his start because of my demand, and he started as a subcontractor under my contract. And when I went to Joe and I said, "Joe, look, I need this and I'll give you the enzyme," and I said, "I need 10 grams of virus about every two months," he said, "No problem," and he delivered it. And we gave him the enzyme. We published the first purification in RT. That's the kind of thing that if the mechanism for underwriting Joe does not exist . . . that would have taken 10 years to do, or maybe even 20, if you have to use piddling amounts of virus. And

> the reason I was able within two weeks after confirming the thing with Rauscher [virus], we confirmed it with nine different viruses. The reason is that I had those viruses available to me.
>
> The Virus Cancer Program, because of its existence, and the level of funding that it had, or that it has, has provided a level of support for one relatively small area of science that's far out of proportion to its total scientific impact. Now, its medical impact you can argue about. I consider that the Virus Cancer Program was a good guess, because if you were going to try to hit the problem of cancer hard with an integrated program that you probably could not have made a better choice than to focus on viruses. Because the outcome, if you were right, if the guess was right, the outcome would be impressive. Yes, it was not as right as maybe we might have thought it was, and so the results have been not as dramatic. They've been scientifically very productive.

Such guarded praise of the Virus Cancer Program only hints at the evils it came to symbolize. It was perhaps the most visible contract program amidst the glaring visibility of the cancer mission, as operationalized by NCI. It was, therefore, the most vulnerable to criticism by the scientific community as well. And criticism–some say a surfeit of criticism–it surely got.

THE VIRUS CANCER PROGRAM AND ORGANIZATIONAL CRITICISM: THE ZINDER COMMITTEE REPORT

In 1974, the report of the ad hoc Zinder Committee, so named for its chairman, Dr. Norton Zinder of Rockefeller University, was submitted to the National Cancer Advisory Board.[12] This committee had been constituted after growing criticism of the Virus Cancer Program (VCP) indicated that an evaluation–not unlike the evaluation of NIH by the Wooldridge committee a decade earlier–was in order. As then-NCI director Rauscher (1978) told us:

> I appointed the Zinder Report, and I called for it. That was my thought. I'll never forget, I talked at coffee with Benno Schmidt, and I said, "Benno, are we going to have to appoint a major group to come in and take a look at this from the outside?" On the way back into the room we talked to Jim Watson and Jim thought it was a fine idea. Before that morning session was over, Jim had walked around my side and given me a slip of paper and given me names that he suggested, and I used most of those names, as a matter of fact, to the chagrin of many of my colleagues in virology.

The committee's comments were generally harsh and pointed:

> First, the committee said, the VCP is too expensive. (It costs about $50 million to $60 million a year and consumes slightly more than 10 percent of the total NCI budget.) Second, the program must be opened up to the scientific community. At present, it is run by a handful of persons who have undue control over large amounts of money, which goes to only a limited number of laboratories. Furthermore, the individuals who award contracts are in a position to award them to each other, which somehow does not seem quite right. The committee called for new management practices and a good stiff measure of peer review by outside scientists [Culliton, 1974: 143].

Centralization of (S)VCP funds was perhaps the most devastating finding of the Zinder report. A few individuals were found to dispense enormous sums of money *annually,* notably $19 million to Robert Huebner (Chief, Viral Carcinogenesis Branch, NCI), $7 million to George Todaro (Chief, Viral Leukemia and Lymphoma Branch, NCI), and $12 million to Robert Manaker (Chief, Viral Biology Branch, NCI).[13]

> It was only natural that when the SVCP was formed [initially to explore the possible role of adenoviruses in malignancy], a small group of investigators was involved—an "in group." It now represents a somewhat larger "in group" of investigators. Administratively its procedures lack vigor, are apparently attuned to the benefit of staff personnel and are full of conflicts of interest. Because the direct targets have become fuzzy since 1964, although the available funds have continued to grow, the program seems to have become an end in itself, its existence justifying its further existence. In doing so, it is eroding what is good in both the grant and contract mechanisms, a fact which may account for the widespread antipathy to SVCP in the scientific community [quoted in Hixson, 1976: 132].

A non-NCI researcher informed us:

> There were clear deficiencies in the VCP . . . because it grew up too fast and things were done that probably would have been done a little bit more rationally, and there were areas of abuse, which should be corrected, and that's essentially what the Zinder report tried to do. I don't think there was any serious question in the minds of the Zinder Committee, and it certainly didn't appear in their report, that the science that was being done by the VC people was

> excellent, and there was no doubt that of all programs that were going on at NCI, as well as the clinical ones, it was the one that was producing the new science for the buck. And so all in all the thrust that was in the report was to correct obvious undesirable features of the VCP. [Administrative?] Administrative, and conflicts of interests which existed between in-house people and out-house research (I use the word *out-house* advisedly)—and so on and so on. I think that's perfectly okay. The Zinder report was a good one and it served a useful purpose . . . because you had to tread on some very powerful toes to get it done, so it took a while. But Rauscher started to move in that direction and Moloney certainly did, and a lot of wings were clipped, not completely—I mean, those things are very difficult to reverse.

Rauscher (1978), in defending the Program, observes that

> When we first got that $10 million in 1966, the Congress said, "You can have the money, but you've got to spend it by contract." That was a mandate, too, incidentally. We had no choice. We couldn't go grants if we had wanted to. . . . And at that time we used some of the money in order to get off the ground very quickly through a sole source contract, some of which was to support what I thought were exceedingly good ideas by in-house investigators. Well, as the dollars became bigger and as these fellows became successful in the sense of publishing many papers, they began to be resented by people on the outside who had to compete for every dollar they had—again, totally predictable. So, yes, when you say that the second criticism[14] was one of administrative arrangement, or of the technique of management, you are absolutely right.

Rauscher also impressed upon us:

> Number one, during much of that program, you could not grant outside of the United States . . . and a major focus was opportunities abroad, so they had to use the contract mechanism. Number two, you cannot grant to a commercial organization. You must use contracts, by law and regulation. Number three, many of our best scientists in this country happen to be in commercial organizations and you want to do work with the best scientists. And that was, I think, overlooked [by critics]. . . . I was there when Mr. Nixon flew out of the sky and said, "You now have Fort Detrick." Not many of us wanted it. I think it was wise to take it, not only for cancer, but for the rest of NIH, as I thought at the time. But, in effect, in getting no more money to take over Detrick, he was saying, "We're going to

> turn swords into plowshares for cancer research; for the public of this nation, you run that facility." We were not given any positions to run it, and we recognized immediately that we would have to contract with somebody to do it–the way Union Carbide runs Oak Ridge–and incidentally, that was the model we used. And, again, I think wisely so. So . . . we're locked in. We, meaning the NCI, are locked into something like $25 to $30 million a year to keep a very good facility with very good people going, but it does not have the same peer review because it cannot, for individual projects, within that $25 million. It's almost like NCI. My people at NCI got their support as a cut off the top. You know, they had to write an annual report and so forth, but in effect their support was guaranteed. They didn't have to write a grant request, contract request, or what have you. Neither do the individual scientists at Litton.[15] When they compete, they compete for . . . a three-year kind of project . . . and for that period of time, they're pretty safe.

Finally, another academic researcher offered this view:

> The difficulty that the Zinder report was talking about was that prime commercial laboratories were getting fortunes to do very little, and they seem to have been too well entrenched to have been touched, at least under the previous administration at NCI. And there you have to look very closely at the power of a single man [Moloney?]. Without a doubt. He determined what was being done and . . . [who to] hire for a position . . . That grated on our self-image and pride, because it was such poor work being funded, such as enormous amount of it, that that gave the VCP a terrible name for producing the worst kind of science at the most cost. But in fact the VCP also supported some of the very best work around the country. And had they been hard-nosed about what they supported, and had they insisted on the principle that you only support good science in the best places . . . they would be in much better shape now.

The administrative upshot of the Zinder Committee review was, in Rettig's words, an

> "opening up" the VCP program specifically through the establishment of an NCAB (National Cancer Advisory Board) oversight committee, a reconstitution of the contract review groups, and the elimination of contract work that was an extension of VCP scientists' intramural research. The NCAB did establish a subcommittee, chaired by Dr. Harold Amos of Harvard Medical School, to monitor

> the program's response to the Zinder Committee's recommendations. The VCP, on its part, has established an advisory committee of nonprogram scientists to provide advice on broad directions of resource allocation, promising lines of scientific inquiry, and means of application of research findings. The contract review process was also modified to increase the rigor of review of individual contract proposals. The Amos subcommittee, in its report to the NCAB of June 1975, indicated its general approval of the program changes [1977: 301].

In addition, NCI has sought to streamline and standardize its procedures for reviewing contract and grant proposals alike, though many of our interviewees doubted the effectiveness, or even the sincerity, of the announced (see Rauscher, 1974) modifications.[16]

The Zinder Committee also concluded, however, that "about 50 percent of the program is supportable at some level" (Culliton, 1974: 144). Hence, the *intellectual* investment of administrators and researchers in VCP may have been politically and organizationally expedient, but reproachable on grounds of knowledge (or ignorance):

> Many of those in administrative control of the VCP are men whose careers are intimately linked to the idea that there is a relationship between certain RNA viruses and human cancer. Much of the research the program supports is aimed at substantiating this idea. VCP support of research on DNA viruses is comparatively small. The committee recommends . . . an integrated program with a built-in series of checks and balances to prevent the special notions of particular individuals from carrying the day. For example, should the first definitive [human] cancer virus turn out to be a papova virus [one of many suspected DNA viruses], the VCP would be in a strange position. It scarcely supports any work in this area and only recently has gotten seriously involved with the DNA viruses such as herpes [Culliton, 1974: 144].

If priorities *within* NCI were scrambled by the cancer war, then we must ask how this mission affected allocations to NIH institutes other than NCI.

NCI and Funding Prosperity[17]

The two major sources of funds in the United States for the support of cancer research have been the American Cancer Society (ACS) and the

National Cancer Institute (NCI). The smooth increase of the ACS curve since 1948 (see Figure 3.2) is no doubt indicative of a set of public beliefs about cancer and its cure. Numerous Gallup polls have demonstrated (e.g., Rauscher, 1974) that cancer is the most feared of diseases in the United States, a fear that translates into contributions to the ACS.[18]

Comparing the amounts of ACS and NCI moneys in Figure 3.2 lends credence to the claim that interpreting shifts in funding is perilous. Had cancer research reached a critical "take-off" threshold of knowledge in 1958 due to the cumulative effects of ACS and NCI funding prior to that year? Was the funding merely part of the overall increase of governmental interest in science stimulated by the Russian Sputnik? Did it stem from the general shift in attitude toward governmental patronage of science in the post-World War II era? Or had the public displaced the responsibility of biomedical progress from private organizations to the federal government?[19]

All of these are plausible, compelling explanations for the steady gain in ACS contributions versus the irregularities on the NCI curve observed in Figure 3.2. Kenneth Endicott (1969), former director of NCI, has argued that the major perturbations are due to the Korean and Vietnamese wars, respectively. Do comparable shifts in priorities obtain when a domestic war has been declared?

With the passage of the Cancer Act in 1971,

> Though separate agency status was not secured, substantial autonomy for NCI was obtained. The new law gave NCI a renewed and expanded mandate, raised the formal status of its director, provided the expectation for vastly increased funds, and in the budgetary by-pass mechanism established a procedure for asserting autonomy. The resolution of the legislative debate left the cancer crusade advocates with much of what they wanted, but gave the opponents the symbolic and material accomplishment of defeating the proposed separate agency recommendation [Rettig, 1977: 291].

Although the "separate and unequal" doctrine was defeated by the act, NCI had become the "I" in NIH. Querying Rauscher about this privileged status, we heard a straining for consistency (that was not very convincing):

Interviewer: Does it matter that the Cancer Institute is inside the NIH fold or outside the NIH fold?

Rauscher: Oh, I always thought it should be inside.

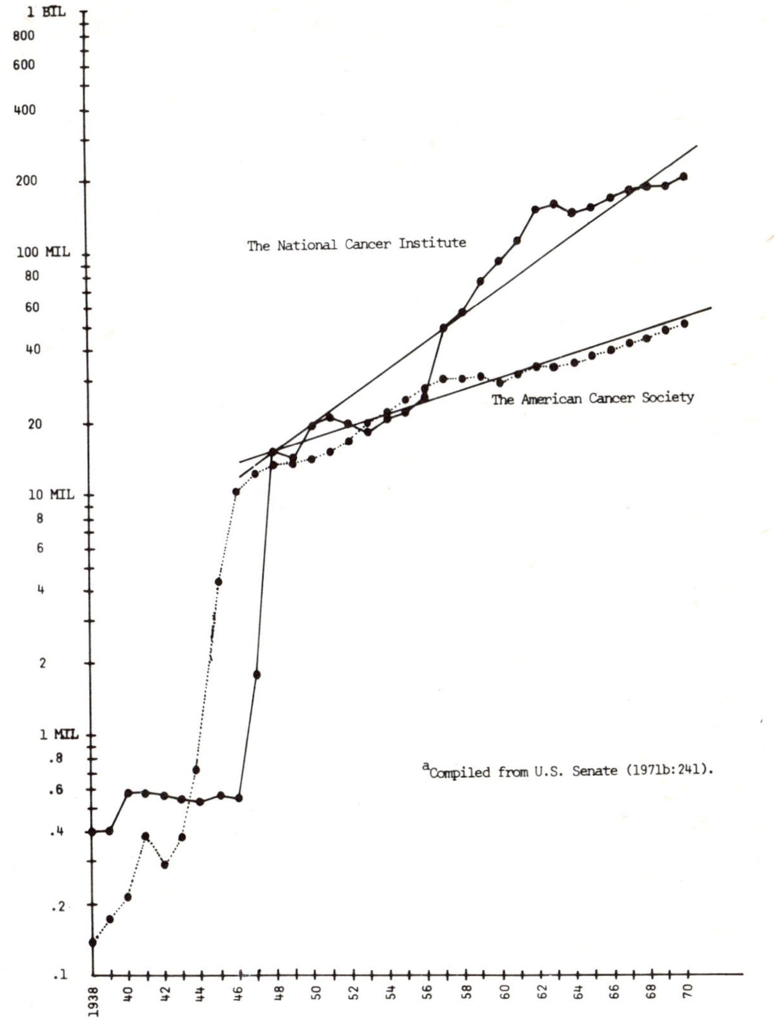

FIGURE 3.2 Amount (in Logarithms) of Appropriations to the National Cancer Institute and Contributions to the American Cancer Society, 1938-1970[a]

Int: But you were a minority on that.

Rauscher: Yeah, I was not very popular when I said that, among some of the outside lobbying groups and pressure people. I was always firmly convinced that in order for the cancer program to be healthy, we needed a healthy NIH. We're part of a family. I wanted our people to be able to collaborate with somebody over in Allergy, or Dental, or what have you.

On the record, Rauscher has maintained that the decrease in funding of other institutes of NIH had little to do with the national mobilization against cancer:

> These reductions cannot in fairness be attributed to the existence of the National Cancer Program, although this would be difficult to prove beyond a doubt. On the other hand, it is just as difficult to prove that the other institutes would have received more funds if the National Cancer Program did not exist. In fact, I am told by people in the Office of Management and Budget that the latter would not have happened in 1972 to 1974 [Rauscher, 1975: 118].

In our interview, however, there is some wavering:

> When I was there [at NCI] I was a member of the Executive Branch, appointed directly by the President. . . . I was fortunate enough to have people like Mary [Lasker] and Benno Schmidt,[20] in particular, and direct access to the White House, so that when I went to a congressional hearing and they said, "But couldn't you use more money," I would be able to say, "Absolutely, my board and panel tell me we can use another 185 million." And, I guess, almost no other director of any other institute had that option.

Elsewhere in our conversation Rauscher remarked:

> You have got to remember the first two years—the critical first two years—of major budgetary increases, that money did not come out of HEW funds. It came out of a pocket that Mr. Nixon had in OMB. So there was no way that we were competing for funds out of the HEW pocket. Very few people understand that point. In later years, that was not true. We *were* competing for what money was available in HEW.

In other words, the conquest of cancer was not entertained publicly as a viable explanation of concomitant decreases in funding for the other institutes. What were "obvious" macro-level explanations in fundings fluctuations when military mobilization was involved are not invoked when the mobilization against cancer is raised. Privately, Rauscher is more sanguine—and less persuasive. His explanations differ in their intuitive appeal depending upon where, when, and to whom he is speaking. His is essentially a nonzero-sum interpretation: "We won but you didn't lose." Yet such an interpretation is plausible if allocations to NCI are seen as independent of the total NIH budget.

Even if the funding of NCI and of the rest of NIH are totally independent events, one must still deal with the whole picture of biomedical organization[21] and support in the United States. In the late 1960s, a tense situation was brewing *within* all of the institutes. As Kalberer observes:

> In the case of NCI, award rates started to fall off dramatically beginning in 1968 as a result of the leveling off of Congressional appropriations. Consequently, there was a steady downward trend in the percentage of traditional grants awarded, particularly new grants, in 1970 the Institute reached its all time low level, awarding only 30% of approved grants. With passage of the Act of 1971 this trend was reversed. Within the last 4 years, at least 50% of all approved new applications have been awarded. [Clearly] the halcyon years, prior to 1964, when NIH, including NCI, was able to fund more than 90% of all approved applications, have passed [1975: 478].

Relative deprivation could thus be felt by some institutes. The new war on cancer did not occur in a vacuum; the basis for a feeling of deprivation was already present, a feeling which Rauscher himself (1975) was trying to defuse.

To illustrate the problem of relative deprivation, Table 3.1 has been constructed. In Table 3.1 the total NIH allocations received by an institute (the six major NIH institutes which have been in operation since at least 1954 are represented) for a given year are shown. By reading across institutes, especially in comparing the "% Δ" columns, one gains a perspective on systematic changes in funding priorities *within* the NIH institute structure.

First, it must be noted that several of the institutes did not come into existence until 1954. The origin years of the six are as follows: National Cancer Institute (NCI), 1937; National Heart and Lung Institute (NHLI) and National Institute of Dental Research (NIDR), 1950; National Institute of Allergy and Infectious Diseases (NIAID), National Institute of

TABLE 3.1 Annual Appropriations with Percentage Annual Increase for Six Institutes of the National Institutes of Health, 1954-1974[a]

Years	Institutes NCI	% Δ	NHLI	% Δ	NIDR	% Δ	NIAMDD	% Δ	NIAID	% Δ	NINDS	% Δ
1954	20.237		15.168		1.740		7.000		5.738		4.500	
1955	21.737	7.41	16.668	9.89	1.990	14.37	8.270	18.14	6.180	7.70	7.600	68.89
1956	24.978	14.91	18.898	13.38	2.176	9.35	10.840	31.08	7.775	25.81	9.861	29.75
1957	48.432	93.90	33.396	76.72	6.026	176.93	15.885	46.54	13.299	71.05	18.650	89.13
1958	56.402	16.46	35.936	7.61	6.430	6.70	20.385	28.33	17.400	30.84	21.387	14.68
1959	75.268	33.45	45.613	26.93	7.420	15.40	31.215	53.13	24.071	38.34	29.403	37.48
1960	91.257	21.24	62.237	36.45	10.019	35.03	46.862	50.13	34.054	41.47	41.487	41.10
1961	110.300	20.87	86.900	39.63	15.500	54.71	61.200	30.60	44.000	29.21	49.600	19.56
1962	142.836	29.50	131.912	51.80	17.340	11.87	81.831	33.71	55.341	25.78	70.812	42.77
1963	155.742	9.04	147.398	11.74	21.199	22.25	103.388	26.34	66.142	19.52	83.506	17.93
1964	143.194	-8.06	127.423	-13.55	19.166	-9.59	107.699	4.17	67.117	1.47	84.471	1.16
1965	150.011	4.76	124.824	-2.04	20.083	4.78	113.050	4.97	69.847	4.07	87.821	3.97
1966	163.768	9.17	141.462	13.33	23.677	17.90	123.203	8.98	77.987	11.65	101.153	15.18
1967	175.656	7.26	164.770	16.48	28.308	19.56	135.687	10.13	90.670	16.26	116.296	14.97
1968	183.356	4.38	167.954	1.93	30.307	7.06	143.954	6.09	94.442	4.16	128.633	10.61
1969	185.149	.98	166.928	-.61	29.984	-1.07	143.888	-.04	96.840	2.54	128.934	.23
1970	190.486	2.88	171.378	2.67	30.809	2.75	146.619	1.90	103.695	7.08	107.365	-16.73
1971	233.160	22.40	194.925	13.74	35.440	15.03	137.986	-5.89	102.368	-1.28	103.502	-3.60
1972	378.794	62.46	232.627	19.34	43.388	22.43	153.337	11.13	109.118	6.59	116.731	12.78
1973	492.205	29.94	300.000	28.96	46.991	8.30	167.316	9.12	113.414	3.94	130.672	11.94
1974	551.191	11.98	302.915	.97	45.565	-3.03	159.447	-4.70	114.000	.36	125.000	-4.34

[a]Compiled from National Institutes of Health (1975).

Arthritis, Metabolism, and Digestive Diseases (NIAMDD), and National Institute of Neurological Diseases and Stroke (NINDS), 1954. That NCI and NHLI enjoyed a comparatively favorable position in 1965 is probably due largely to the fact that they had been in existence for a period, were therefore well-entrenched, and had acquired funding momentum.[22]

Second, recognize that changes in appropriations may derive from several types of organizational shifts. An example is the change in NIDR 1956-1957 fostered by an unusually large appropriations increase (177%, Table 3.1). In contrast, the precipitous decline of NINDS in 1970 is no doubt a result of the creation of the National Eye Institute (1968), a spinoff from NINDS (with independent budget status in 1970).

Our primary concern, however, is the realignment of the institute structure in the 1970s, for this is the period of disjunctive, selective funding shifts. The stability observed from 1964 to 1969 dissipates markedly in the 1970s. Although some of this may be accounted for by the reorganization and separation of new institutes from established ones, the general tendencies seem to follow economic exigencies, new orientations to basic and applied research, and policy decisions based on these views. From 1970 forward, the allocations of funds to NCI, NHLI, and NIDR stand in striking contrast to the allocations of funds to NIAMDD, NIAID, and NINDS. The patterns of percent increase per year are salient in this period; the concentration of funds, especially in NCI but also in NHLI and NIDR, greatly depresses the relative positions of the remaining groups.

But the National Cancer Institute also had reasons to feel slighted in the years *prior* to the Cancer Act. Figure 3.3 displays the percentage of NCI grants, both in numbers and in dollars, of all NIH grants from 1946 to 1974. The Shannon years (1955-1968) were years of decreased cancer funding relative to the growth of NIH. Numerous new institutes had been formed during these years and their funding demands had cut into the percentage of biomedical funds devoted to cancer research. Given the broadened institute structure and the shifts in funding priority during the 1950s and 1960s, it is quite understandable why the funding policy changes in the 1970s should create tension. With more institute "mouths" to feed, combined with an overall decrease in biomedical research allocations, noncancer research was threatened by the war on cancer. Even those institutes which were experiencing increases in their funding allocations during the 1970s were not increasing as rapidly as NCI. Absolute and relative deprivation were being felt by all except those involved with cancer.

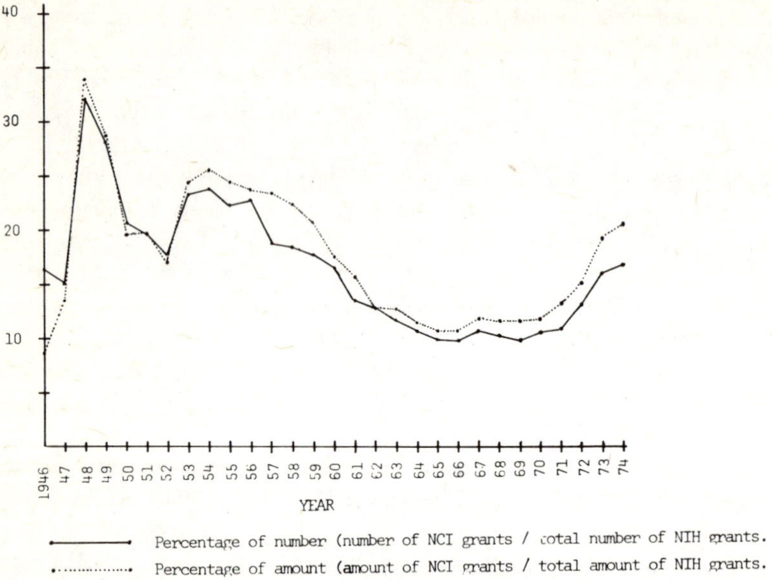

[a]Compiled from National Institutes of Health (1975:117).

FIGURE 3.3 Percentage of Number and Percentage of Amount of the National Institutes of Health Grants Awarded by the National Cancer Institute, 1946-1974[a]

KNOWLEDGE FROM MISSION MONEY?: DOUBTS ABOUT CONTRACT RESEARCH

Within the cancer research community, the decade of prosperity enjoyed by NCI brought to a head the philosophical clash over strategies for funding biomedical research. To contract or not to contract for knowledge: That is the question. For some, the steady rise of "contracted" projects within NIH signalled a major intellectual shift and, therefore, an encroachment on biomedical research. Longo (1973), for example, has pointed out that from 1971 to 1972, contracts in NIH increased by 47% but research grants by only 19%. The concentration of this funding mode in the new mission-oriented programs (46.4% of NCI and 27.7% of "heart" funds administered in 1973 through contracts) was particularly alarming to this critic. Why?

> Forty-seven percent of NCI contracts were with *profit* making organizations in 1972. Route 70S near Bethesda, MD, is rapidly developing into a biological Route 128 composed of industrial contractors nourished by NIH.... It is clear, however, that well-motivated scientists must provide for themselves and that they can find reasons to shift allegiances toward contract funding, especially if the squeeze is tight enough and long enough. Contract research, which is largely for product delivery or procurement purposes, has *the potential of undermining a scientist's commitment to patient, systematic and often frustrating discovery-oriented basic research* [Longo, 1973: 2080; italics added].

While the trend has clearly been toward more contract research, NCI spent virtually half of its external research moneys on contract research, a rate almost five times greater than for the rest of NIH. This coupled with the fact that by 1974 NCI accounted for 40% of all NIH contracts and 55% of all research money expended through contracts reveals the basis for concern. The war on cancer thus precipitated a more rapid shift toward contract research than would have occurred through more gradual evolution. As one of our interviewees put it:

> The whole Cancer Institute ... grew too fast, and without any decent quality control. It turns out a lot of people knew that and knew what they were doing: which was simply taking advantage of a positive political climate in order to get as much as they could. And when you get it, you have to spend it. If you give it back, they are not going to give you as much again. So they were quickly finding ways to spend lots of money. And what [present NCI director Arthur] Upton's got to do now,[23] and I think he recognizes that, is revamp things so that the amount of money that they have can now be utilized better, effectively building on the political clout or threat of his predecessors to restructure the institute so that it uses that money effectively. Because we're under an enormous amount of pressure.

NCI's mandated commitment to fund nonacademic research (recall Rauscher's statements above) was a major source of "pressure." Some of its largest contractors were private laboratories. Microbiological Associates, a subsidiary of Dynasciences Corporation which in turn is a subsidiary of Whittaker Corporation, has been very active in developing and producing tissue cultures as well as reagents for viral and immunological research for the cancer effort. Flow Laboratories, which dominates the European market of "biological products" through its laboratory in Scotland, has long been a "commercial leader in the virology field" so that it could easily shift when the war on cancer began to "studying the role of cancer viruses as potentially causative agents in human cancer" (Monaghan, 1974: 19).[24]

If the contract mechanism *did* signify a shift in organizational focus of biomedical research, then NCI can legitimately be given credit for hastening the shift by emphasizing nonacademic contract research. Contract research was rapidly becoming a symbol of targeted research executed outside the academic setting by quasi-governmental research laboratories. The NCI and its war on cancer was perhaps the single most important instrument for establishing this new organizational image for biomedical research.

For the biologist, however, such research was a violation of cognitive norms, of epistemologies ("how do I know, learn, and discover within biomedicine") which, in turn, implicate some fundamental etiological understandings about the biological world. The etiological conflicts seem to be a particularly resilient bone of contention, for if one acknowledges that biological existence is an evolving, systematic phenomenon, then the quest for *any* causal explanation (as is often latent in mission-oriented research) can lead to a kind of "sectarian" science, for example, the "pill concept" (Pigman, 1973) or some other quick technological fix, that can distort and perhaps hamper the development of research programs in biomedicine (Zubrod et al., 1966). NCI's discouragement of research on the viral induction of cancer in 1938 and its official reinstatement with the establishment within NCI of the Laboratory of Viral Oncology in 1971 are excellent illustrations of changes in etiological emphasis. Whatever the merits of this emphasis (as embodied in the Viral Cancer Program), some regard the vast sums of support for a viral etiological explanation of cancer as the epitome of sectarian science.

REORDERING CANCER PRIORITIES

With Rauscher's retirement as NCI director in 1977, a cloud of doubt hung over the future place and value of virus research in the cancer program. Some (Culliton, 1977) predicted a change in emphasis to environmental carcinogenesis research and a corresponding de-emphasis on viral oncology. Others lamented that with Moloney's ouster, the VCP would slowly be dismantled. On the fate of the Virus Cancer Program, ACS Executive Vice-President Rauscher hopes that

> it increases and expands. Again, recognizing that it's not the Virus Program that it was in 1966. . . . Rather than detract from that Program, they ought to increase it. I know of no other way even conceivable right now in which we can prevent many cancers in common denominator ways despite the fact that we're breathing carcinogens right now and we're going to continue. . . . There's no doubt about the fact that the environment out there will continue to be contaminated for some time. We're not going to do away with the automobile, the asbestos in its brake linings, very quickly. So it's good to try and to talk about cleaning up the environment, cutting down on emission, and so forth. I'm very much for that, but . . . we're also talking about a hundred different diseases that people call cancer. . . . [We] cannot, it seems to me, look for a hundred ways of preventing these diseases. We've got to look for some common denominator ways of preventing cancer (despite the fact that we're going to continue to be exposed to carcinogens for our bad habits). . . . The identification of pieces of the virus, of RNA viruses, or of genetic information, and the only thing that can code for that, as far as we know in all of biology, is an RNA tumor virus.

The switch from broad-based support of basic research to the concentrated betting on certain cures or causes creates tensions for scientists with cognitive orientations to cancer other than those which currently enjoy popularity and political power. Given the necessity of explicit policy decisions in a national mobilization effort such as the war on cancer, there is also a danger that organization will lead to the perception of out-right "governmentalization" or the "politicization" of science[25] in the form of privileged research traditions or approaches. As Rettig recently stated in testimony before the Senate Subcommittee on Nutrition:

> The research effort that came after 1971 legislation looked very much like the effort that preceded it. Only it was on a grander scale. Though an internal planning effort of substantial proportions was undertaken, that effort had relatively little connection with the resource allocation processes and did little to set priorities for a period of resource scarcity. Programs that were important before the Act remained important afterwards. But concern for environmental carcinogenesis, for instance, emerged forcefully only in the mid-1970s after the identification of and attendant publicity about

> asbestos, vinyl chloride, and other chemicals as occupational and environmental hazards of cancer-causing potential. And that concern emerged primarily from sources outside the national cancer program rather than from within it. It is my impression, furthermore, that the concern for the relationship of nutrition and diet to cancer shares a similar history [1978: 4].

Today, we hear echoes of the same allegations made about organizational priorities in 1974:

> Bad feelings about the VCP exist because there are a lot of virologists who share the same goals. The ones in the VCP were very rich. The others, who are just as good, were very poor [Watson in Culliton, 1974: 144].

Watson, an outspoken proponent of funding for basic research,[26] draws qualified support for his position from two unlikely sources—the "fortuitous" cancer war team of Schmidt and Rauscher:

> We need to have a cadre of very good scientists just following their noses and not worrying about relevance. I felt very strongly about that, too; and I had no opposition, therefore, from many of my people, certainly not from the Congress. So there's a place for an ivory tower, but not at the expense of transferring technology that might benefit people. . . . The thing that I feared most was that as funds became tight and as there was a reaction against the cancer establishment because of its privileged status—this was absolutely predictable five or six years ago—the first thing that Congress would do, I think, would be to attack the image of an ivory tower privileged government laboratory, and they would delete funds from our own in-house organization or operation. I felt that would be devastating, really, to the national program, not only to NCI. So now that NCI is involved in technology transfer, in cancer control programs, I don't think there are many in the Congress who could say, "Those guys out there just want to be left alone; they want to be funded simply because they are scientists; and they don't give a damn about Johnny with leukemia out in my district." They can't say that because there's an honest-to-God commitment on the part of most of those people to help in various aspects of the national program, be it review, site visiting, advice to the Director, advice to people on the outside, advice to the Congress, for that matter. They're heavily involved, more so than any other institute, and I think that's healthy [Rauscher, 1978].

Even more telling is the language of Schmidt's fifth report to the President on the National Cancer Program:

> There is no question that there has been during this period an enormous extension of our science base and our knowledge as a result of the vast amount of highly excellent fundamental basic research that has been supported. But this extension of our knowledge only underlines how vast are the areas of ignorance which remain. Just as the past five years have brought a greatly enlarged science base, they have also brought important improvements in the clinic in dealing with cancer, but here again our progress only serves to emphasize how far we have to go. . . . [We] cannot afford not to support basic research. . . . For we are, in truth, profoundly ignorant about the real nature of cancer [quoted in Rettig, 1977: 319].

The promise of 1971, fortified by massive mission money, has carried the Cancer Act to reauthorizations (as mandated by law) in 1974, 1977, and 1978. Since fiscal 1972, NCI appropriations have cumulated to over $5 billion, but the rhetoric *has* subsided. Today, Schmidt's report is restrained; Rauscher speaks of "over-promising" and "over-expectancy," and a reverse transcriptase researcher comments on the politics of cancer:

> The whole Yarborough Committee operation that set in motion the war on cancer occurred before the RT was known. . . . RT fit very comfortably into their idea that there was new progress in cancer research that was exploitable. . . . It was certainly, then, used politically a lot. There is no question. And, in a sense, appropriately, because it did represent the first opportunity to deal with a class of viruses that everybody knew were important, and no one knew how to deal with. And up to the time that we discovered RT, the amount of sensible work on RNA tumor viruses was miniscule. . . . And just by providing a tool, never mind about providing a concept, it changed (overnight) the whole ability of handling these viruses. And since Huebner had imbued everybody with the belief that these were the key to cancer, there was no question that this was an enormous political, as well as scientific, breakthrough. The tough thing is to really say to what extent it mattered.

Conclusions

If 75% of all biomedical research carried out in U.S. medical schools and over 40% of all university research is funded by NIH (Gustafson,

1975), then through shifts in policy such as that embodied in the war on cancer NIH can exert tremendous pressures on the selection of research topics.[27] And scientists *will* pursue the opportunities which increased funding makes possible.[28] But there is more. For by listening to criticisms by scientists one can quickly ascertain their concerns qua researchers. The norms to which they appeal are cognitive norms of argumentation within biomedicine.

Accordingly, by weighing both the discovery processes within areas such as cancer research and the criticisms which scientists have directed toward organizational tensions, sociologists of science can rethink their research tasks. The structure of reasoning can be pivotal in defining areas for study, while the search for violations of cognitive norms can translate the criticisms which scientists articulate into vital research questions about their "vocabularies of justification." For what we have here is not just Big Biology and contract research; what we have is ideology. And in Gouldner's words:

> It is one of ideology's essential social functions—of considerable cognitive relevance—to stand outside of science itself, and to reject the idea of science as *self*-sufficient or *self*-grounded. In other terms, ideology's critique of science, its refusal to let science be the only judge of itself, its public exposure of science's selfishness, . . . and the *limits* of science, mean in effect that: ideology functions as an epistemology of everyday life [1976: 36].

For the biomedical researcher, science policy has created a new rhetorical vocabulary to vouchsafe the epistemology of their everyday science.

Postscript to Part I

If the organization of science can distort and even thwart the development of science (as numerous scientists quoted above seem to think), then how can one ever know what the biological argumentation process *should* be? By considering the possibility that the development of science should *not* be equated with the development of the social system of science, one begins to fashion a realistic theory of scientific growth which captures the force of knowledge. Knowledge seems to develop *in spite of* its formal and informal social structures. This can occur because of the "predominance of cognitive orientation" (Boehme, 1975: 241) which scientists share and which shapes the parameters of their intellectual work.

By recognizing the predominant knowledge function of science, a norm is established by which a meaningful analysis of science can proceed. Sociologists must learn to recognize organizational "distortions" of science. But first, they must inform themselves of the scientists' "cognitive orientation"; only then can they speak forcefully to science policy questions, making the "is" of the scientific reasoning process the "ought" of science policy and research organization.

Through a series of arguments the theoretical groundwork has been installed for the following chapters. First (Chapter 1), the unfolding of a research tradition, cell transformation, and the confluence patterns which precede discovery were discussed. Second (Chapter 2), by demonstrating how meaningful "slices" of biomedical research can be isolated for sociological analysis, it was seen that biomedicine features a "structure of relevance" or distinctive rationality for the formation and study of problem domains, including the perceptions of researchers who were instrumental in the establishment of those domains. Third (Chapter 3), we examined how scientists routinely separate the organization of science from the structure of argumentation which advances their research, and how funding policy creates a research mission that can facilitate, deter, but surely alter the production and recognition of knowledge claims.

With these perspectives in place, we are prepared to survey the intellectual history of reverse transcriptase, a domain of research within viral cell transformation, and then analyze quantitatively the various local, sectoral, and international configurations of collaboration and research organization within this cancer community. This is the challenge of Part II: to bring the biomedical rationality we have discerned to bear on the interpretation of growth and specialization of a problem domain.

NOTES

1. The widely acknowledged architects of that policy—a coalition working from within and without the government in behalf of the cause—were prime congressional movers John Fogarty and Lister Hill, National Institutes of Health Director James Shannon, and the tireless champion in the private sector (notably the American Cancer Society), Mary Lasker. For an assessment of Lasker's role see Rettig (1977: especially Chapter 2).

2. The National Cancer Act of 1971, Public Law 92-218, 92nd Congress, Senate 1828, December 23, 1971. This was followed by the National Cancer Act Amendments of 1974, Public Law 93-352, 93rd Congress, Senate 2893, July 23, 1974.

3. As Jesse Steinfeld, then Surgeon General, testified before the Senate health subcommittee deliberating on S.34 (the blueprint for the Conquest of Cancer Act), "Scientists are like other people, they tend to go where the funds are, where the opportunities are, and it is conceivable that if we spend an enormous amount of money in the cancer program that people who might be more productive in other programs would move to cancer programs" (U.S. Senate, 1971a: 55).

4. The National Heart and Lung Institute did not have long to wait, however, before it would also be singled out for special funding. In 1972 the President signed the National Heart, Blood Vessel, Lung, and Blood Act (U.S. Senate, 1972; see Culliton, 1973).

5. Again, in the words of Rettig:

> The conflict between the fundamental research strategy and the categorical disease strategy, then, actually masks five closely related issues. What kind of research is to be supported or favored–basic or clinical? What instrument of support is to be used–the grant or contract? Who is to make the authoritative decisions allocating support–the external scientific community, the professional staff of an institute, or the advisory council to an institute? Who is to be supported–university scientists or industrial researchers? What is to be the extent of formal research planning–limited, significant, or very extensive? This potpourri of issues was basically rolled into one in the debate over the National Cancer Act of 1971. The overarching issue concerned the most appropriate strategy of research management for conducting the war against cancer [1977: 14].

Specifically, the 1970 report of the Panel of Consultants called for a "comprehensive national plan" for cancer. Toward this end, then-NCI director Carl Baker initiated an effort to develop the National Cancer Program. As Louis Carrese, then Baker's assistant and now Associate Director for Program Planning and Analysis, describes it:

> We brought together the whole scientific community, 250 people selected out of two thousand names submitted by every professional society in the country. Then we had 40 planning sessions to develop the National Cancer Program plan. The people who were there doing it were fighting the process. During the very time they were doing it [over a four-month period], they were fighting it. . . . It's like the drowning person who says "Dear God (if there is one), save my soul (if I have one) from hell (if there is one)." So some of these guys were saying, "I'm going to participate in this national planning session, but I will maintain my integrity as a scientist. You know, if the plan is fine, all right. If it isn't I've knocked it enough." This process is, well, one of the most fantastic things I've ever witnessed. We turned it over to the community; we were very low profile by design.

In Rettig's view,

> The plan, though the object of much concern and criticism, has proved useful in explaining the cancer program to the Congress and the public and in providing general directions for NCI. It has not been used to any significant degree in governing the actual day-to-day management of various NCI programs. Neither Schmidt nor Rauscher have displayed more than mild support for the management importance of the plan itself [1977: 300].

6. As Carrese (1978) told us:

> Our major problem here was to convince people that, first, in addition to the traditional support of many bench investigators, we should try other things. The cancer problem is certainly large enough to accommodate more than one approach to try and solve it, and these would not supplant or replace things, but these new approaches would be complementary and supplementary, and introduce ways for us to think on how best to distribute and invest the total resources we've got across a whole spectrum of activities. Not just basic research, but other kinds of research, other kinds of developments, and now cancer control, with the passage of the act.

7. Indeed, as Rettig points out, the AAMC and FASEB (the Federation of American Societies for Experimental Biology) "did most of the work mobilizing the academic medical-scientific community to oppose S.34."

8. Schmidt has been the chairman of this panel since its creation in 1971.

9. Speaking at a "retrospective" on the Cancer Act of 1971 in 1976, Harold Amos, an NCI stalwart in the academic sector, put it this way:

> All investigators in the biological sciences are agreed that serendipity is their most valuable ally. What emerges unexpectedly in experiments is often the most critical information obtained in the experiment and those findings are especially pertinent to new directions in approach and understanding, throwing new light on old questions. It is imperative that the state of mind of the investigator be such as to perceive the unexpected for what it may ultimately be worth. Program relevance dictates a selection in registering of observations that may categorize as worse than useless a contradictory finding [Amos, 1977: 262].

10. Mulkay (1976) stresses this very point in recognizing that the rhetoric of scientists' pronouncements or "vocabularies of justification" vary with the audience they are addressing. Such a strategy serves multiple purposes, for example, maintaining distance between the scientist-experts and the lay public and promulgating the search-for-truth ideology as a rationale for decrying impediments to the flow of research dollars.

11. Testifying before the Rogers subcommittee, Baltimore himself argued that

> Cancer should not be separated from the rest of biomedical research, and a crash program atmosphere should not be created, because . . . the American people should not be misled into thinking that a cure for cancer is imminent [quoted in Rettig, 1977: 235].

In view both of the rhetorical excess surrounding the cancer legislation and the political side of the debate with which the American Cancer Society was aligned, it is ironic, as Baltimore (1978) commented to us, that

> The American Cancer Society has an extremely honorable record supporting basic science, from way back. And lots of people . . . who do work on bacteriophages and general problems of molecular biology will tell you that the key support that they got was from the American Cancer Society at a time when NIH wouldn't touch them. The Cancer Society has had very far-reaching effects, very good panels, and has very good luck with its approach toward its goal of research; in fact, more so then than now, now that they are caught up in the climate of "Let's get cancer cured."

12. It appears, however, that this *Report of the Ad Hoc Review Committee of the Virus Cancer Program* was never officially *accepted* by the board. As late as February 1978, the report was not catalogued in the National Library of Medicine. So its status remains somewhat of a mystery to us, although it is cited as "submitted" in draft and final report forms as November 1973 and March 1974, respectively, in Rettig (1977: 369). The reports we secured through the courtesy of Dr. Rauscher's office at the American Cancer Society bear these same dates.

13. Todaro and Huebner were quick to deny any wrongdoing in this policy or their role in implementing it when we queried them—separately—about it.

14. The first criticism we suggested to Rauscher was an intellectual one, essentially that mentioned in the draft of the Zinder report itself:

> It was the assumptions that were wrong. There did not, nor does there, exist sufficient knowledge to mount such a narrowly targeted program. Basic ignorance of the mechanism involved in the cancer process, even in animals where a viral etiology is definitively established, is so profound that it is difficult to be certain where to begin, much less organize a focused attack.

15. Litton Bionetics "manages" the Frederick Cancer Center at Fort Detrick for NCI. There is more than a little ambiguity as to which researchers are on which payroll, a problem Rauscher and other of our interviewees readily acknowledged.

16. Again, in justifying the past, but assessing the present situation (now as an ex-NCI spokesperson), Rauscher (1978) confides:

> One other reason, incidentally, we use the contract mechanism so strongly in our own Viral Oncology Program, is we were able to award contracts in something like 2 or 3 months, with peer review. Right now, it's taking the NCI something like 12 months to award a grant, and almost 16 to 18 months to award a contract. Nobody wants a contract anymore. The people at NCI don't want to manage contracts. It's just too much regulatory red tape. But we could use contracts at that time to abet a congressional decision to give us money to get on with the virus cancer research. You couldn't do that with a grant.

17. For a good survey of shifts in funding policy as well as levels of funding within NCI after the National Cancer Act, see Kalberer (1975). For a comparable analysis of the whole NIH for the decade *preceding* the act see Kennedy et al. (1972).

18. This fear has also been translated into massive Mary Lasker- and Ann Landers-inspired letter-writing-to-your-congressman campaigns, as that which was urged when S.34 was nearing a vote in April of 1971.

19. The role of the American Medical Association during the gradual displacement of private support of governmental programs for biomedical research is of particular interest; the AMA remained aloof. With the passage of the National Cancer Institute Act four decades ago, the AMA warned that "The danger of putting the government in a dominant position in relation to medical research is apparent." On the AMA's "neutrality" toward medical research, Strickland states:

> For a long time it was as though the organization which represented most of the thousands of practicing physicians had vacated the field of medical research policy. . . . Ultimately, the Association came to realize that there was a major and ironic incongruity in the fact that the organization claiming as a cardinal tenet the advancement of good health for all citizens had had nothing

to do with the greatest effort of the century to make possible the attainment of that goal [1972: 154].

20. Commenting on the Schmidt-Rauscher team as a "fortuitous" combination, one NIH official has said:

> Rauscher could cause a convulsion in NIH if he tried. A director who wished to exercise the full range of authority could beg a hell of a large degree of autonomy from NIH. But Rauscher had played it very carefully [quoted in Rettig, 1977: 298].

21. For example, several of our NCI interviewees stressed that the *laboratory* is the basic unit of the Cancer Institute (and all of NIH, for that matter), whereas the *program* is more flexible and perhaps more ephemeral in carrying out specific parts of the mission at various times. Rauscher (1978) agrees with this distinction, and that accurately reflects NCI planning.

22. Along with mental health, cancer and heart (which is now called Heart, Lung and Blood) are also the only institutes with statutory obligations for disease control.

23. After 27 months as NCI director, Upton resigned in December 1979 to become head of the environmental medicine department at New York University's medical school. He criticized the widespread conception that billions of dollars spent on cancer in the last 30 years had accomplished little, citing an epidemic of lung cancer as obscuring real gains.

24. It is noteworthy that an NCI-Litton Bionetics team, Gallo (NCI), Yang, and Ting (Litton Bionetics) were the first to find the enzyme reverse transcriptase in human leukemia patients (see Anonymous, 1970a). The wedding of the private and the governmental laboratories has (as shall be seen in Chapter 5) created distinctive collaborative patterns within cancer research.

25. Even the most gradual policy shifts can politicize a research problem by establishing a reward system which is out of touch with the present scientific realities (see Haberer, 1969; Ezrahi, 1971). A recent example is the NCI's bioassay program which has suffered from charges of negligence and mismanagement (see Smith, 1979).

26. More recently, Watson has severely criticized those scientists who advocate a moratorium on recombinant DNA research (see Nelkin, 1978).

27. Gustafson estimates that "proposals to NCI now account for roughly half of all applications to NIH" (1975: 1063).

28. This is, of course, an "externalist" view of history (introduced in Chapter 1). It would be useful to know if researchers have actually changed their research programs or merely altered their rhetoric to fit under the umbrella of the cancer program. See van den Daele et al. (1977) for a discussion of such "relabelling" in science and Lowenstein (1979) for a journalistic view.

PART II: REVERSE TRANSCRIPTASE

CHAPTER 4

REVERSE TRANSCRIPTASE:
An Intellectual History

> The viral etiology of cancer in animals suggests that the genetic information of oncogenic RNA viruses could be involved in human cancer. The impressive progress of the past three years in understanding the molecular events during the replication of oncornaviruses and the mechanisms of cell transformation by these viruses, and the new technology developed during the course of this work, has motivated investigators to analyze human cancers for oncornavirus-specific base sequences and RNA→DNA polymerase activity. . . . The exciting results of these studies appear like science fiction in the context of our scientific knowledge and concepts of three years ago.
>
> Green and Gerard (1974: 261)

> The awarding of the Nobel Prize to Dulbecco, Temin, and Baltimore marks the convergence of lines of research which at one time were thought to be quite separate. It now seems clear that the DNA tumor viruses and the RNA tumor viruses operate, at least in part, by a common pathway. They become part of the genetic material of the cells they transform. To what degree they resemble each other in the mechanisms by which they affect cell growth regulation is a fascinating question for the future.
>
> Eckhart (1975: 714)

A Prelude to Analysis

The recognition that the sites of intellectual activity culminating in research and research advances are not the traditionally defined disciplines was long in coming, especially considering Price's (1963, 1975) reminders that Invisible Colleges form the "frontguard" of scientific progress. Social scientists have now generated a plethora of case studies which chronicles the birth and unfolding of research and knowledge claims in subdisciplinary units.[1] Some of these studies emphasize intellectual history, while others detail social organization and patterns of influence. Most suffer, as Edge and Mulkay (1976) suggest, from a common malady: idiosyncrasy. Idiosyncrasy would seem to plague many examples of the case study approach; whether this is a necessary feature of such research is debatable (see Lemaine et al., 1976).

If units lack comparability, then replication of "specialty" research is all but foreclosed. But what constitutes comparability?

> We do not know whether two things are to be regarded as the same or not unless we are told the context in which the question arises. However much we may be tempted to think otherwise, there is no absolute unchanging sense to the words "the same" [Winch, 1958: 27].

In other words, what one means by similar or comparable specialties or problem domains depends to a great extent on the type of questions one wants to ask. As we argued earlier (Chapter 2), the difficulties of specialty definition will recede in importance as the sociologist shifts research interest to the knowledge functions of science. If the complex of problems surrounding a topic, keyword, object, method, and so on can be understood *at all,* then it is a meaningful research unit for the sociologist of science. The point of comparison and the basis for replication in the sociology of problem domains thus reside in the ability of the researcher to grasp the context of argumentation, the unity of the scientists' cognitive efforts within an area. This is, in effect, what creates a problem domain for the scientist and provides a point of comparison for the sociologist.[2]

A problem domain can be seen as a cognitive region around which scientists gather and through which they eventually pass. Its best approximation in the sociology of science literature is Edge and Mulkay's (1976) "transient network," Whitley's (1974) "research area," and Mulkay et al.'s (1975) "problem area" and "research network." The danger, however, is that certain types of networks, for example, highly connected networks, may be assumed to be an identifying characteristic of problem domains. Indirectly, in other words, a *social* criterion would be utilized to define the viability of a research unit. It would seem, however, that it is the responsibility of the sociologist to specify the nature of the flow of ideas and researchers and not to make assumptions about necessary social conditions of knowing. Thus, the concept of a "problem domain" must seek clarification by others, for example, historians, philosophers, and psychologists, because it represents a nexus of research interests without assuming the cognitive or social structure of those interests.

The study of the cognitive orientation of scientists is, therefore, not an afterthought to social analysis of scientific growth and development. The discussion of reverse transcriptase research which follows is needed not merely to *illuminate* but also to *criticize* the networks discussed in later chapters. By using multiple approaches[3] to analysis of a problem domain, a view of the affinity and rapprochement (see Spiegel-Roesing, 1977) of various levels of analysis becomes possible. The following recounting of focuses of reverse transcriptase research makes no attempt to "typify" the problem domain. Instead, what we seek to reveal, as in Chapter 1, are the confluences that allowed progress to occur. This contemporary problem domain emerges as part of the fabric of cell-transformation research; what must be seen is how reverse transcriptase research is a result of this larger historical effort. Later we examine in detail patterns of coauthorship and cocitation within reverse transcriptase (RT), but only after we trace the intellectual unfolding of events and perspectives in this problem domain.

Research Foci of the Reverse Transcriptase Domain

THE PREDISCOVERY PERIOD

The intellectual activities associated with the discovery and advancement of RT research have been recounted in numerous places.[4] But if one were to select a single event which helped to shift the focus of cancer research onto viral cell transformation, it would be Peyton Rous's (1959) strongly worded article on "Surmise and fact on the nature of cancer." This article represents a head-on confrontation with the dominant theory of cancer etiology in the 1950s, namely, Boveri's (1929) somatic mutation hypothesis. Boveri's views had been reiterated at an international cancer congress (see Reif, 1958) and Rous felt compelled to respond:

> A hypothesis is best known by its fruits. What have been those of the somatic mutation hypothesis? It has resulted in no good thing as concerns the cancer problem, but in much that is bad. It has led within the year to an authoritative statement, in the lay press, that

> since cancer is certainly due to somatic mutations, the possibility of having it is "inherent"; and that this being so, the most man can ever do is to palliate such malignant tumours as may have become disseminated in the body and to avoid new carcinogens as well as the old.
>
> Here is fatalism to blast many a hope and effort. Fortunately, the public, now empowering large-scale attempts to cure cancer, are [sic] a hard-headed generation. They have learned the lesson of the antibiotic substances that do deeds transcending all medical preconceptions.
>
> Most serious of all the results of the somatic mutation hypothesis has been its effect on research workers. It acts as a tranquilizer on those who believe in it, and this at a time when every worker should feel goaded now and again by his ignorance of what cancer is [Rous, 1959: 1361].

The time seemed ripe, the public seemed to believe in a possible cure for cancer, and for Rous and others[5] the place to begin was with the known carcinogenic viruses, chemical compounds, and radiation. In retrospect, this research strategy was an uncanny choice. For the shift from inherited characteristics and somatic mutations to viruses as the focus of research was to lead in the next two decades back to the somatic mutation theory (see Temin, 1971). A "reconciling assumption" (Potter, 1964) was developing which would bring the viral and the somatic mutation theories closer together; but before the synthesis of the two traditions could occur, much research had to be done. The effect of Rous's argument was to shift research to an area, viral carcinogenesis, in which there were immediately researchable questions.

The problems of inheritance were also being greatly clarified in the 1950s. The work of Hershey and Chase (1952) had already demonstrated that viruses inject DNA into cells, and Crick and Watson (see Watson, 1968) had discovered in 1953 the double-helical model of DNA structure. Such research clearly demonstrated that it was DNA which acted as the template of heredity. It was soon discovered (Kornberg et al., 1956; see also Kornberg, 1959, 1961) by studying *Escherichia coli* that a DNA enzyme exists which assists the transcription of DNA strands. When the strategy of viral infection became known and the enzymatic mechanism of DNA replication was discovered, it became possible to begin a new chapter in enzymology which would eventually revolutionize virology.[6]

The discovery (see Potter, 1964) that mammalian cells contain a DNA-dependent DNA polymerase (Bollum and Potter, 1958) and a DNA-dependent RNA polymerase (Geiduschek et al., 1961; Weiss, 1960) firmly established the mechanism of inheritance. From the perspective of the ongoing life of the normal cell, these two polymerases seemed sufficient. Given only these polymerases, one could argue what was apparently Watson's (1965, 1970) version of the Central Dogma of molecular biology, "RNA never acts as a template for DNA."[7] The anomaly, of course, was the existence of RNA viruses; more enzymes must exist which explain viral RNA replication. Potter (1964) argued at an early date that the strong (later to be Watson's) version of the Central Dogma was not what Crick had intended.[8] Crick's statement of the Central Dogma stipulated:

> that once "information" has passed into protein *it cannot get out again.* In more detail, the transfer of information from nucleic acid to nucleic acid, or from nucleic acid to protein may be possible, but transfer from protein to protein, or from protein to nucleic acid is impossible. Information means here the *precise* determination of sequence, either of bases in the nucleic acid or of amino acid residues in the protein [1958: 152].

Thus, the Central Dogma concerned the role of protein within biological systems and not the interaction of RNA and DNA. Crick's unspecified "nucleic acid," Potter contends, allowed for more possible transcription processes to occur than the most obvious types found within normal cells.

The early 1960s were a time of questioning, a time when the impact of the momentous findings associated with DNA and RNA were being digested by the biologist. Whereas virologists knew the importance of viruses in oncogenesis, the replication process of the oncogenic DNA (see Dulbecco, 1976) and RNA viruses[9] were not yet known. In the early 1960s, however, research began to suggest that there did exist RNA-dependent RNA polymerases (Franklin and Baltimore, 1962, experimenting with actinomycin D) and an RNA-directed DNA polymerase (see Temin, 1976) which were important in viral replication. The atmosphere of the era was characterized thusly:

> This is a time for steady nerves and abiding faith in the ethics and methods of our scientific community. As oncologists we are on a collision course with an army of molecular biologists, biochemists, embryologists, microbiologists, immunologists, cytologists, and many others. I believe that the possibility of a general understanding of the nature of the cancer problem may be very near at hand or even already published [Potter, 1964: 1088].

Usage of the phrase "collision course," with all its negative connotations, seems also to imply a good omen. The confluence of traditions of research seemed to foreshadow a major breakthrough in cancer research.[10]

Temin's outline of the major steps that led to his discovery of the RNA-directed DNA polymerase[11] gives one an overview of how the collision course was being charted in the 1950s and 1960s:

> The major scientific concepts required to understand the behavior of RSV [Rous sarcoma virus] were that genetic information was contained in and transferred from nucleic acids, developed especially by Avery, MacLeod, and McCarty [1944], and by Watson and Crick [1953], as well as the concept that viral genomes could become part of cell genomes, developed especially by Lwoff [1972]. The major technical tools required were those of quantitative virology and the study of animal viruses in cell culture, developed especially by Delbruck [see Cairns et al., 1966], Enders, Robbins, and Weller [1964], and Dulbecco [1966] [1976: 1075].[12]

Of immediate importance to Temin's research with Rous sarcoma virus was the line of research which demonstrated how viral genomes become incorporated in cells. Lwoff's (see especially 1953, but also Lwoff, 1962, 1966) research on lysogenic bacteria had demonstrated that bacteriophage genomes (prophage) become incorporated in the genetic material of the bacterium. Thus the prophage can be transmitted at cell division to new cells and, under certain conditions, can be induced to produce complete bacteriophages. In this situation, that which exists "before (pro) the phage" is concealed in the genetic material of the host. Temin's research with RSV showed that cells transformed by the virus could produce other cells with the same morphological characteristics. Something was being inherited from the virus. The genes of the virus had altered the genetic structure of the host and "transformation was a conversion analogous to lysogenic conversion" (Temin, 1976: 1075). If the incorporated phage genome was called prophage, then the genetic unit of viruses which was transmitted from cell to cell should be called provirus.

As of yet, Temin had little idea as to the nature of the RSV provirus. Some had suggested by 1962, however, that certain RNA viruses produce RNA intermediaries (proviruses) which were capable of producing proteins and other RNA viruses (Franklin an Baltimore, 1962; Barry et al., 1962). But when Temin experimented with Rous sarcoma virus he was unable to replicate these experiments using DNA inhibitors, concluding that,

> These results suggest that actinomycin does not affect the replication of RSV and the production of other RNA viruses in the same manner. Since the effect of actinomycin depends upon interaction with DNA, the effect on RSV production is probably mediated through DNA. It appears (Temin, 1979) that the treatment prevents formation of viral RNA. Therefore, it is suggested that the template responsible for synthesis of viral nucleic acid either is DNA or is located on DNA [Temin, 1963: 582].

By 1964 Temin (1964b) was fairly certain that the provirus *was* DNA for Rous sarcoma virus. The problem was that he still could not locate either the provirus or the enzyme that created it in any of the infected cells. If a cellular host was capable of incorporating a viral genome, why could the mechanism not be found?

The key to the problem was discovered in 1967 (Kates and McAuslan, 1967; Munyon et al., 1967) when a simple fact was uncovered: DNA-dependent RNA polymerase was "*in* purified infectious vaccinia virus." The next year saw the isolation of the RNA-directed RNA polymerase *in* reovirus (Borsa and Graham, 1968; Shatkin and Sipe, 1968). The Baltimore group then found an RNA-dependent RNA polymerase *in* vesicular stomatitis virus (Baltimore et al., 1970) and *in* Newcastle disease virus (Huang et al., 1971). It was becoming "obvious" that if the RNA-dependent DNA polymerase (RT) was to be found, then the analogy to the other viruses must be pursued.

THE DISCOVERY: SUPPORT FOR PROVIRUS

The background for the simultaneous discovery (Baltimore, 1970; Temin and Mizutani, 1970) of the RNA-dependent DNA polymerase, has been duly reported.[13] Temin notes:

> In 1969 Satoshi Mizutani came to my laboratory [as a postdoctoral student]. He demonstrated that no new protein synthesis was required for the synthesis of viral DNA during RSV infection of stationary chicken cells, and, therefore, that the DNA polymerase that synthesized viral DNA existed before the infection of the chicken cells. This work was never published completely for in December 1969, we decided that the experiments indicated that RSV virions contain a DNA polymerase, and we decided to look for the virion polymerase first [1976: 1077].

In the case of Baltimore:

> The discovery of the RNA polymerase in virions of vesicular stomatitus virus was the impetus . . . to search for an RNA-directed DNA polymerase in virions of an RNA tumor virus. By analogy, it seemed likely that if the RNA tumor viruses carried out a transfer of information from RNA to DNA as an early step in replication and transformation, they might bring the necessary enzyme into the cell as part of the virion [Temin and Baltimore, 1972: 133].

Baltimore (1970) was successful in discovering the polymerase in Rauscher mouse leukemia virus,[14] and Temin and Mizutani (1970) discovered the polymerase in Rous sarcoma virus. Later when Baltimore discussed various viral genetic systems, he would underscore the lesson learned in the research leading to the discovery of RT:

> The existence of an RNA-dependent DNA polymerase in the virions of the RNA tumor viruses had led us to the concept that, *whenever the first function performed by virion nucleic acid after its introduction into the cell is the transfer of its information to another nucleic acid, the enzyme responsible for this transfer is likely to be found in the virion* [1971: 237].[15]

After the fact, the discovery looked deceptively easy; was it not merely a problem of looking in the right spot? But the right "spot" for the oncologist *is* ostensibly the cell and the transformation process, and the prediscovery period greatly enhanced understanding of viral-cell interactions (see Temin 1976). The growth of evidence concerning the difference between normal and transformed cells, for instance, made rapid exploitation of the RT assay possible after the discovery.

Perhaps the discovery of RT did occur later than it had to[16] (see O'Connor, 1973), but there appears to be no definite rationale for the unfolding research strategy. The argumentation process within molecular biology had elevated the unidirectional transfer of information (from DNA to RNA to protein) to the status of Central Dogma. Thus, Temin presented his DNA provirus hypothesis in 1964 (to the International Conference on Avian Tumor Viruses at Duke University) only to find that, "at this meeting and for the next six years this hypothesis was essentially ignored" (Temin 1976: 1076). It was ignored, on the one hand, because a very fruitful hypothesis of molecular biology was at stake, the Central Dogma,[17] and, on the other hand, direct evidence was lacking. The cognitive ("evidential") norms demanded more than Temin could deliver in the mid-1960s,[18] despite the mounting evidence concerning genetic systems of oncogenic RNA viruses:

> There are two classes of evidence [presently available] which point to a DNA intermediate. One is the data accumulated by using metabolic inhibitors and other perturbations of events in cells [Bader, 1967; Temin, 1967, 1970a]. The measured variable in these experiments is production of virions or morphological transformation, or both criteria which are distant from the affected biochemical process and which have therefore provided circumstantial but not convincing evidence. The second class of evidence is the demonstration of an RNA-dependent DNA polymerase in virions of the RNA tumor viruses [Baltimore, 1970; Temin and Mizutani, 1970]. This has been taken as strong evidence for a DNA intermediate, but, in fact, it shows only how the DNA intermediate could be formed if it is formed. A third form of evidence, and potentially the most powerful, would be the direct demonstration of the postulated DNA in infected cells; however, aside from a few suggestive reports [Baluda and Markham, 1971; Baluda and Nayak, 1970], strong evidence has yet to appear [Baltimore, 1971: 238].

Both Baltimore and Temin were utilizing actinomycin in the mid-1960s to demonstrate the plausibility of the DNA provirus (see above). But plausibility was insufficient in the face of a general suspicion of inhibitor research; inhibitors "were widely suspected of producing artifacts"[19] (Eckhart, 1975: 714).

Baltimore's second class of evidence is, of course, the discovery of RT. But even here he is hesitant to suggest that this is the final proof of the existence of a DNA provirus. It only shows that it "could be formed if it is formed." He awaits the "direct demonstration" that the DNA homologous to the viral RNA actually exists (see Watson, 1965, 1970). When Baltimore wrote in 1971 this was still problematic,[20] but shortly thereafter the third class of evidence was forthcoming (those cited by Temin, 1976; including Neiman, 1972; Hill and Hillova, 1972; Varmus et al., 1974; Shoyab et al., 1974; Cooper and Temin, 1974). Hill and Hillova put virtually all doubt concerning the DNA provirus theory to rest. They took DNA from cells which were known to be infected with avian sarcoma viruses (an RNA virus), placed them in uninfected cells, and new avian sarcoma viruses were produced. The strong evidence for the DNA provirus of RNA oncogenic viruses had been found.

Thus, from what was basically a genetic hypothesis gradually emerged the theory of the DNA provirus (Temin, 1964b). Temin's evidence, until the 1970 discovery of RT, was essentially from research on inhibitors of Rous sarcoma virus. But the data that Temin (1964a) initially cited in support of the provirus hypothesis came from a hybridization experiment which, according to Spiegelman (1978),

> was so weak, in terms of the number of counts you see and so on, that people simply discarded it and they discarded the hypothesis with it. Both were thrown down the drain. [Were you incredulous at that time?] Well, I was not willing to accept the data that were proposed. I mean, that's a field I know a hell of a lot about. I would never have published that kind of data as support for anything. [But apart from the data, other people have suggested that it was just unwarranted speculation.] No, that I disagree with. That's a perfectly valid idea. The fact that I did not find it when I looked for it in the RNA phages didn't mean that it wouldn't be adopted as a solution by some other kind of RNA virus. That has to be recognized, and the fact that you have viruses which in fact do induce permanent genetic phenotypic changes in the cell—that is, RNA viruses which do that—demands that you provide a mechanism for explaining a permanent genetic modification by means of an RNA virus, and that the straightforward simple explanation is still Temin's. You make a piece of DNA, stick it in the genome, and you've got it. But we know that DNA viruses do this. The transducing viruses have been known for years. They go in, insert themselves into the genome, and that's it. An RNA virus can't do that directly, but it can if you solve the problem of making a DNA copy. I think the speculation of Howard's was brilliant. I think the experimental support he first proposed was not very good. . . . I must say this, I think that Temin's finding was the result of an intellectual ethic. It was preceded by defiance, but also he had the guts to stick to it for a number of years, and I think he deserves credit for that.

We shall return later to provirus and Temin's dogged defense of it. Presently, it is more appropriate to consider other contributions to a general theory of oncogenesis which intersected with Temin's provirus framework. One intersecting tradition in particular seemed to have its roots in a medical orientation to viral oncology. Furthermore, its participants (especially Huebner and Todaro) were researchers associated with the National Cancer Institute rather than academic researchers such as Baltimore and Temin and tended to emphasize the role of viruses in *cancer.* Their impact on the RT domain was considerable, while the status of their theory and (apparent) research program remains controversial.

THE ONCOGENE THEORY

Central to Temin's thoughts regarding the DNA provirus hypothesis was the infection of a cell by an RNA virus. The "cause" of the provirus was the RNA virus; it entered the cell, was transcribed by an enzyme, and placed a homologous DNA provirus into the cellular genetic structure. In this model, if a prevention of RNA-induced cancer was to be found, then one should attempt to block the synthesis of the DNA provirus (see Temin, 1964b; Temin and Baltimore, 1972). In other words, a typical "infectivity" model formed the basis for Temin's early work. Although this model was very instructive in directing research, other models of viral oncogenesis were also presented prior to the discovery of RT. For these theories, RT would be assigned a different, almost incidental, level of importance.[21]

In "Oncogenes of RNA tumor viruses as determinants of cancer," Huebner and Todaro first proposed that "the viral information (the virogene), including that portion responsible for transforming a normal cell into a tumor cell (the oncogene), *is most commonly transmitted from animal to progeny animal and from cell to progeny cell in a covert form*" (1969: 1087; italics added). Although Bittner had shown how mouse mammary carcinoma was transmitted in the milk, the theory Huebner and Todaro proposed was a much bolder extrapolation. Essentially their theory argued that viruses had entered the germ cells in the distant past (nothing seems to be stated about the origin of viruses) and become manifest in cells as C-type (cancer-inducing) particles. These particles are genes which, under certain conditions, are expressed as cell-transforming agents. "Carcinogens, irradiation, and the normal aging process all favor the partial or complete activation of these genes" (Huebner and Todaro, 1969: 1087). One of the keys to this theory, therefore, is the "derepression"[22] of the cancer genes:

> This hypothesis implies that the occurrence of most cancer is a natural biological event determined by spontaneous and/or induced derepression of an endogenous specific viral oncogene(s). Viewed in this way, ultimate control of cancer will therefore very likely depend on delineation of the factors responsible for derepression of virus expression and of the nature of the repressors involved. We believe that the hypothesis provides a rational basis for a unifying theory and is consistent with the phenomena of radiation and chemically induced cancer as well as the stochastic occurrence of spontaneous cancer. The availability of *in vitro* test systems to study the derepressed virus in cells in culture should make it possible to analyze this

> phenomenon at the cellular and molecular level [Huebner and Todaro, 1969: 1092].

It is very clear that this theory outlines a specific research program. It incorporates data from epidemiology, namely the "stochastic occurrence" of cancer (see Huebner et al., 1970), and from repressor theory (Jacob and Monod, 1961; also see Stent, 1967) and fashions a genetic theory of cancer. It is already evident that the oncogene theory goes beyond a narrow focus on viruses and extends in some interesting ways back to the somatic mutation theory of cancer.[23] The dread disease in this conceptualization, it would seem, has once again become hereditary.

The Huebner and Todaro model intersects the Temin provirus model at various points. The oncogene hypothesis suggests that the DNA provirus, the oncogenes, exists in most cells and when it is derepressed it forms C-type particles resembling RNA viruses. But if such is the case, reverse transcription from the RNA virus to the DNA provirus pales in importance because the cellular infection supposedly occurred in the distant past and thereafter sustains itself via normal cellular genetic transfer (see Temin and Baltimore, 1972). Perhaps the most important function of RT within the Huebner and Todaro schema is its use as an indicator of the presence of natural oncogenic C-type viruses (see Todaro and Huebner, 1972).

With these considerations in mind, it is obvious that Huebner and Todaro, while developing a similar theory to that of Temin, are approaching the problem from a very different perspective. In contrast to the virologist Temin, Huebner and Todaro represent what may be called a tumor or pathology tradition[24] within viral oncology. They have arrived at their position based on a series of studies demonstrating the presence of C-type particles in tumors.

> Numerous studies, some of them only recently completed, have established these viruses as significant causes of cancer in mice, chickens, cats, and probably also in hamsters. The C-type RNA-virus particles have also been observed by electron microscopy in tumors of guinea pigs, rats, swine, snakes, and humans; thus, three classes of vertebrates are now known to have at least some natural expression of viruses of this class [Huebner and Todaro, 1969: 1088].

Of particular importance to this line of research is the work of Aaronson et al. (1969) on "Mouse leukemia virus: 'spontaneous' release by mouse embryo cells after long-term *in vitro* cultivation." The problem which the oncogene hypothesis was designed to explicate had been developing in the NCI laboratories over a period of years:

> In the [earlier] report describing the tumorigenic properties of the BALB/3T3 and BALB/3T12 cell lines [Aaronson and Todaro, 1968] it was noted that one line of BALB/3T12, began to release mouse leukemia virus (MuLV) [Huebner, 1967] after many cell generations in culture although the original embryo culture and earlier transfer generations of this BALB/3T12 line were negative for virus. In the present study we have analyzed the cell lines derived from the BALB/c embryo culture and the original Swiss embryo culture for the production of mouse leukemia virus antigen and infectious murine leukemia virus after many months in culture, and the data to be presented strongly suggest that the virus and/or the capacity for virus production is present in the original embryo cells. Certain cell culture procedures favor the appearance of viral antigen and infectious virus, while other conditions prevent or retard their appearance [Aaronson et al., 1969: 87].

Once this experimental context for the oncogene hypothesis is understood, its implications are seen to differ from those flowing from the provirus theory. If the provirus theory suggested the disruption of the transcription process to impede virally induced cancers, the search for protein repressors of the normal cell oncogenes was now viewed as the object of cancer research. If the provirus theory sent researchers searching for traces of RT, the oncogene hypothesis pointed toward more research on activation (derepression) of cells. It was soon discovered that C-type particles were found in chick embryos which had no opportunity for exogenous infection. But these C-type particles did not appear to be carcinogenic in such embryo cells (see Todaro and Huebner, 1972). The nature of the viral expression in different stages of the differentiation process would thus become an area for future research. The ability to induce C-type particles by using chemical means, for example, using bromodeoxyuridine or iododeoxyuridine (Lowy et al., 1971), also seemed to confirm the oncogene hypothesis and stimulated further research. Derepression indeed seemed to occur under controlled circumstances.

Nevertheless, the status of the oncogene hypothesis remains in doubt. A diversity of opinion was voiced by our interviewees as to the empirical support for the theory. Indeed, the question of its testability was raised repeatedly by some, while others spoke matter-of-factly about its confirmation. Juxtaposing these opinions, it is hard to believe that the *same* theory is being described. An anonymous representative sample illustrates not only the lack of unanimity but also the covert bond between intellectual content and the politics of science:

> Well, I think it [oncogene] served many purposes. But the one thing it did *not* serve was to attract the admiration and approval of molecular biologists, because it was just a lot of nonsense. The verbiage was confused; we didn't know really what the hell they were talking about; and things kept shifting from virogene to oncogene; and one never knew what the hell was going on. I can recall at meetings people getting up, like Zinder getting up and asking Huebner, "For God's sake, will you tell me what the hell you mean by an oncogene! Where *is* it?" You know, he'd get irritated after a while with all this nonsense. It was an attempt by people who were not really familiar with molecular biology to begin to use the terminology of molecular biology, but they coined their own terms. It has great political advantage, you see. Intellectually, it had no impact on the field at all, at least from where I stood. It served a very useful purpose for the proponents, because, as you sort of implied, people identified this whole area of activity with this slogan, you know, and that was the banner that was flying over NCI.

> Well, I liked it because many of the data, that is, the stochastic data on cancer, and many other things, seemed to fit into that oncogene theory. Now remember, the oncogene theory has been modified as new information comes in, so the oncogene theory you talk about today is a relative but not an identical kind of thing with what Huebner and George [Todaro] proposed at the time they proposed it. Also at the time, Howard [Temin], as you know, was talking about a provirus which was subtly different, and I think the jury is still out today as to which one was a better predictor of what we might find in the next 5 or 10 years. I also liked it because it was testable by any scientist. The thing that you like in a hypothesis was its testability. And I think much of what Wally Rowe [and others] have done in showing that every cell of every animal contains virus information is in part, at least, confirmation of the original ideas that Huebner had.

> The oncogene theory was never even formulated well enough to be tested. . . . Not only wasn't it testable, but it was never really well defined. Because I could never really tell if they were talking about a virus gene or a cell gene. I don't think *they* ever knew whether they were talking about a virus gene or cell gene. They mix up the two all the time. And they tried, by combining the two ideas, to make it seem like it was understandable, but to me it has never been understandable, and I've read through that stuff any number of times. They were pointing to very important experimental observa-

tions–experimental observations of parent genetic transmission of virus and experimental observations of the parents of virus and cells that apparently have never been infected. Those were clear-cut phenomena of great importance, and the oncogene theory served to highlight those experiments, and focused a lot of attention on those experiments and therefore that area went forward very rapidly. But the oncogene theory itself was never explicit enough to be a statement of anything. . . . Furthermore, almost all the viruses that Todaro isolated were nononcogenic. To this day, most of the viruses he isolates are nononcogenic. So none of them have to do with oncogenes. So not only has Todaro not proved the oncogene hypothesis, but (1) I don't think it was ever formulated into a form which could be proved and (2) I don't think we know enough now to know what genes cause cancer.

There were not too many people who dared to say that oncogene was nonsense. Because, you know, Huebner was a powerful force. . . . But Maurice Green was able to expand his operation by agreeing with Huebner about oncogene. I thought that was too bad.[25]

Theories probably are, I think, virtually proven concerning the oncogene. In other words, there are genes in cells whose expression can result in cancer. That's certainly proven in the mouse system, the cat system, the chicken system. And that these genes are normal genes and that they are inherited. And the thing that is incredible, that's been shown because we have RT, is that virtually all primates, except man (and man probably won't be an exception), have endogenous viruses, RNA tumor viruses. It's not shown that they cause cancer. We're not sure what their role is, but in the last year in Todaro's lab, he and his colleagues have found about five different primates–Old and New World monkeys–and it might take about seven months, but they can get out specific virus never before seen. It's likely that we have such viruses. I think it's likely that it's involved in collagen diseases such as Lupus and connective tissue disease. Those diseases are much more important than cancer.

Theories develop on the basis of scientific evidence. On the oncogene thing, I think that probably if he had left it at simply genetic transmission of a group of viruses of which we really are not sure what they do, that would have been perfect, tremendously in keeping with current thinking. I think that they probably went one step further because again of Huebner's thrust–that it was something that did everything. It was not only genetically there, but that it did everything. And that had not to be true. And for awhile it was frustrating to people, because not only was it sort of intuitively not

> likely to be the case, but they had set it up in such a way as how in the hell would you ever show that it wasn't true. I mean, it was a tough one to grapple with. It just was frustrating—that latter part of it—that the oncogene was there and that anything you added, chemicals, or this, or that, worked through this final common pathway of this oncogene, which was associated with this genetically transmitted virus. . . . But it was a reasonable concept at a reasonable time. It was stimulating. It caused discussion. But nobody who had any brains, I think, would become over-sold or over-imbued, to the point where they are not able to look at their data and decide what, hopefully on an objective basis, what are the facts.

Thus, like the provirus hypothesis, the oncogene theory was met with incredulity, serving as a kind of Rorschach test for RT researchers.[26] Lest your score-keeping has been keen, our tally indicates the "cons" exceeding the "pros" by a slim margin; furthermore, opinions do not align simply along an NCI versus non-NCI continuum. As for the political character of oncogene, Rauscher (1978) demurs:

> I think, contrary to its being handy, it was pretty complex as a matter of fact. When you get down to the molecular aspects of what's going on . . . that's not easy to talk about to the Congress or the public. I don't think it was used as a political tool. I would have used it had it been useful.

Of course, politics can be waged with various audiences and in various arenas, as Chapter 3 aptly demonstrated. Further evidence emerges with the entry of the protovirus hypothesis in the history of RT.

THE PROTOVIRUS HYPOTHESIS: MORE THAN A FOIL TO ONCOGENE?

Within a few months after the discovery of RT, Temin once again entered the discussion. He was now developing what he called the "protovirus" hypothesis. However, this was no hastily developed hypothesis in response to Todaro and Huebner's oncogene theory. Since the early 1960s Temin had believed that viruses alter the host genome (see Potter, 1964). The oncogene hypothesis was essentially epigenetic, not genetic (see Temin, 1971), and it relied upon "switches," or derepression of the oncogenes, to trigger cell transformation.

In the protovirus hypothesis, we are informed that a *normal* RNA to DNA to RNA transcription process becomes altered so that incorrect information is encoded. Perhaps the most important feature of protovirus is that it encompasses much more than an explanation of cancer. Again, Temin's research seems to be clearly governed by a perspective different from that of Huebner and Todaro. In Temin's own words, "This protovirus theory was derived *a priori* from consideration of the origin of RNA sarcoma viruses" (1971: vi). The protovirus hypothesis incorporates the normal process of cellular genetic development into a theory of viral origin and evolution. This new hypothesis is a natural outgrowth of the provirus hypothesis which specifies the possibility of RNA to DNA synthesis, although the earlier hypothesis did not specify why such a mechanism would ever need to be established within biological evolution. What selective advantages would be found in the RNA to DNA transcription process? To assume that such a process is a normal part of the genetic structure of the cell would portray viruses as extensions of this normal process. The protovirus would be part of the genetic makeup of cells and, according to such a theory, would be identifiable with a region of the normal DNA strand. But why would this be advantageous to the evolutionary process? Temin believes that because

> there is great genetic instability in this type [RNA→DNA] of information transfer, variants would appear and wholly new DNA sequences would be formed. . . . In the development of an organism, information transfer from DNA→RNA→DNA would allow variability and amplification; information transfsfer from DNA→DNA would allow stability and storage [1971: iv].

It is therefore the relative instability of the reverse transcription process which allows for evolution, in all its forms, according to the protovirus hypothesis. It provides the dynamic for a cell to alter its own structure through one transcription process (RNA→DNA) and yet maintain its stability through another process (DNA→DNA). It is this possibility for shifts in the genetic map of a cell which provides, in turn, a basis for further theorizing about the origin of viruses and carcinogenesis:

> The normal physiological evolution of the protovirus-derived DNA's would fall within a pattern predetermined by the rest of the cell genome and by the state of the cell and of the developing organism. Integration of protovirus-derived DNA, specifying some polymerases, for example, next to a region controlling membranes or other aspects of the cell surface could affect surface specificities of the cell. Integration next to a region controlling cell multiplication

> could affect multiplication control of the cell. Continued evolution along these lines could put together in a contiguous region of the chromosomes the information necessary for formation of an enveloped virion [Temin, 1971: v].

If viruses have evolved in this manner, it is not difficult to suppose that at a later date they could recombine with information in the cellular DNA. The RNA viruses that are known to cause cancer would thus be capitalizing on the normal cellular processes by which they were created. Chemical carcinogens would also be seen as disruptive of this normal cellular process by creating a "misevolution of protoviruses" (Temin, 1971).

Whereas the oncogene hypothesis suggested that research should focus on switching mechanisms and derepression, the protovirus hypothesis recommends a research program to characterize the structure of normal cellular processes of information transfer. In Todaro's (1978) words,

> I think the theories have merged so much data. I mean, they are really not basically different at all. It's not very clear which one is more right. I think it's very clear now that the basic virogene idea, that almost all species have the genetic information, so they can use viruses—it's part of their cellular information. And something about these viruses, I'm still convinced, is involved in cancer causation. And the argument, I think, centers around whether it really is a strictly normal set of cellular genes that are turned on, or whether they have to be modified somewhat. And that almost becomes semantic. . . . I think that the main point is that the potential information is already there is the cells and that there isn't a contradiction between the genetic theory of cancer and the virus theory of cancer—that they are aspects of the same thing.

Though conciliatory, Todaro readily acknowledges the political dimension of his theory:

> My frame of reference, in writing the paper with Huebner, was almost as much to tell the people working in the Cancer Institute that if one is dealing with a situation where the genes, where the information is already present in the cellular DNA and gets expressed, and gets expressed as a function of age, and carcinogens turn it on, and genetics are factors, then one is dealing fundamentally with a very different situation than a classical infectious virus situation, and the kinds of approaches that one should be thinking about are really quite different. And this was at a time when, I think, most of the focus was a very simple, over-simplistic,

> focus, of, okay, we'll have a crash program, we'll find the virus, we'll make a vaccine, we'll wipe out cancer. And we were saying very much that it wasn't going to work that way. . . . But I think, in 1969, when we did propose it, we succeeded also in alienating probably all the chemical carcinogenesis people, because we were also saying, "Look, we know it's not an infectious thing, but a virus is still involved." And I'm really quite satisfied that we've turned out much more right than wrong about that, because we alienated the carcinogenesis people; we spent a lot of time checking their samples and saying, "I checked it and I didn't find any virus in it. Therefore, it must be wrong."

NCI's Aaronson concurs, almost verbatim, with Todaro's impression:

> If anything it antagonized people on the outside more. I mean, how do you feel if you are a chemical carcinogen worker? This is again the politics of it, and Huebner is going around saying, "Hey, you guys are wasting your time, it's all mediated through the virus."

Meanwhile, Temin had begun to specify the first phase of research on the protovirus hypothesis:

> The most immediately testable prediction of the protovirus hypothesis is the existence of RNA to DNA information transfer in normal cells. The existence of such a mode of information transfer could most easily be established by finding an RNA-dependent DNA polymerase like that found in virions of RNA tumor viruses [1970b: 24].[27]

During the next few years Temin's laboratory (Kang and Temin, 1972, 1973) would demonstrate the presence of "RNA-directed DNA polymerase activity in uninfected chicken embryos."[28] And during the early 1970s intense research activity began to clarify the differences between normal and viral polymerases. It became clear that even endogenous C-type particles were sometimes associated with an RT similar to that found in C-Type viruses (see Hill and Hillova, 1974). Just as the discovery of RT in 1970 only demonstrated the possibility of RNA to DNA transcription, so once again more evidence was needed to show that a homology existed between cellular DNA and C-type particles. The Hill and Hillova (1972) demonstration that proviral DNA of Rous sarcoma virus could transcribe complete viruses when placed in previously uninfected chicken cells[29] had emerged from a tradition of research on the cellular uptake of DNA by animal cells (see Hill and Hillova, 1974; Zhadnov and Tikchonenko, 1974). Now it had to be shown that the proviral DNA could not be distinguished from the cellular DNA–seemingly contrary to the oncogene hypothesis–and that the cellular DNA was homologous to the RNA in viruses and C-type particles. The research effort associated with these questions has itself spawned further extensions of the basic protovirus hypothesis. Two examples furnish a sense of the direction of this research front.

In 1974, Hill and Hillova were convinced that experimental results had demonstrated that "infectious proviral DNA of PR-RSV [Prague strain Rous sarcoma virus] cannot be separated from large chromosomal DNA even under conditions which readily separate viral or exogenous DNAs from the cellular genome" (1974: 36). The problem became one of explicating the mechanism by which virus replication could take place. Difficulties seemed to arise when the proviral DNA template seemed to be shorter than that required for the viral RNA. They responded to this problem with a new model featuring the "circularization of proviral DNA before its insertion into the cellular chromosome" (Hill and Hillova, 1974: 38).[30] The Hill and Hillova model was designed to solve a puzzle generated, in effect, by their earlier proof that the DNA provirus *could* transcribe new RNA viruses. The strong evidence (see above) for the DNA provirus hypothesis had created a problem domain of its own.

Many other laboratories, too, were actively deciphering the relationship between cellular DNA and viral RNA with the hope of discovering the origin of viruses and the nature of cancer. The work of Gillespie and Gallo (1975), for instance, not only reviews this research but also attempts to formulate a new model of virus origin and evolution.[31] First they postulate a genetic "hot spot" (Gallo, 1974), which is essentially a "readily mutable or frequently recombining genomic DNA site that, when altered, can affect the regulation of expression of viral genes or the action of viral gene products" (Gillespie and Gallo, 1975: 807). When alterations occur within a hot spot, the potential for creating RNA viruses increases; or when an RNA virus is present, the reverse transcription and insertion of DNA at a hot spot is possible. In this regard it seems essentially compatible with Temin's protovirus hypothesis. Next, however, Gillespie and Gallo suggest a mechanism for viral transcription, namely, "paraprocessing," which goes beyond protovirus:

> We propose that the type of RNA processing ("paraprocessing") that leads to the formation of an RNA tumor virus genome involves

> relatively little RNA cleavage in the nucleus. We further suggest that paraprocessing is a form of RNA processing used normally for the expression of particular genes during early stages of differentiation but normally in mature adult cells [Gillespie and Gallo, 1975: 802].

In the normal adult transcription of RNA from DNA, the RNA is segmented within the nucleus and appears in the cytoplasm as shortened messenger RNA. In paraprocessing, it is theorized, the RNA escapes into the cytoplasm without the normal cleavage into messenger RNA. If, of course, such paraprocessing occurs, then the molecular biologist should be able to demonstrate homologies between certain normal DNA sequences and RNA viruses. What Gillespie and Gallo demonstrate is that RNA viruses can be divided into two groups: Class 1 virus genomes whose nucleotide sequences are demonstrably homologous with the normal cellular DNA and Class 2 virus genomes whose nucleotide sequence diverges from the normal ordering. If paraprocessing of normal cellular DNA is the mechanism to be credited with the creation of new viruses, then one should be able to read from the homology of the viral RNA and cellular DNA the evolutionary history of these viruses and cells.

> If bacteriophages did originate from cellular genetic information, the genetic elements of the phage itself and those of its host have since diverged to the extent that they no longer share most nucleotide sequences. The situation with the RNA-containing animal tumor viruses is different. Evidence from molecular hybridization experiments suggests that the RNA genomes of these viruses have nucleotide sequences found in DNA of normal cells. This indicates that RNA tumor viruses can probably be measured as having occurred within the last tens of millions of years. Biological experiments indicate that the viruses are still being generated from cells [Gillespie and Gallo, 1975: 802].

The theory of paraprocessing is not merely a further specification of Temin's protovirus hypothesis; rather, it is designed to elicit experimental research along new paths. Paraprocessing provides a focal point for seeking diverse types of data and specifies how they are *relevant* for the exploration of a specific problem. RT is still systematically part of the problem, but it is increasingly taken for granted as research shifts to other "unknowns" in the biological system.

Reverse Transcriptase: Current Status, Future Promise

The gradual elucidation of RT has greatly enhanced its relevance to the biomedical research community at large. Its relevance has become more diffuse at the same time that the problem domain in which it was discovered and characterized has become more secure in its findings. RT research has reached a stage where the enzyme can now assume a "reagent status." As Temin has stated:

> The avian RNA tumor virus DNA polymerases are stable and easy to solubilize and study. Numerous workers have purified these enzymes, especially from avian myeloblastosis virus, and this DNA polymerase has become a standard reagent for molecular biologists. It is especially useful because it has no deoxyribonuclease activity, but it does have ribonuclease H activity (Ribonuclease H activity degrades the RNA strand of an RNA-DNA hybrid molecule, but not single stranded RNA.) [1976: 1077].

This new status allows RT to be the "constant" in molecular biological experiments, just as earlier, actinomycin D (as an inhibitor with known properties) could be used to clear the path for the provirus hypothesis and the discovery of RT.

When asked about current uses of RT, Temin (1978) was indeed quick to invoke the actinomycin parallel:

> In the '60s actinomycin was first used in cancer chemotherapy. It was also used in biochemistry. And then it was used, and still is used, as a tool in virology. The biochemistry there defined its action as DNA-directed RNA synthesis (10 micrograms block DNA synthesis). Because of that knowledge, it could be used. Baltimore was one of the second generation of people to use it, to log those kinds of syntheses, and uncover RNA directed RNA synthesis in animal cells. But that didn't really feed back to the biochemists; the biology didn't feed back to the people interested in cancer chemotherapy. It became a very valuable tool in biology both as a way to uncover the poliovirus and the other ordinary viruses, and as a tool to further the idea that two viruses were different. Based on that you have cancer chemotherapy. . . . People can be interested in it as a polymerase enzyme. Then there are people who are interested in polymerase as an important component of viral replication and as a marker for RNA tumor virus appearing in humans. And then as a by-product of this we can use it as a tool to make DNA.

Baltimore's (1978) response to the question of current uses of RT is equally lucid:

> First of all, the study of RNA tumor viruses from any point of view you wish . . . because it's the simplest to assay—the virus. It's a 1, 2, accurate fast assay, so almost everybody uses it when they want to know if they have virus or not. So it's just a simple detection. Secondly, as a key to understanding the life cycle of the virus, it remains indispensable. Thirdly, in the manufacture of reagents for studying the virus, the C-DNA probes and now full-length DNA which we are making to do heteroduplex analysis and to do infectivity studies, all sorts of things. It's all made in vitro RT. And so it provides the best way of doing that. Then outside of tumor virology, it is a way of making C-DNA from any message and so it is at the heart of most cloning procedures. I can remember Phil Leder[32] coming up to me a couple of years ago and saying how important the discovery of the RT was to his work, and yet he doesn't work on viruses at all.

As Kolata recently concluded,

> Since viruses are easy to manipulate genetically and easy to obtain in large enough quantities that their products can be detected in host cells, most investigators agree that viruses have only begun to exhibit their potential as tools in cell biology research [1977: 418].

It is because the integration of the genetic information of RNA viruses into the host cell genome requires transcription into DNA (the provirus) that the enzyme RT is so indispensible. For example, even RNA viruses that lack the enzyme have been found to produce proviruses in persistently infected cells. Evidence of DNA copies of the RNA genome has been detected for respiratory syncitial virus and for measles virus (the latter by V. M. Zhadnov, the chief Russian among the visible foreign biologists elaborating on the RT discovery).[33] Thus, the information from the viral genome may be harbored in a noninfectious form in certain cells, as research with reovirus and visna virus, among others, has suggested (Marx, 1977). However, the question persists: Do these transformations observed in animal disease occur in *human* disease? Through 1977, direct support for this notion was lacking.

In 1978, however, two developments were reported which hold future promise. One concerns genetic studies showing that avian (or Rous) sarcoma virus contains a gene, designated *src* for sarcoma, that codes for a protein product which *must* be produced in order for cell transformation to occur.

> The function of the *src* gene and its products may not be limited just to transformed calls, however. Normal cells contain DNA sequences related to the RNA sequence of this gene, according to Harold Varmus, J. Michael Bishop [and colleagues at] . . . the University of California at San Francisco. . . . They find that calls from all the vertebrate species they have examined–ranging from fish to primates–have one or at most a very few DNA sequences related to the *src* gene [Marx, 1978a: 162].

Not only is the *src* an advance toward unraveling the transformation process (see Marx, 1978b) but also the protagonists of this research program bear a striking affinity to pre- and post-RT discovery domains. The identifiers of *src* are Peter Duesberg of California–Berkeley, Peter Vogt of UCLA, and Hidesaburo Hanafusa of Rockefeller University.[34]

But there is another affinity between *src* and the RT domain, namely, that the two hypotheses ("which are not necessarily mutually exclusive," according to Marx, 1978a: 163) about the origin of the genetic information that transforms a cell, making it cancerous, are the oncogene and the protovirus theories:

> Aspects of the new work with ASV [avian sarcoma virus] and the murine sarcoma viruses suggest that an oncogene may actually be present in cells. However, Varmus and Bishop say that not all of their findings with ASV are consistent with the predictions of the theory. Neither are they totally consistent with the predictions of the protovirus theory, although certain aspects of the work are reminiscent of this hypothesis, too [Marx, 1978a: 163].

Once again, whether the results of these animal systems will prove applicable to human cancers is uncertain, though "mice and men are more closely related than mice and chickens" (Marx, 1978a: 164).

Finally, a press release in September 1978 (Atlanta *Constitution,* 1978) trumpeted that "The Epstein-Barr [E-B] virus is the frontrunner in the race to be elected the first human oncogenic (cancer-causing virus)." The new evidence is based on an epidemiological study begun in 1971 involving 42,000 children in an area of Uganda where Burkitt's lymphoma is relatively common. The research group, led by Guy de-The of the International Agency for Research on Cancer, found support for the hypothesis that "cancers developed only after long and heavy exposure to the virus."

It also reinforced the long-standing belief that another factor *besides* severe virus infection—in this case, malaria—must be present if the cancer is to develop. "If the strongly suspected link between Burkitt's lymphoma, E-B virus and malaria is valid, a drop in the frequency of that kind of cancer should become evident during the next several years."

If the link between E-B or some other virus and a cancer is confirmed,[35] the import of discovering RT—even though E-B does not contain RT—will be further enhanced. Similarly, the expectations raised by the pre- and postdiscovery research we have recounted will be realized, while the much-maligned resource allocation policies of the NCI will, at least in part, be vindicated. This is not to say that the present justifies the past; rather, new developments recast historical events to illuminate connections that were either imperceptible or intellectually distinct. With future confluences, RT may reveal an even longer and richer history.

Conclusions

This chapter has traced the intellectual history of theoretical and experimental developments within, and outgrowths of, RT research. Indeed, the theoretical statements of provirus, oncogene, and protovirus identified problems as "belonging" to protein chemistry, enzymology, virology, and such, so that the proper evidential norms could be applied to the research process. Such identification demarcates the types of evidence needed and suggests how previous research is relevant to the problem at hand.

Problem domains so delimited are not necessarily homogeneous in theory or research program. Thus, they embody the various intellectual, for example, disciplinary, inputs to the domain.[36] In the discovery and elaboration of RT, the RNA-dependent DNA polymerase fulfilled an array of experimental and theoretical functions. Even when the enzyme appeared somewhat peripheral to the discussion, for example, in the oncogene theory, research still contributed, perhaps often inadvertently, to the elucidation of reverse transcription. The problem domain has been and continues to be approached from numerous perspectives, out of many motivations; most concern viruses and some concern cancer. All highlight interplay between ideas and a foraging or testing of them. As two of our interviewees affirmed:

> I (and some other people) am a strong believer that the hypothesis is the important thing, that facts without a hypothesis to give them meaning don't really exist [Temin, 1978].

> I'm always suspicious of consensus. My experience has been to try to look for alternate explanations. But I don't think one can study virology in the absence of knowing about carcinogenesis [Todaro, 1978].

If theories do represent an expressed rationale for doing the kind of research that one is doing, then we can predict a complementarity of the research efforts in various academic, government, and private laboratories. A consensus on theory allows localized research units to proceed without unnecessary argumentative disruptions. Indeed, Boehme (1975) has asserted that "explicit controversies in science are rare," thereby making the scientific argumentation process difficult for the analyst of science to perceive. But this may be so because the analyst has chosen to focus on theories and theory groups rather than upon the problem structure of research. In any case, one can easily recognize the outworking of the argumentation process in the protovirus hypothesis as it confronts the oncogene hypothesis. We recall Temin arguing that:

> The major problems with the [oncogene] model are (a) it does not approach the question of origin; (b) it requires 100% efficient initial infections of the germ lines of all ancestors of present-day chickens, cats, and mice; (c) it requires many different infections to explain the different types of endogenous ribodeoxyviruses and the multiple, distinguishable, endogenous representatives of some of them; and (d) it has no mechanism for the maintenance and evolution in these inactive proviruses of structural genes for many functional virion structural proteins, for example, a DNA polymerase distinct from host-cell DNA polymerases (The viral DNA polymerase is needed only for horizontal transmission of proviral or protoviral information. The other cellular DNA polymerases take care of vertical transmission of the provirus.) [1974: 172].

The fruits of these criticisms are revealed in a closing remark from Todaro et al.:

> The ubiquitous presence of endogenous type C viruses among vertebrates and their preservation throughout millions of years of evolution suggest that these genes express normal physiologic functions which provide a selective advantage to the species [1975: 1167].

This conclusion, on the one hand, must certainly be credited to a long line of careful research reviewed and accomplished by the authors. On the other hand, it speaks to many of the criticisms which Temin has leveled against the oncogene theory.

The argumentation process, incorporating the experimental evidence gained over a period of years, tends to approximate a "consensus of rational opinion over the widest possible field" (Ziman, 1968: 9). Consequently, we have rehearsed emerging evidence that (1) reverse transcription is part of normal cellular function, (2) evolutionary theory will be important for elucidating the nature of cancer, (3) embryological studies are needed to strengthen understanding of the differentiation processes that are altered with maturity, and (4) chemical induction of transformation must be studied from a genetic perspective.

The drive toward consensus is thus a drive toward the proper formulation of research questions. The argumentation process helps specify where one can expect a "legitimate" confluence of ideas to occur.[37] Temin was betting on the benefits of understanding viral origins in relation to normal cellular processes. Once the question is so formulated, channels are opened for a flow of research information from a perspective that Huebner and Todaro did not immediately define as relevant. Likewise, the repressor theory which Huebner and Todaro called upon has exerted much influence on the definition of problems worth considering, for example, derepressors such as 5-Bromodeoxyuridine (Margalith et al., 1975). What might have been considered incommensurable theories at an earlier date have so interacted that biomedical science has progressed both in its understanding of biological reality and in its ability to formulate researchable hypotheses for future research.

Finally, to conclude that the growth of its reagent status is but one, and not *the,* culmination of RT research is to recognize some important consequences for future studies of biomedical problem domains as the primary site for the production and negotiation of knowledge. First, as the enzyme is utilized for understanding ribonuclease activity, its own properties will be better elucidated. These refinements of understanding will naturally feed back into the theoretical structures which we have discussed; these theories will follow the "reagent" into an expanding body of molecular biological literature. Second, the reagent status or RT can be expected to create an expansion of the literature which deals with the enzyme. In particular, the keyword system which we used to retrieve the literature of the domain will display both the growing and the changing uses of the enzyme. It would be premature, if not incorrect, to suggest, therefore, that such growth is an artifact of a data collection technique or that the domain has "peaked," been displaced, or been swallowed by other larger problems (see Mullins et al., 1977).

The problem is one of understanding the compass of our techniques and knowing *how* they influence our perceptions (i.e., reconstructions) of the ongoing research process. We conclude that if the growth in the utilization of RT were not deployed as a guide to sociological analysis, then the process by which knowledge is *accumulated* within biomedicine would be incomplete, if not misconstrued. We conclude, too, that technical literature, no matter how comprehensive, tells only part of the story. Written history is a social form that is rhetorical and self-serving (Mulkay, 1976; Gilbert, 1977). Oral history is no less rationalizing, vulnerable to poor memory and recollections that juxtapose or blur detail (Woolgar, 1976b). But the key to reconciling written and oral history is not to discard the memoir and the interview as hopelessly myopic. These are perspectives on scientific reality as seen by participant-observers.[38] Just as the path to the double helix was traveled by Watson, Olby, and Sayre (see Bernstein, 1978; also see Mullins, 1972), we have traveled (hitch-hiked?) to and through the RT domain in several vehicles–posing questions here, comparing observations there, relying on textual material throughout. We alight now to experience other modes of travel in Chapters 5 and 6. En route, however, we shall retain an orientation to biomedicine anchored firmly *not* in social structure, but in the intellectual history–the process and content–of knowledge claims.

NOTES

1. It is interesting that the *death* of such units is rarely recounted. For a pair of prime exceptions, see Fisher (1966, 1967).

2. Boehme's (1975) typology of solidarity within scientific communities is quite suggestive, but perhaps overgeneralized. Although he does emphasize the structure of the context of argumentation, can the integration of a scientific group be founded simply on a solidarity of method, purpose, theory, or research object (Boehme, 1975)? The question is not whether these are exhaustive categories. Of course they were not meant to be. The difficulty is that the "logic-in-use" (Kaplan, 1964) within science "synthesizes" these analytical categories in distinctive ways. Reverse transcriptase, as will be seen, can function as a method, a common purpose, a theory, and as a research object. The argumentation process within biomedicine interweaves such categories as Boehme would isolate and it creates the distinctive textures of various problem domains. By focusing on the structure of the argumentation process in all its "region-specific patterns" (Boehme, 1975) instead of isolating typologies, the sociologist can avoid constricting the cognitive as well as the social dimension of a problem domain. Just as one must forestall the bias of choosing only those specialties which

meet certain social criteria, so too the premature establishment of cognitive typologies can be detrimental to analysis. Such typologies can lead to an ad hoc approach (Comroe and Dripps, 1976) to analysis which suppresses the diversity of cognitive orientations found in science.

3. Multiple approaches to scientific specialties, however, tend to transform the nature of the research task. The "discrepancies" seen by various orientations to specialties suggest that no single research tool, method, or theory is sufficient unto itself. The focus, as a consequence, necessarily shifts from providing simple sociological answers to that of providing clear statements as to what is perceived by using different methodologies and orientations to questions. The policy maker must then weigh and choose rather than expect legitimation of decisions from any single approach. The process is one of approximation and negotiation of reality.

4. The following discussion is based on a reading of numerous technical and review articles on RT. Those articles which are of particular importance for gaining an overview of the area are: Baltimore (1976a, 1976b), Culliton (1971), Dulbecco (1967, 1973, 1974, 1976), Eckhart (1972, 1975), Furth (1959), Gallo (1972), Gallo and Ting (1972), Gillespie and Gallo (1975), Green and Gerard (1974), Hill and Hillova (1974), Huebner and Todaro (1969), McAllister (1973), Maugh (1974b), O'Connor (1973), Potter (1964), Temin (1970b, 1971, 1972, 1974, 1976), Temin and Baltimore (1972), Todaro and Huebner (1972), and Zhadnov and Tikchonenko (1974).

5. We must note here that among the RT protagonists whom we met in Chapter 3 and from those we shall hear in the present chapter, the calling to cancer came much later than 1959. Most denied an *active* interest in linking their research to cancer cure and prevention. A notable exception is Huebner, whose immunological approach was matched by an unflagging optimism in the ability to inoculate against cancer, as he had done in developing vaccines against conventional viral and rickettsial diseases during his early "Public Health Service days at [the National] Institute of Allergy and Infectious Disease." The other exception is Spiegelman (1978), who told us:

> In 1968, I made the decision that I was going to turn my attention to the cancer problem. Now I'm directed–not because I really feel like I know it all now, I don't need any more information–but really because at that time I had already reached the age of 55 or 54. . . . Anyhow, it was clear to me that if I didn't switch now, I just wouldn't have enough time to do anything significant on the cancer project, and so I made the break then. And at that time, I also made the decision to move [to Columbia] because of the decision to change. And when I changed, I also decided that I wanted to work on human cancer, not on animal cancer or cell model cancer, or so on, because I felt that if I find anything, I want to be able to transfer it directly to the patient, because that was the only reason I went for it.

As Spiegelman (1978) and Temin (1978) each reminded us, the discovery and elaboration of RT were *not* indebted intellectually to the war on cancer.

6. Enzymes are catalytic *proteins.* Just as the assertion of the importance of viruses would lead back to the somatic mutation theory, so too the discovery of DNA would eventually lead to the problems of proteins. Crick states, "Watson said to me, a few years ago, 'The most significant thing about the nucleic acids is that we don't know what they do.' By contrast the most significant thing about proteins is that they can do almost anything" (1958: 138).

7. However, Watson was aware of Temin's work on Rous sarcoma virus: "Now data are being collected . . . that have suggested to some (but not all) scientists working with RSV that the RSV genome becomes part of one of the host chromosomes (a provirus stage), where it replicates as if it were a set of host genes" (Watson, 1965: 466). After rehearsing the evidence from inhibitor and homology experiments with RSV, he states,

> The concept of a DNA provirus for an RNA virus is clearly a radical proposal. If true, it overturns the belief that flow of genetic information always goes in the direction, DNA to RNA, and never RNA to DNA. Much more evidence must be presented before it could gain general acceptance. On the other hand, if true, it offers an even greater variety of ways for cells to exchange genetic information. Considering the enormous complexity of biological systems, it would not be surprising if this device should be uniquely advantageous in some situations [Watson, 1965: 466].

In the second edition of *Molecular Biology of the Gene,* Watson (1970) restates in precisely the same words the Central Dogma. In a footnote, however, Watson asserts that "this statement holds for normal cellular RNA, it does not hold for cells infected with certain RNA viruses." Later, Watson (1970) even cites and discusses the discovery of RT. Perhaps his book was in press and he could not alter the statement of the Central Dogma, or perhaps he saw the Central Dogma as a heuristic device for students approaching molecular biology for the first time. But he may still have believed in the essential correctness of the Central Dogma. It appears that the latter was true. Although he saw RT as a "radical departure," it did overturn the basic tenet of the Central Dogma; nevertheless, in his thought the newly discovered enzyme seemed to function as the "exception to the rule." Watson's view seems to be that the Central Dogma obtains for normal cells. The real threat to this formulation of the Central Dogma is therefore not the discovery of RT in Rous sarcoma virus, but rather the latter (albeit disputed) contention that RT can be found in normal cells (Kang and Temin, 1972, 1973). If this is a correct interpretation of Watson's views, it suggests the existence of a hiatus between the molecular biologists and virologists. While the molecular biologists were studying the "rule," the viral oncologists were studying the RNA viruses which could prove the "exception to the rule." But, as will be seen, even the virologists and oncologists would be reluctant to accept the early formulations of Temin's provirus hypothesis, presumably partly because they also accepted the strong version of the Central Dogma (but see Note 20 below). It is interesting to note, however, that in the third edition of Watson's text, his views have been moderated: "Their [RNA molecules'] relation to DNA and protein is *usually summarized* by the central dogma, a flow scheme for genetic information first proposed some twenty years ago" (1976: 281; italics added).

8. Crick (1970), after the discovery of RT, reiterated this point.

9. In the following we will concentrate on oncogenic RNA virus-related enzyme research. As Temin has stated, "The name *RNA tumor viruses* describes the oncogenicity of some of the members of the virus group. It does not mean that all of the viruses that belong to this group cause tumors. RNA tumor viruses are also called leukoviruses, rousviruses, oncornaviruses, retraviruses, retroviruses, ambiviruses, rnadnaviruses, oncoviruses, and ribodeoxyviruses" (1974: 155). The nomenclature is further complicated by the existence of so-called A-, B-, and C-type viruslike particules discovered by electron microscopy in various neoplastic tissues (see Bern-

hard, 1958, 1960). In general "The RNA viruses contain a single stranded RNA with a molecular weight of 10^7 daltons which normally sediments at 70S and some other smaller RNA molecules which sediment at 35S, 28S, 18S and 4-5S" (Wu and Gallo, 1974: 148).

10. Potter *was anticipating* a confluence of research onto a new set of problems prior to its actual occurrence. This suggests that the scientist's perception of the relevance of previous research to emerging problem domains is based on a broad systemic orientation to biological phenomena. Without this orientation it would be difficult, for instance, to make the jump from bacteriophage research to mammalian viruses (as did Spiegelman). The power of broad systemic principles such as evolution and presently DNA theory is that they allow the biologist to anticipate fruitful "collision courses."

11. RNA-directed DNA polymerase was apparently first called RT by a correspondent to *Nature* (Anonymous, 1970b). This reference is incorrectly cited by Baltimore (1976a, 1976b), a fact he (Baltimore, 1978) admitted to us. The fact that the adjective *reverse* was used to describe the enzyme reflects the strength of the Central Dogma during the period, that is, it stated the "forward" transcription process. But the etymology of the term, in some sense, remains a mystery.

12. The references within this quotation have been reported as given by Temin. They do not, in most cases, refer to discovery dates but rather to reviews of the discoveries and the techniques used.

13. As usual, numerous between-the-lines observations have escaped the light of print. In the forthcoming commentary derived from our interviews, we seek to broaden the one-dimensionality that characterizes intellectual histories based solely on public documents. The insights to which we became privy through our conversations are shared in the *need* to augment, correct, and refine the public record.

14. Baltimore first attempted to find the polymerase in Rous sarcoma virus and failed. Then, after discovering it in Rauscher mouse leukemia virus, he returned to RSV and found it there also (see Baltimore, 1976b). Such early difficulties in locating the enzyme point up the gradual emergence of the techniques required for a precise RT assay. As Baltimore (1978) recalls:

> the first experiment that I did was to look for an RNA-dependent RNA polymerase because I *wasn't* convinced and that was the thing that we had in our hand–it was the easiest thing to assay. And so we tried that first.

Perhaps Spiegelman (1978) put it most succinctly:

> He [Baltimore] found the enzyme as a control. He wasn't looking for that. He was looking for an RNA-directed RNA polymerase. He threw in the deoxyribocides just as a control for his incorporation. And he found those were the ones which incorporated.

The other previously untold story concerns the way Baltimore obtained the Rauscher virus in which the enzyme was discovered:

> Well, that was a most bizarre situation. I had this idea and I had no previous experience with either RNA tumor viruses or with the Virus Cancer Program–I didn't even know the Virus Program existed. But I was an old friend of George Todaro. We went to college [Swarthmore] together. And so I knew he was interested in these things, and so when I decided I wanted to look for the DNA polymerase, by then I had kind of used up the virus that Peter Vogt had

> sent me to look at for RNA, I called George and I said, "Where would I get a lot of virus from?" I guess George believed in me, so he said that there's a whole program that's got lots of virus; its fantastic; why don't I get some? So he put me in touch with someone . . . and about a month later he wrote back that they had the virus and they could ship it up to me and asked how they should ship it. . . . [Todaro's and Rauscher's recollection accords with this account.] He says, "Well, I think it is worth $10,000. Maybe we should send it by courier." I said, "Well, it sounds like for that amount of money maybe you should send it by courier." But I was really flabbergasted. I later discovered that was a gross underestimate; it was probably worth a million dollars. . . . They had actually been stockpiling this stuff. Nobody had ever wanted it for anything, so this Program in effect existed for that one shot of virus that I got, but no one had ever needed bulk virus before. There was nothing you could do with it. In fact, the stuff that they produced was crummy; luckily, the enzyme was very stable. . . . I assayed for it and there was nothing there; and so I spun down a whole lot of it together since I didn't have anything else to do with it and assayed that—and there it was. It was as simple as that [Baltimore, 1978].

Baltimore's initial use of informal channels certainly contrasts with Bader's woeful experience (see Chapter 2) in trying to secure virus through formal NCI channels and failing because of his position *outside* of Viral Oncology (though *within* NCI). Together, the Baltimore and Bader experiences provide a lesson in coping with Big Science bureaucracy.

15. Baltimore commented further to us that:

> The nicest experiment, almost—the experiment that I remember quoting myself before (I guess I must have been teaching it before) was the Duesberg and Vogt experiment—another *PNAS* paper, about 1969 [1969]—where they showed that each virus had to make its own provirus. And that's in fact what the experiments showed. What they showed was that the DNA synthesis phase was required even if the cell was already infected with one virus in order to establish the second virus. It was a very impressive experiment. It's not widely recognized.

16. According to one of our interviewees, the activity of an RNA-directed DNA polymerase *was* detected years before the Temin-Baltimore discovery, but never reported as such. Spiegelman (1978) assured us that:

> To people working in the field of DNA duplication and DNA transcription, the chemistry of using an RNA template to make a DNA copy is essentially the same as making an RNA copy from a DNA template. It's nothing. And so, we all entertained that as a possibility and when I began to work on the RNA viruses in 1960, the first experiment I did was to ask the question, "Do the RNA viruses I was working with—do they use the pathway of going into a cell and then going to DNA and then using the cellular transcription and the whole business?" That was always one way out—to explain the life cycle of the virus. . . . After Kornberg came out with the DNA polymerase—it was '53 . . . maybe '54—some other people then began to work on it. There was one very strange character who came up with a series of remarkable observations, many of which were similar, but nobody paid any attention to it because he was the kind of guy that only made someone else—you always get—suspicious. . . . He came out with a study of the Kornberg DNA polymerase and he showed that, in fact, the Kornberg polymerase would accept R-poly-RU. This is an alternating polyribonuclear type—RU, RU, RU, that it would accept that as a

> template to make poly DADT. Now that's reverse transcription. Indeed, this is years before RT, and in fact, it was the common practice in biochemical laboratories. Whenever they wanted to make a good supply of poly DADT, that was the easiest way to do it. They used the Kornberg enzyme, and gave it this RNA template. So, I mean, RT–now, nobody when that came out said, "Oh, my God, this is a violation of this and that." People simply accepted it, and used it, and that was that. [The man's name?] Cavalieri. . . . I cited it in the [1971] Royal Society [paper]. Lee-Huang and Cavalieri, 1964 *Proceedings of the National Academy*. I say, "Finally, and most concretely, Lee-Huang-Cavalieri in 1964 demonstrated that a DNA polymerase preparation employed would accept an AU polymer as a template for the synthesis of the DADT polymer." Now, that's a perfectly straight story. And so that's six years before, right? And nobody made a big fuss. . . . So the point is that the discovery by Cavalieri and Huang was really discovery of an RT reaction. There's no doubt about it. I used the same enzymes to do a really proper job. So this says already that even if RT had never been found, we could still reverse transcribe. [With the Kornberg enzyme?] Yes. The trick, as we found here, is really just adjusting the ratio of enzyme to the template. That's all. It's as simple as that.

Remarking to Bader that Spiegelman mentioned someone working with the Kornberg enzyme and that *this* was reverse transcription, we were told:

> There was a guy named Cavalieri, Liebe Cavalieri, who has always done funny kinds of experiments, it seems, and he had shown that there was an enzyme in cells, which was probably regular DNA polymerase, which under certain conditions synthesized DNA using an RNA template. That's the only thing I have ever seen in the literature which made a point of that. [Then others were saying that RNA to DNA, and DNA to RNA were both possibilities?] There was nobody else saying that. . . . Just me and Howard Temin. And that was *it*. Because if Sol Spiegelman had had an inkling that that was the case, he would have had guys working on it. There was no question. He had a big operation.

This perception coincides with the overwhelming majority view of our interviewees.

17. The hypothetical and speculative nature of the Sequence Hypothesis and the Central Dogma was clearly stated:

> The direct evidence for both [hypotheses] is negligible, but I have found them to be of great help in getting to grips with these very complex problems. I present them here in the hope that others can make similar use of them. Their speculative nature is emphasized by their names. It is an instructive exercise to attempt to build a useful theory without using them. One generally ends in the wilderness [Crick, 1958: 152].

As Watson's (1965) strong version of the Central Dogma became widely accepted, the very fruitfulness of the hypothesis, it would appear, made alternatives look more and more like "wilderness."

18. As Temin (1978) explained to us:

> I'm a virologist, and the experiments I did were, as far as I'm concerned, sound virologically, and therefore led to an unmistakable conclusion. It was something where I believed the data were conclusive long ago, just the virological phase. Now the virological experiments are, first, very complicated, because you're working with biological systems with many variables; the biology is very complicated, so (1) they were not really accessible to a lot of people, and

(2) you had to understand the whole thing before they were convincing. There were relatively, as I told you before, in the '70s, very few people in this area. Now there were some in this area, like Harry Rubin, who could not understand for other reasons and rejected it; but people like Peter Vogt and especially Peter Duesberg had more luck in their reviews that they wrote before we discovered the enzyme. . . . Peter Vogt could follow the virology, but there were just a very small number of people. The biochemists could not follow this pattern.

19. Two of our subjects elaborated on this suspicion:

There was an uneasiness about what conclusions one could draw. But if the experiments were properly done and properly controlled, certainly one could make determinations. For example, if you have a control situation in which you know all cellular RNA synthesis is inhibitive (that's with actinomycin D) and Sendai virus or vesicular stomatitis virus are cytolytic viruses fully capable of growing in those cells–and then by the same conditions Rous sarcoma cannot grow–then I think that is an appropriately controlled experiment and it says that at least under conditions where other RNA viruses grow, Rous sarcoma virus does not. Now to say that it required RNA synthesis or the participation of DNA, that's extending it a little bit. Suggesting that participation of DNA was required, one could certainly not talk about viral DNA intermediates. All you could talk about was differences between the viruses at that point and it appeared from the mechanism of action of the inhibitor that participation of DNA was required as well [Bader, 1978].

Inhibitor experiments always have a problem, which is, if they fit into the concepts that are ongoing and you can bolster them by other kinds of things, then they make sense. Standing by themselves, everybody is itchy. You don't know enough about the inhibitor to interpret the experiment. And Howard was broadly criticized on that ground, unfairly. But you can't take an inhibitor experiment any further. You can't show that you are right, unless you can go at it by an orthogonal new mechanism. And that's what the RT did. But the problem was that up until the Spring of 1970, no one had an orthogonal way to go at it. And so it just stayed around and was knocked about [Baltimore, 1978].

20. It must be remembered that in 1964 Temin had published an article entitled, "Homology between RNA from Rous sarcoma virus and DNA from Rous sarcoma virus-infected cells." In other words, Temin thought that he had already given the "direct demonstration" which Baltimore demanded. Baltimore (1977) states, however, that Temin

had done his own hypothesis an enormous disservice. In 1964 he published a paper [Temin, 1964a] which purported to show that there was Rous sarcoma virus-specific DNA in infected cells. In fact the paper showed almost as much DNA in uninfected cells as infected cells but because Howard [Temin] was so stuck on his hypothesis he interpreted the small difference as supporting his ideas. The scientific community being what it is, the reaction was extremely negative. People felt that if that was the best data the hypothesis could support then the hypothesis was probably wrong. Much later it became clear that there is in fact Rous sarcoma virus-specific DNA in uninfected cells and that Howard's data were not bad but that was only after the provirus hypothesis was widely accepted.

21. It was seemingly the infectivity model which stimulated much of the early enthusiasm after the discovery of RT. If the synthesis of this enzyme could be blocked, then perhaps cancer could be cured. Huebner (1978), in a private communication, stresses this enthusiasm and its waning:

> Cancers in man especially are clearly due to direct transcription, but it [RT] represents an interesting discovery and presumably is an important factor in certain animal cancers caused by infectious retraviruses. Its importance has been overblown in relation to cancers. Its presence in viruses of animal cancers, however, did provide opportunities for studying the evolution of animal oncornaviruses [Todaro and his colleagues].

22. Earlier it was seen that Temin's research owed much of its inspiration to Lwoff's (1953) research on prophage. It would appear that Huebner's and Todaro's research is similarly indebted to the work of Jacob and Monod (1961) on operons and repressors (see Huebner et al., 1970).

23. Todaro (1978) claims that the oncogene theory "grew out of the data, rather than being purely theoretical." He continues:

> One of the objections to the theory early on was that aspects of it were very hard to test. And it's come to be that it's not so hard to test [this is still hotly contested, as is revealed below]. They are being tested, and they are being confirmed, certainly the idea that the genes are there–they pre-exist in the cells–and there are multiple copies. So a fair amount of the experiments that we have been doing really did grow out of the theory. There is a lot of recent stuff about evolutionary relationships in anthropology now, but most of it comes out of the theory–and I may be somewhat more willing to go into unusual approaches to things, or new areas. But I think that the frame of reference has been that of a medical researcher interested in the cancer problem. And genuinely interested, not because of where I was located.

24. Although Huebner and Todaro represent a pathology tradition in cancer research, other theories have also arisen from this tradition. Burnet's (1968) "immunological surveillance" theory, for instance, rejects the viral theory of tumors and proposes that immunological responses of the body normally keep in check the cancer-producing mechanisms. In a recent address, Huebner echoes this view, stating that

> Immunoprevention of a variety of infectious viral diseases had not only proved to be a tremendous boon to humanity, but clearly established that one of the chief advantages of successful immunoprevention of disease was that it also provided the highest order of information concerning etiology [1977; 4].

25. Being an alumnus of St. Louis University Medical School, Huebner has always kept closely in touch with Green's operation there. And Green (1978) considers

> the most gifted and propetic and moving force I've seen in any area–Bob Huebner. He's made discoveries in DNA tumor viruses. He discovered all of these [e.g., T-] antigens, these proteins that are transforming proteins, many years ago. The oncogene–I thought this was a very worthwhile hypothesis. It was correct. And he's made monumental contributions. . . . In the early 70s . . . every paper that came out he had several girls go through, screen, bring them to him. He would read them all, make notes, and send copies of the papers to everybody with suggestions on what might possibly be done. And that's very valuable. That's communication. That's how progress is made informally.

26. This is reminiscent of the acrimonious private testimony Mitroff (1974) elicited from his elite sample of Apollo moon scientists regarding theories of origin and change which were to be resolved by analysis of specimens recovered from exploratory lunar missions.

27. Perhaps Baltimore (1978) put it best when he said:

> This whole business of balancing the oncogene theory against the protovirus theory strikes me as just pure foolishness. I have never heard a productive discussion along those lines in my life. . . . I think the oncogene theory is as much public relations as it is anything else. The protovirus idea is the workings of Howard's very imaginative and fertile brain. . . . It's not like when Francis Crick said, "If you are going to build a code, the simplest way is out of three letters and that was it." Elegant statement of simple theories. None of these things fall into that category.

28. The latest "textbook wisdom," however, notes that "despite some claims of reverse transcriptase-like DNA polymerases in uninfected cells, no convincing evidence for the existence of such enzymes has been provided" (Luria et al., 1978: 388).

29. As Baltimore (1978) told us:

> In a real sense, they provided the key observation that said everything was right. Had they done it before the RT, they would have made the RT a confirmatory piece of evidence. Absolutely. [That's how the Nobel prize could have shifted?] Oh yes! Because the kind of evidence that they were able to provide was so totally incontrovertible–it's DNA and it does it; there it is. And if anyone today wants to give a single key observation to a class of students that says that RNA tumor viruses make themselves into a DNA chain, the evidence is that you take the DNA out of cells and it's infective. What better evidence could there be? Enzymes are only enzymes. You can make enzymes jump through hoops for you. So the fact that you can make an enzyme copy RNA doesn't mean that the function of the enzyme is to copy RNA. You've got to show it. In fact, 95 percent of the scientific community upon hearing that we found it said, "You guys have shown it." The fact of the matter was that we hadn't shown it. We had only provided the kind of evidence that people are very comfortable with and therefore they accepted it. But you can't get out of it the proof.

30. Note that the protovirus hypothesis had begun to generate new problem domains of its own. It was now functioning as a backdrop for the further growth and development of molecular virology. Yet at the same time, the demands of laboratory research as it followed the systemic paths through the virus-cell complex were serving to elucidate further the place of reverse transcription within cellular systems. The result was the postulation of new models which again had to be submitted to the evidential norms of the newly defined problem.

31. The hypothetical and speculative nature of their work would probably not be denied by Gillespie and Gallo. Their work is cited here primarily as an example of the type of research and thought which has become possible *because of* the discovery of RT. Other uses are discussed below.

32. A recombinant DNA researcher formerly at NCI and now at NICHD, Leder has applied techniques developed to isolate specific messenger RNAs for specific proteins and then locating the nucleotide sequences of certain genes. Using RT, one

makes a complementary DNA from a messenger RNA and then locates the gene in the chromosome.

33. It has been noted by every biologist who commented on this chapter that the work of Zhadnov is not replicable.

34. All of these researchers were postdoctoral students under Harry Rubin at Berkeley. Duesberg also worked with William Robinson who himself had done postdoctoral work under Rubin. It is Rubin who worked in Dulbecco's lab at California Institute of Technology. Dulbecco, of course, shares the 1975 Nobel prize with RT codiscoverers Temin (who was a Dulbecco student) and Baltimore, Apparently, Dulbecco's lab—as Bader implied in Chapter 2—was a source of much intellectual inspiration.

35. As claimed in a recent review:

> In spite of the fact that all the indirect criteria for linking a virus to a human cancer have been satisfied for the Epstein-Barr virus, uncertainty remains about the exact role of the virus. . . . Indeed, a final proof to everyone's satisfaction may never be attained. For those willing to accept the indirect evidence, however, the Epstein-Barr virus is the foremost candidate for being the first known human cancer virus [Henle et al., 1979: 59].

36. These inputs are less a selective borrowing from extant ideas and literature (see Schon, 1963) than the presence within a cognitive region, to use once more Boehme's (1975) spatial metaphor, of concepts manipulable by those "inhabiting" that region, producing new ideas, and reading that literature. Methods of demarcating and, therefore, anticipating the intellectual composition of a region, are sorely lacking, of course—a problem discussed in foregoing chapters.

37. Schaffner (1974) has suggested a Bayesian (subjective probability) approach to understanding the scientist's choice of models within biological science. This indeed may be a useful avenue to explore, but analyzing the scientist's "educated guess at the probability of discovering the possible experimental outcome" (Schaffner, 1974: 138) should not be seen as a substitute for understanding the confluence structures that made the "educated guesses" possible.

38. Historian of biology Goodfield (1977) recently called for direct observation of scientists "at the bench" as a means of reducing the cognitive distance between the nonscientist observer (e.g., social scientist) and the source of his/her data. Goodfield's clarion call should resound to sociologists for reasons of empathy, access, and insight which they, as outsiders, should crave but seldom seek due to their positivistic inclinations (see Whitley, 1972).

CHAPTER 5

REVERSE TRANSCRIPTASE RESEARCHERS:

Patterns of Organization, Coauthorship, and Careers

If I have seen a little further it is by standing on the shoulders of giants.

Newton

In the sciences, we are now uniquely privileged to sit side by side with the giants on whose shoulders we stand.

Holton (1961: 807)

Introduction

One of the most convenient and enlightening points of entrée into a problem domain is through its literature. Literature is more than a public record of knowledge claims; it is a source of data (Chubin, 1975) on the monitoring of cognitive and social structures of a research area by "gatekeepers" (e.g., Crane, 1967). Journals therefore exercise the cognitive (evidential) norms of a domain. Just as such norms "stylize" ideas, they reveal other dimensions of research that demand clarification. To wit, intellectual development and quantitative indicators of that development are rarely isomorphic (see Thackray, 1977). Time lags and measurement errors thus recommend a strategy of data collection and analysis which allows a problem domain to "speak" in its various structural terms. What will emerge in the present chapter, then, is a shifting of analytical focus—from individuals to institutions, coauthorship to laboratories—and back again. Where one begins is less important than one's capacity to shift to another perspective and visualize structure in yet another way.

The Bibliographic Data

As a prelude to analysis, we highlight several features of the RT article set which has been compiled from *Index Medicus, Biological Abstracts,* and the *Source Index* of the *Science Citation Index.* The stage upon which the RT drama has unfolded can be seen in the summary statistics which describe the literature growth of this domain. This literature also provides a broad spectrum of relationships against which the protagonists of the research can be viewed. For if the organization of biomedicine reflects the complexities of its cognitive objects, we must analyze biologists with an eye toward understanding how they organize around and interact with these objects.

The 656 articles on RT,[1] for instance, point to numerous structural features which aid in understanding the growth curves of the domain. Table 5.1 represents a decomposition of the growth curve (Figure 5.1) of the RT literature. It suggests how scientists are distributed across employment sectors and how funding is acknowledged within the research domain. This is where the social parameters of development intersect with the political and institutional features of research in particular ways. When coauthorship relations are discussed, they must be seen as further decompositions of the social structures which should aim to provide the social matrix in which the confluence of lines of research has occurred within biomedicine. That is, before assuming that cognition and institutionalization interact in a particular fashion, for example, to produce a degree of codification (see Zuckerman and Merton, 1972), one must entertain approaches to the data which allow that events "could have been otherwise."

One of the most promising tools presently in use and under investigation by science analysts is citation analysis.[2] It is common practice to couch such analysis in terms of social and intellectual structures. Thus, from viewing the scatterplots of Figures 5.2 and 5.3 of journal frequencies and citations to journals within the RT data set,[3] we can orient analysis toward questions concerning the structural properties of publications and citations. Of course, someone sometime must choose the references to be included in an article, but those choices, however motivated on the individual level (see Chubin and Moitra, 1975; Moravcsik and Murugesan, 1975), create patterns that can be structurally analyzed.

The fact that the journal *Nature (New Biology)* was created as an entity separate from *Nature* in 1970, when RT research was expanding rapidly, points to shifts in organizational structure and its manifestation in the

TABLE 5.1 Distribution of Employment Sectors of Reverse Transcriptase Authors and Their Acknowledged Agencies of Funding Support[a]

Employment Sectors:	n	%[b]
University Dept. or Lab.	202	39.0
Hospital or Medical School	154	29.7
Government	180	34.7
Private Company	148	28.6
Foreign	158	30.5
Agencies of Support:		
Virus Cancer Program (VCP)	104	20.1
National Cancer Institute (NCI)	255	49.2
National Institutes of Health (NIH)	178	34.4
Public Health Service (PHS)	95	18.3
Other Government	42	8.1
American Cancer Society	53	10.2
Other Foundation	53	10.2
Foreign Support	59	11.4

[a]Data are for the Index Medicus subset (n = 518, 80 percent of the set) only. Information concerning employment sector was deduced from the authors acknowledged location at time of publication. Funding support was, likewise, obtained from acknowledgments in the articles.

[b]Percentages do not sum to 100 because the location of each author was coded (mean authors = 3.5; S.D. = 1.9; sole authorship is rare) and multiple sources of support are common.

[c]Eighty-one percent of the articles acknowledge PHS funding at some level, i.e., PHS, NIH, NCI and/or VCP.

literature. In Figure 5.3, comparing citations to articles within the set with those to articles outside the set, *Nature* and *Nature (New Biology)* shift in their relative positions within the literature. Likewise, the position of the *Proceedings of the National Academy of Sciences* is more imposing in Figure 5.3 than in Figure 5.2. If one is dealing with a fast-breaking area of science, the dominance of *PNAS* may be explicable in terms of its rapid turnaround time, a phenomenon which telegraphs the scientific innovation process. If one wants to know how the published literature cuts across subject areas, then study of the contents of, for example, *Nature* or *PNAS*

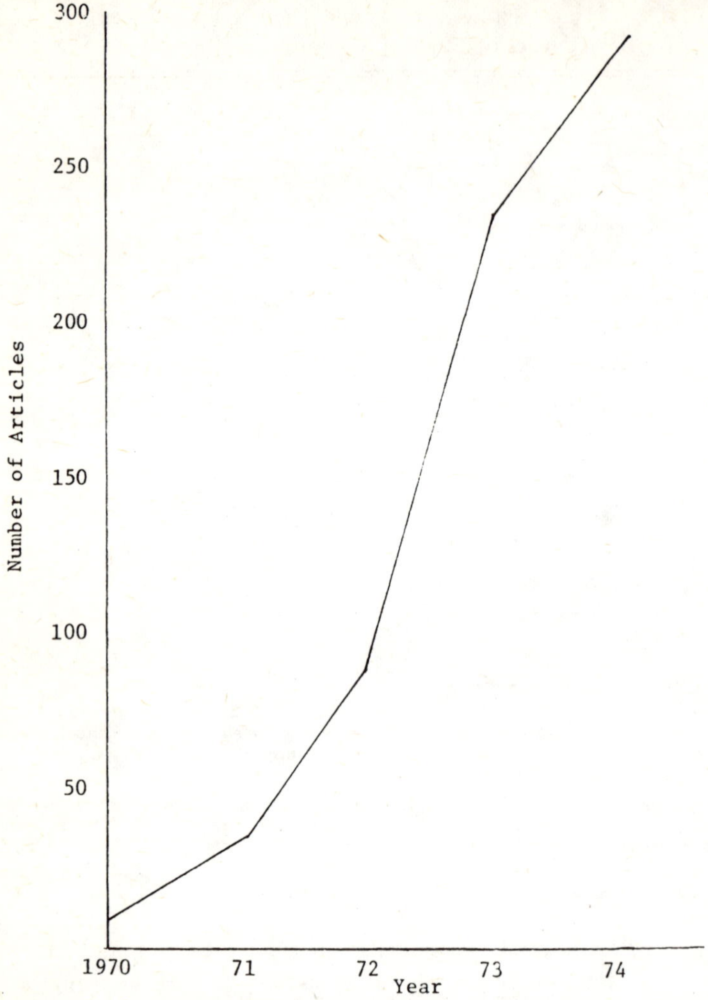

FIGURE 5.1 Frequency Distribution by Year of Reverse Transcriptase Articles (N = 656)

may provide an important clue to the confluence of subjects into specific journals.

Finally, our analysis of characteristics reflected in the scatterplots in Figures 5.2 and 5.3 leads us to network representations which portray the

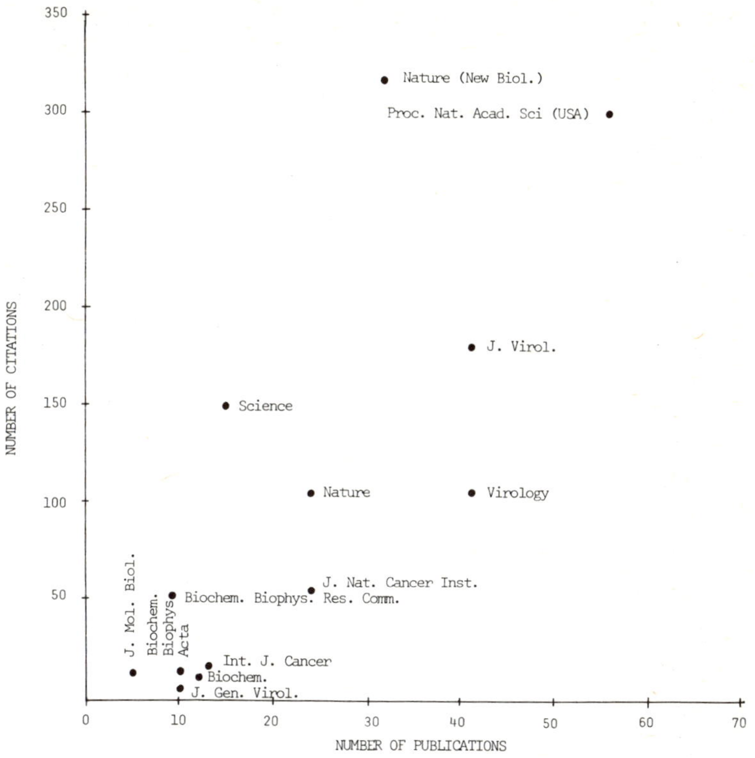

FIGURE 5.2 Scatterplot of Journal Location in Reverse Transcriptase by Citations and Publications Within the Article Set, 1970-1974

skeletal social structure of the domain. Taken together, these network structures will force us away from the stereotyping of research as methodological versus substantive or from facile explanations based on the routinization of paradigmatic structures. The present structures impel us to ask questions concerning historical details which accumulate in one's mind to form a composite picture of the unfolding problem domain.

The In-House Coauthorship Network

By looking at the domain of RT as a totality, without controlling for individual years within its lifetime, we can form an initial impression of its

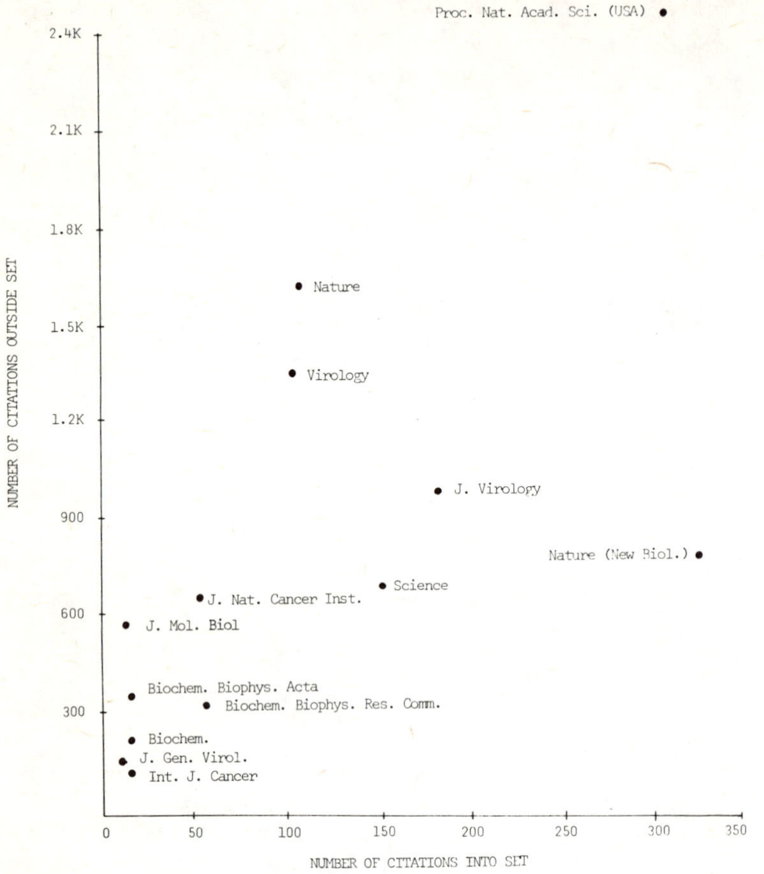

FIGURE 5.3 Scatterplot of Journal Location in Reverse Transcriptase by Citations Outside and in the Article Set, 1970-1974

research organization. In Figure 5.4 is displayed a coauthorship network of the 16 authors who have published at least 10 articles on RT (i.e., more than two standard deviations above the mean published articles per author) from 1970 through 1974. Although other authors (i.e., the seven others in Table 5.2) satisfied this publishing criterion,[4] they were not linked into this network of coauthorship. This, of course, suggests that many important researchers, notably Temin and Baltimore, are not tied

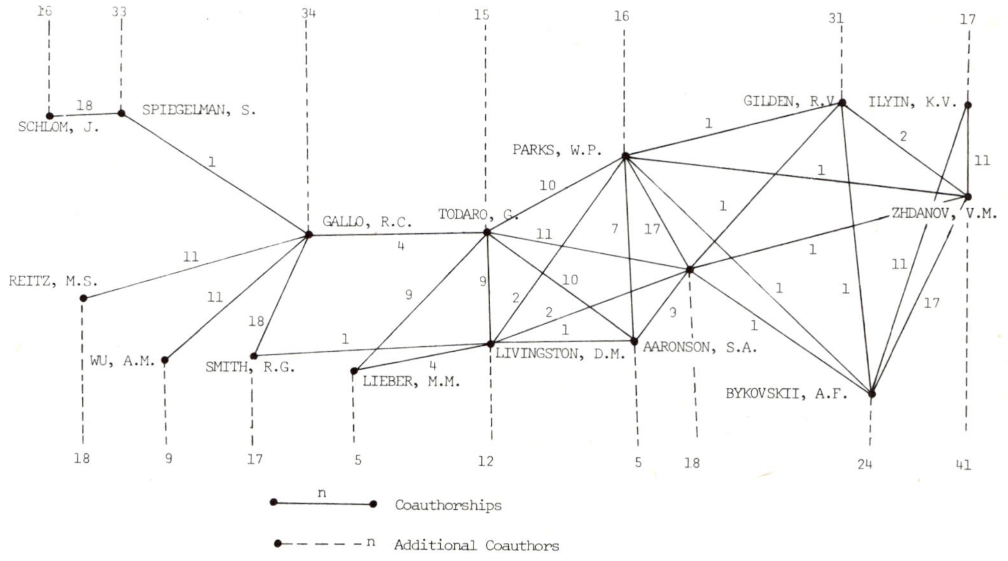

FIGURE 5.4 Cosmopolitan Network of Reverse Transcriptase Coauthors, 1970-1974

TABLE 5.2 Articles and Average Citations per Article for the Highly Published Authors of the Reverse Transcriptase Literature

Cosmopolitan	Articles	Citations/Article
Gallo	53	10.9
Spiegelman	49	15.9
Todaro	31	15.8
Zhadnov	24	1.5
Scolnick	23	19.4
Parks	19	11.6
Gilden	18	3.8
Schlom	18	22.0
Smith	18	9.2
Aaronson	17	18.2
Bykovskii	17	2.1
Livingston	14	5.2
Wu	12	2.8
Ilyin	11	1.7
Reitz	11	13.0
Lieber	10	4.4
all	345	
unique article n	268	
% of total set	39.0	

Other	Articles	Citations/Article
Green	19	11.7
Temin	15	23.1
Verma	13	8.1
Baltimore	12	36.3
Moser	11	0.3
Paul	11	2.9
Rainer	11	0.3
all	92	
unique article n	71	
% of total set	10.3	

into the network. The exclusivity of this network–both in terms of productivity[5] and the affiliation of most of the Americans with laboratories of NCI–prompted our labeling this the "in-house" network. The existence of this network suggests the operation of a distinctive social structure at one front, and perhaps *the* front, of the problem domain.

The nature of the coauthorship relation, however, is not straightforward as it might first appear. For what does "authorship," the placement of a name on the title page of an article, really mean? It can indicate intellectual contributions, technical assistance, principal investigator status, laboratory affiliation, and so on. In a word, coauthorship is a more ambiguous relationship than has been suggested heretofore. Although the nodes or authors are known in such an analysis, the linkages are defined over many different relationships. Connectivity in such a situation requires adequate decomposition so that the constituent relationships implied by signatory status become apparent.

By focusing momentarily on the Russians (Bykovskii, Zhadnov, Ilyin) who met the criterion for inclusion in the authorship network, one glimpses some of the difficulties of this type of network analysis. All of the lines connecting them with the rest of the network are composed of *one* coauthorship. What is not known, of course, is how many articles are represented in the six linkages with their respective weights of one. The answer is that only *one* article created this set of pairwise interrelationships. The article, "Mason-Pfizer virus characterization: a similar virus in a human amniotic cell line" (*Journal of Virology,* December 1973), was coauthored by W. P. Parks, R. V. Gilden, A. F. Bykovskii, G. G. Miller, V. M. Zhadnov, V. D. Soloviev, and E. M. Scolnick. With a little calculation, it can be seen that there is a possibility of 21 different pairwise coauthorship relationships that can be generated by this one set of authors. The number of the total authorships of articles in RT has led to the inclusion of the Russians (Table 5.2), but it was only *one article* that linked them to the U.S. contingent of researchers (Figure 5.4).

The question is, of course, is it deceptive to connect individuals on the basis of such a seemingly tenuous link? What one sees here is the meeting of two international communities, "united" through the coauthorship of one scholarly product.[6] And this meeting is between elites, recognized as worthy and capable of working on a cooperative venture of international science. They are not only confirming "the presence of virus particles in five different human cell lines." They are also part of an "investigation of several human cell lines and viruses [which are] being conducted as part of a joint agreement between cancer virologists in the U.S.A. and the USSR" (Parks et al., 1973: 1540). It is this research that brought together not only seven men but also NCI, Flow Laboratories, Gamaleya Institute of Epidemiology and Microbiology (Moscow), and the D.I. Ivanovsky Institute of Virology (Moscow). Thus, what at first seems to be a set of tenuous relationships begins to take on meaning as we consider the historical events which have led to the network configuration. Why, we can ask, were the specific men chosen for this cooperative task, how did this interaction come about, and what does coauthorship mean in this context?

An equally interesting connection can be found on the left side of Figure 5.4, between S. Spiegelman and R. C. Gallo. As we have seen and shall again later, these men are both central researchers in the domain, but they seldom write articles together. Spiegelman's location at Columbia and Gallo's at NCI have created two institutionally divergent paths of research. They are connected by one article/letter within our data set, and this leads us to ask, "What caused the exception to the rule?" The coauthorship connection is due to an editorial in *Lancet* (Anonymous, 1973: 542) suggesting that there was a discrepancy between the results of experiments performed by Spiegelman's and Gallo's respective research teams. They state in their response that the earlier article,

> described a "discrepancy" between the experimental data of our respective laboratories relative to reverse transcriptase in leukaemic cells. It states that the work of Gallo et al. shows hybridisation of the DNA product made with human leukaemic reverse transcriptase to the 70S RNA of avian myeloblastosis virus (AMV), whereas Spiegelman et al. did not observe hybridisation of the DNA products with AMV 70S RNA, but only to RNA of mouse leukaemia between the two sets of experiments. Gallo et al. examined the response of the reverse transcriptase *purified* from the cytoplasmic particulate fraction from human acute leukaemic cells to *added* AMV 70S RNA and MLV 70S RNA. . . . [In the Spiegelman et al.] experiments the DNA was made from the endogenous reverse transcriptase reaction—i.e., one using the resident RNA of the cytoplasmic particle in human leukaemic cells. . . . At the moment there are no significant discrepancies between the results of our respective laboratories nor with any of the laboratories seriously working on these questions [Gallo and Spiegelman, 1974: 1117].

The reason for surmounting institutional boundaries in this instance of coauthorship is therefore apparent. In response to a misinterpretation of their collective efforts, they coauthored a letter bringing their separate efforts into proper focus. The sparseness of their collective effort in terms of coauthorship rightfully can be seen as an extension of their institutional affiliations, and this is all the more reinforced by the exception to the rule.

As the Gallo-Spiegelman response, there often occurs the et alia shorthand for the string of authors assembled on an article. The coauthorship relation has thus become arranged around the "superior" member of the research staff. It is "their" laboratories, it would appear, which they personify. Thus, the et alia relationship (signified in Figure 5.4 by the numbers of other coauthors at the ends of the broken lines) raises many questions as to the "authority structures" represented in coauthorship networks. Could it not be that our criterion for inclusion in the network, namely, having published at least 10 articles on RT, has brought to the fore a set of researchers who occupy "authority" positions within large laboratories? In short, they may be the fixed point around which numerous lesser (as measured by number of coauthorships) members orbit.

VISIBILITY OF INDIVIDUALS AND LOCAL ORGANIZATION

To pursue analysis of this problem, Table 5.3 has been constructed to reveal the structure of authorship "strings" for the 22 individuals included in Table 5.2. What we discern are traces of a scientific etiquette system which orders the authors. If collaborative authorship were always simply an alphabetic ordering, Aaronson would appear first on every article he coauthors. But such is not the case. Of course, name ordering on articles is often determined by location, all of the individuals from one laboratory grouped together for ease of attribution of location (especially in *Nature*). Nevertheless, it would seem that groups themselves could be so arranged that the most important laboratory would appear first, and likewise the most important individuals first within the group. But then why do individuals such as Gilden pale in importance when only first authorships are taken into account? These explanations may obtain. First, perhaps there is observance of *noblesse oblige* (Zuckerman, 1977)—those who have "made it" in the scientific community (e.g., Nobel laureates) defer to their lesser colleagues, allowing them to be placed in the forefront through publication. Second, perhaps those who receive tremendous amounts of research moneys[7] have their names placed on articles due to their principal investigator/administrator status, rather than to their playing the research role. Third, perhaps the ordering is determined according to the amount of work actually invested in the final article/research product.

Predictably, the whole tradition of personal attribution of responsibility for intellectual contributions has been greatly altered by the large

TABLE 5.3 Number of Articles, Name Order, and Coauthorship Among Reverse Transcriptase Cosmopolitan Authors[a]

Authors	Total No. Articles	No. Articles Coauthored	No. 1st Authorships	Percent 1st Authorships	No. Different Coauthors
Aaronson, S.A.	17	15	2	13.3	8
Baltimore, D.	13	12	1	8.3	17
Bykovskii, A.F.	17	17	2	11.3	26
Gallo, R.C.	55	49	7	14.3	40
Gilden, R.V.	18	18	0	.0	34
Green, M.	19	19	5	26.3	21
Ilyin, K.V.	11	11	2	18.2	18
Lieber, M.M.	10	10	3	30.0	7
Livingston, D.M.	14	13	4	30.8	18
Moser, K.	11	11	1	9.1	9
Parks, W.P.	19	17	4	23.5	22
Paul, J.	11	11	1	9.1	13
Rainer, H.	11	11	8	72.7	10
Reitz, M.S.	11	11	3	27.3	21
Schlom, J.	18	18	7	38.9	14
Scolnick, E.M.	23	22	6	27.3	23
Smith, R.G.	19	19	5	26.3	21
Spiegelman, S.	50	49	6	12.2	37
Temin, H.M.	16	11	3	27.3	4
Todaro, G.J.	32	31	7	22.6	21
Verma, I.M.	13	11	8	72.7	13
Wu, A.M.	12	12	9	75.0	12
Zhdanov, V.M.	24	24	12	50.0	44

[a]This table was constructed from the entire reverse transcriptase data set covering all years since the discovery of the enzyme.

laboratory tradition that has grown up during the highly funded, especially post-1971, cancer war period. When a coauthorship network involves a Gilden, Spiegelman, and Gallo, men who have coauthored with numerous individuals during a short (four-year) span, we must hypothesize that authorship measures not only personal research attributes but also laboratory, bureaucratic, and authority structures as well. The ordering of signatories on an author string reflects these complexities.

What becomes necessary to understand the nature of the coauthorship network is further disaggregation until historical, institutional, and personal facts are able to inform the larger structure. For instance, it can be readily seen in Figure 5.5 how such a micro-level coauthorship network for 1972 and 1973 aids in understanding the Spiegelman group. In terms of coauthorship, this group is not connected for these two years to any other group; it forms a disjoint subset of coauthors (see Appendix C for a discussion of disjoint subsets and the derivation of the network representations which follow).

At this level of analysis it becomes more evident that the institutional affiliation of coauthors is not as homogeneous as one might expect. The sphere of influence extends through the mobility of doctoral students, postdoctoral fellows, visiting scholars, interlaboratory research, and government contracts and grants. But there is little doubt that Speigelman's grants (especially, CA-02332, 1973 = $1.1 million) and contracts (especially, 70-2049, 1973 = $.4 million), and CP-33258, 1973 = $.6 million) were a strong magnet for attracting students and researchers. His was a big operation. And the concentration of Spiegelman's coauthors on these three grants and contracts is as telling as their acknowledgements of him as a coauthor of their articles. Inevitable questions arise at this point, for example, Does the laboratory have some explicit policy concerning coauthorship? Is it a "one-man"[8] laboratory dominated by Spiegelman's personal research interests?[9]

The general coauthorship networks have not led, in the above discussion to the construction of equally general indicators of scientific organization but, on the contrary, have led to further disaggregation. In the present situation, the network generator to which we appeal in our disaggregation implies social consequences that make for structural ambiguities in the domain. Authorship, in short, is *not* a homogeneous network generator. Hence, other factors relating to coauthorship networks must be utilized to evaluate the nature of the linkages between individuals. If the coauthorship linkage is ambiguous, then it would be wise to define a relationship which will measure similarity-dissimilarity. Thus, we shift the focus from authorship per se to that of another bibliographic relationship defined over

FIGURE 5.5 Local Reverse Transcriptase Coauthorship Networks, 1972 and 1973

1972

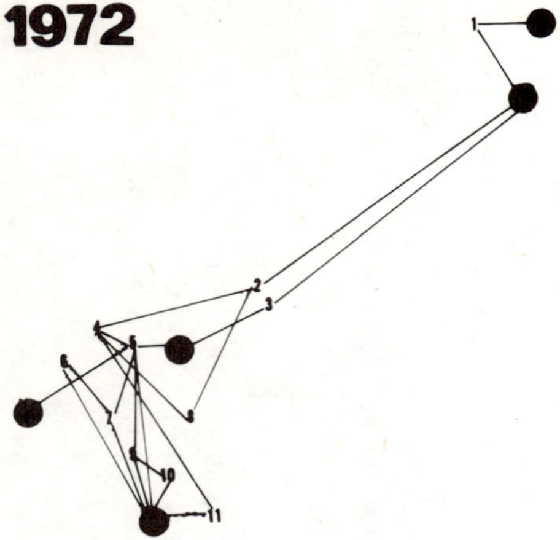

AUTHORS

1. Aoki, T., Inst. Med. Res., Camden
2. Sarkar, N.H., Inst Med. Res., Camden
3. Nowinski, R.C., Inst. Med. Res., Camden
4. Moore, D.H., Inst. Med. Res., Camden
5. Spiegelman, S., Columbia
6. Gulati, S. C., Columbia
7. Axel, R., Columbia
8. Dion, A.S., Inst. Med. Res., Camden
9. Baxt, W., Columbia
10. Hehlmann, R., Columbia
11. Schlom, J., Columbia

OTHER NETWORK CHARACTERISTICS—1972

Articles published 10

Mean citations/article 8.9

Other locations (present address, home institution, etc.) attributed to authors

Sloan Kettering
McArdle Lab., U. of Wisconsin
Inst. Pathol. Anat. U. Paduva, Italy
Vir. Leuk. and Lymph. Br., NCI

Acknowledged sources of funding

Special Virus Cancer Program, NCI
National Cancer Institute
State of New Jersey

Research awards, number of articles acknowledged in, and principal investigator

CA-02332	4	Spiegelman
70-2049	4	Spiegelman
7 others	1	

1973

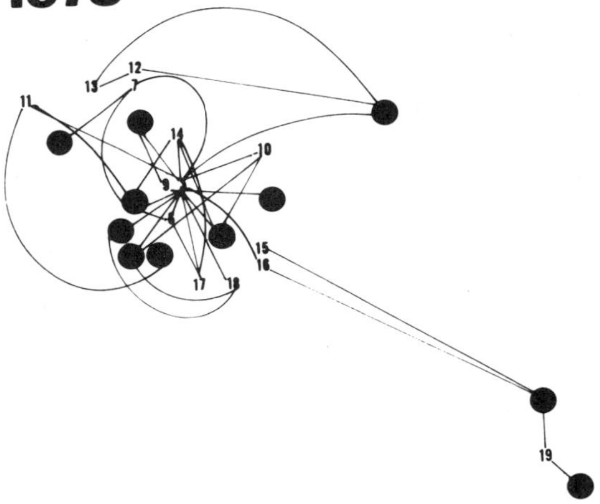

AUTHORS

12. Bank, A., Columbia
13. Marks, R.A., Columbia
7. Axel, R., Columbia
11. Schlom, J., Columbia
14. Burnv, A.. Columbia
10. Hehlmann, R., Columbia
9. Baxt, W., Columbia
5. Spiegelman, S., Columbia
15. Goodman, N.C., Columbia
16. Ramirez, R., Columbia
17. Yaniz, A., Columbia
18. Kufe, D., Columbia
19. Deinhardt, F., Columbia

OTHER NETWORK CHARACTERISTICS—1973

Articles published 16

Mean citations/article 3.4

Other locations (present address, home institution, etc.) attributed to authors

Rush Presbyterian Hosp., Chicago
U. of Illinois Med. Center
Uganda Cancer Inst.
Lab. Mol. Biol., NIAMDD

Acknowledged sources of funding

Special Virus Cancer Program, NCI
National Cancer Institute
National Institute of Neurological and Communicative Disorders and Stroke
National Institutes of Health
Public Health Service
National Science Foundation
American Cancer Society

Research Awards, number of articles acknowledged in, and principal investigator

CA-02332	10	Spiegelman, S.
70-2049	8	Spiegelman, S.
CP-33258	3	Spiegelman, S.
CM-14552	2	Marks, P.A.
RR-05477	2	Lepper, M.H.
11 others	1	

the same set of individuals–citations–and undertake an assessment of the intracitation and intrareferencing patterns among the 16 individuals in the in-house network.

THE IN-HOUSE INTRACITATION NETWORK

What we seek here is to ascertain relationships established through the practice of referencing articles within this small set of authors. However, when one wants to shift the unit of citation analysis from articles, which are the typical units, to that of individuals, some difficulties emerge. An example will clarify the major difficulty. If individual A writes an article and is *referenced* by individual B, then A is said to have received one *citation.* But what if an article is authored by more than one person, say A, B, and C, and this article is later cited by an article authored by D and E? When the citations are distributed to A, B, and C, each receives *two* citations. Coauthorship, in other words, creates overlapping citation patterns among individuals. One's count increases the more one is referenced by articles with multiple authors. What is needed is a means of examining the citation and referencing *profiles* of individuals that is impervious to the multiplier effect of citation counts. The most common measure of the strength of the linear relationship between two variables which discounts scale effects is the Pearson product-moment correlation coefficient. Because it is a well-known and easily interpretable measure of association, we will use it to measure the degree of similarity between citation and referencing profiles.

What is needed for the analysis is a 16 X 16 matrix of individuals connected by their referencing patterns. Reading across rows one sees how a particular author references (chooses) other authors, while reading down columns one discovers the way that the respective authors are cited (chosen). In terms of correlation analysis, we recognize three possible perspectives from which we could proceed. First, we could correlate the columns of the matrix and discover the intercorrelations of the citation vectors, namely, how the profiles of being chosen by others compare (Table 5.4). Second, we could correlate the rows of the matrix and discover the similarities of the referencing vectors (Table 5.5). Third, we could compare the referencing vectors with the citation vectors, creating an asymmetric matrix of correlations (Table 5.6).[10] This last technique, while not often utilized (see Bearden et al., 1975), is of great assistance in comparing an individual's self-perceptions as chooser with those of his colleagues.

From Table 5.4 it appears that there are distinct choosing patterns among the 16 authors. The situation noted earlier between the work of

Gallo and Spiegelman is strikingly reflected in the dissimilarity of their citation vectors. Of all of Gallo's and Spiegelman's coauthors, their mutual relationship is by far the most fragile, that is, r = .1834. They are not being chosen by others in the same proportions as are their respective other coauthors, for example, Gallo and Reitz, and Spiegelman and Schlom, who have virtually identical profiles. This is due, in large part, of course, to the citation overlaps stemming from coauthorship discussed above. High correlations can stem from substantial intersection of the two cited article sets, that is, when two authors have written virtually all of their articles *together.* What is of interest is the departure from perfect correlation of such profiles for coauthors, that is, Spiegelman and Gallo, and the high correlations for those not directly linked via coauthorship.

The outstanding finding is that the Spiegelman-Schlom group does not project a profile similar to any of the others within the network. Members of this group are neither chosen (Table 5.4) nor do they choose the other highly published authors with a similar profile. Their profile is truly divergent from the NCI research workers. The same can be said, predictably, of the Russians Bykovskii, Zhadnov, and Ilyin. Their work is not chosen, nor do they choose, in a fashion that conforms to the research programs of the NCI scientists.

In the case of Gilden, however, a comparison of Tables 5.3 and 5.4 suggests that there is an imbalance in his citation and referencing patterns that places him on the periphery of the in-house network. Although Gilden references in a fashion similar to those Americans with whom he is connected (e.g., Parks and Scolnick, although this link is not strong in terms of coauthorship count, which is one), he also shares a similar referencing pattern with Aaronson and Lieber. The latter two are, respectively, two and three steps removed from Gilden in the coauthorship network. Gilden also shows a strong referencing relationship with Todaro and Livingston, both correlations hovering around .5. When one turns to Table 5.4 to see how Gilden's citation pattern compares with the rest of this group, no strong relationships can be found. This imbalance between the referencing and citing vector correlations suggests a peripherality to the central NCI group. This differs, for instance, from the profiles of Spiegelman and Schlom. Unlike Gilden, Spiegelman and Schlom do not appear to be drawing their intellectual sustenance from NCI research. Gilden (then director of Flow Laboratories) appears to enjoy a symbiotic relationship with the NCI in a manner that Spiegelman does not.[11]

To generalize beyond the relationships of the 16 coauthors is unwarranted at this juncture. For purposes of the present analysis, the 16 coauthors comprise a closed system; of course, they are not a closed

(text continued on p. 163)

TABLE 5.4 Correlation of Cosmopolitan Person-to-Person Citations[a]

	GALLO	TODARO	SPIEGELMAN	PARKS	REITZ	SCOLNICK	SMITH	SCHLOM	LIVINGSTON	ZHADNOV	BYKOVSKII	LIEBER	AARONSON	ILYIN	WU	GILDEN
GALLO	1.0000	0.6544	0.1834	0.0583	0.9911	0.0644	0.9866	-0.0121	0.5611	-0.3327	-0.3327	0.4080	0.2609	-0.3075	0.8761	-0.1183
TODARO	0.6544	1.0000	-0.0868	0.6737	0.6611	0.6679	0.6317	-0.1980	0.9331	-0.4181	-0.4181	0.9040	0.6629	-0.4257	0.4940	-0.0117
SPIEGELMAN	0.1834	-0.0868	1.0000	-0.2279	0.2611	-0.2254	0.0862	0.9621	-0.1688	-0.1814	-0.1814	-0.1955	0.0003	-0.1655	0.0706	-0.1325
PARKS	0.0583	0.6737	-0.2279	1.0000	0.0779	0.9898	0.0248	-0.2284	0.5279	-0.2243	-0.2243	0.5762	0.7857	-0.2748	0.0304	0.2952
REITZ	0.9911	0.6611	0.2611	0.0779	1.0000	0.0826	0.9647	0.0630	0.5613	-0.3490	-0.3490	0.4049	0.2828	-0.3221	0.8265	-0.1088
SCOLNICK	0.0644	0.6679	-0.2254	0.9898	0.0826	1.0000	0.0336	-0.2289	0.5445	-0.1705	-0.1705	0.5836	0.7221	-0.2254	0.0372	0.3525
SMITH	0.9866	0.6317	0.0862	0.0248	0.9647	0.0336	1.0000	-0.1013	0.5585	-0.3180	-0.3180	0.4085	0.2369	-0.2925	0.8530	-0.1001
SCHLOM	-0.0121	-0.1980	0.9621	-0.2284	0.0630	-0.2289	-0.1013	1.0000	-0.2517	-0.2360	-0.2360	-0.2501	-0.0550	-0.2209	-0.0839	-0.0479
LIVINGSTON	0.5611	0.9331	-0.1688	0.5279	0.5613	0.5445	0.5585	-0.2517	1.0000	-0.3770	-0.3770	0.9420	0.4531	-0.3679	0.3857	0.0411
ZHADNOV	-0.3327	-0.4181	-0.1814	-0.2243	-0.3490	-0.1705	-0.3180	-0.2360	-0.3770	1.0000	1.0000	-0.3361	-0.4096	0.9863	-0.2726	-0.0376
BYKOVSKII	-0.3327	-0.4181	-0.1814	-0.2243	-0.3490	-0.1705	-0.3180	-0.2360	-0.3770	1.0000	1.0000	-0.3361	-0.4096	0.9863	-0.2726	-0.0376
LIEBER	0.4080	0.9040	-0.1955	0.5762	0.4049	0.5836	0.4085	-0.2501	0.9420	-0.3361	-0.3361	1.0000	0.4921	-0.3425	0.2532	-0.0345
AARONSON	0.2609	0.6629	0.0003	0.7857	0.2828	0.7221	0.2369	-0.0550	0.4531	-0.4096	-0.4096	0.4921	1.0000	-0.4461	0.1394	-0.1142
ILYIN	-0.3075	-0.4257	-0.1655	-0.2748	-0.3221	-0.2254	-0.2925	-0.2209	-0.3679	0.9863	0.9863	-0.3425	-0.4461	1.0000	-0.2571	-0.0394
WU	0.8761	0.4940	0.0706	0.0304	0.8265	0.0372	0.8530	-0.0839	0.3857	-0.2726	-0.2726	0.2532	0.1394	-0.2571	1.0000	-0.0872
GILDEN	-0.1183	-0.0117	-0.1325	0.2952	-0.1088	0.3525	-0.1001	-0.0479	0.0411	-0.0376	-0.0376	-0.0345	-0.1142	-0.0394	-0.0872	1.0000

[a]Pearson correlation of columns (citations) of data matrix of person to person citations and references. Data contain self-citations. Underlined (——) correlation coefficients represent individuals connected in the cosmopolitan coauthorship network. Wavy underlines (~~~) indicate high correlations (≥ .5) between individuals who are not connected in the cosmopolitan coauthorship network.

TABLE 5.5 Correlation of Cosmopolitan Person-to-Person References[a]

	GALLO	TODARO	SPIEGELMAN	PARKS	REITZ	SCOLNICK	SMITH	SCHLOM	LIVINGSTON	ZHADNOV	BYKOVSKII	LIEBER	AARONSON	ILYIN	WU	GILDEN
GALLO	1.0000	0.3168	0.1453	-0.0772	0.9819	-0.1369	0.9842	-0.0688	0.2734	-0.3004	-0.2995	-0.0320	-0.0686	-0.2408	0.9685	-0.2322
TODARO	0.3168	1.0000	-0.1061	0.7760	0.2296	0.7546	0.3937	-0.1526	0.9765	-0.2343	-0.2167	0.8921	0.7787	-0.3563	0.1487	0.4941
SPIEGELMAN	0.1453	-0.1061	1.0000	0.0785	0.2357	0.0370	0.0605	0.9643	-0.0976	0.1207	0.0510	-0.2582	-0.0643	0.1237	0.0774	-0.2287
PARKS	-0.0772	0.7760	0.0785	1.0000	-0.1027	0.9918	-0.0533	0.1073	0.7673	0.0745	0.0782	0.6776	0.9109	-0.1337	-0.2054	0.7051
REITZ	0.9819	0.2296	0.2357	-0.1027	1.0000	-0.1616	0.9463	0.0123	0.1864	-0.2421	-0.2468	-0.1462	-0.1091	-0.1824	0.9441	-0.2334
SCOLNICK	-0.1369	0.7546	0.0370	0.9918	-0.1616	1.0000	-0.1116	0.0779	0.7446	0.1085	0.1172	0.6720	0.9157	-0.1036	-0.2609	0.7156
SMITH	0.9842	0.3937	0.0605	-0.0533	0.9463	-0.1116	1.0000	-0.1437	0.3553	-0.3382	-0.3325	0.0641	-0.0197	-0.2772	0.9379	-0.2151
SCHLOM	-0.0688	-0.1526	0.9643	0.1073	0.0123	0.0779	-0.1437	1.0000	-0.1362	0.1315	0.0609	-0.2239	-0.0385	0.1104	-0.1270	-0.1623
LIVINGSTON	0.2734	0.9765	-0.0976	0.7673	0.1864	0.7446	0.3553	-0.1362	1.0000	-0.2845	-0.2687	0.8892	0.7742	-0.4065	0.1055	0.4845
ZHADNOV	-0.3004	-0.2343	0.1207	0.0745	-0.2421	0.1085	-0.3382	0.1315	-0.2845	1.0000	0.9971	-0.2059	-0.1196	0.9710	-0.2810	0.0280
BYKOVSKII	-0.2995	-0.2167	0.0510	0.0782	-0.2468	0.1172	-0.3325	0.0609	-0.2687	0.9971	1.0000	-0.1855	-0.1062	0.9656	-0.2770	0.0505
LIEBER	-0.0320	0.8921	-0.2582	0.6776	-0.1462	0.6720	0.0641	-0.2239	0.8892	-0.2059	-0.1855	1.0000	0.6792	-0.3095	-0.1845	0.5052
AARONSON	-0.0686	0.7787	-0.0643	0.9109	-0.1091	0.9157	-0.0197	-0.0385	0.7742	-0.1196	-0.1062	0.6792	1.0000	-0.2966	-0.1969	0.6009
ILYIN	-0.2408	-0.3563	0.1237	-0.1337	-0.1824	-0.1036	-0.2772	0.1104	-0.4065	0.9710	0.9656	-0.3095	-0.2966	1.0000	-0.2035	-0.1442
WU	0.9685	0.1487	0.0774	-0.2054	0.9441	-0.2609	0.9379	-0.1270	0.1055	-0.2810	-0.2770	-0.1845	-0.1969	-0.2035	1.0000	-0.2901
GILDEN	-0.2322	0.4941	-0.2287	0.7051	-0.2334	0.7156	-0.2151	-0.1623	0.4845	0.0260	0.0505	0.5052	0.6009	-0.1442	-0.2901	1.0000

[a]Pearson correlation of rows (references) of data matrix of person to person citations and references. Data contain self-citations. Underlined (——) correlation coefficients represent individuals connected in the cosmopolitan coauthorship network. Wavy underlines (〰) indicate high correlations (⩾ .5) between individuals who are not connected in the cosmopolitan coauthorship network.

TABLE 5.6 Asymmetrical Correlation[a] of Cosmopolitan Person-to-Person References and Citations[b]

	GALLO	TODARO	SPIEGELMAN	PARKS	REITZ	SCOLNICK	SMITH	SCHLOM	LIVINGSTON	ZHADNOV	BYKOVSKII	LIEBER	AARONSON	ILYIN	WU	GILDEN
GALLO	0.93682	0.74567	0.21415	0.24460	0.96460	0.24067	0.89235	0.02102	0.61711	-0.36809	-0.36809	0.48307	0.39831	-0.35062	0.74299	-0.12636
TODARO	0.07278	0.66458	-0.12010	0.84299	0.10686	0.80448	0.00526	-0.14866	0.50502	-0.23527	-0.23527	0.57584	0.71620	-0.28262	0.01910	-0.14030
SPIEGELMAN	0.08746	-0.12483	0.95948	-0.22321	0.16918	-0.23224	-0.00662	0.98474	-0.19333	-0.32041	-0.32041	-0.20551	-0.02622	-0.30010	-0.01581	-0.08407
PARKS	-0.25599	0.23398	0.08134	0.70705	-0.23201	0.66741	-0.31491	0.11038	-0.00514	-0.04785	-0.04785	0.16928	0.65664	-0.11556	-0.19616	-0.14371
REITZ	0.91132	0.64635	0.30935	0.17218	0.95243	0.17181	0.86630	0.11248	0.50618	-0.34644	-0.34644	0.37345	0.35512	-0.32871	0.68137	-0.09942
SCOLNICK	-0.31185	0.17907	0.04210	0.67380	-0.29151	0.63328	-0.36612	0.07428	-0.05255	0.01049	0.01049	0.13190	0.61665	-0.06403	-0.24073	-0.15771
SMITH	0.91115	0.83102	0.12747	0.32043	0.93643	0.31261	0.87589	-0.06065	0.72668	-0.37311	-0.37311	0.60135	0.46469	-0.35587	0.68956	-0.13816
SCHLOM	-0.10800	-0.25382	0.88242	-0.25159	-0.03961	-0.26113	-0.18445	0.97067	-0.29331	-0.27579	-0.27579	-0.27528	-0.09500	-0.26309	-0.16494	-0.05668
LIVINGSTON	0.04104	0.63202	-0.11175	0.83213	0.07597	0.78513	-0.02227	-0.13219	0.48867	-0.31059	-0.31059	0.53281	0.77214	-0.35264	-0.00916	-0.17492
ZHADNOV	-0.28355	-0.46818	0.27712	-0.33560	-0.26709	-0.30045	-0.31602	0.20564	-0.48330	0.86752	0.86752	-0.43088	-0.33206	0.86541	-0.26326	-0.26406
BYKOVSKII	-0.28219	-0.45422	0.21355	-0.31451	-0.27057	-0.27961	-0.30970	0.13573	-0.47031	0.89512	0.89512	-0.41619	-0.32280	0.89068	-0.24620	-0.26490
LIEBER	-0.24108	0.51368	-0.30073	0.78451	-0.22371	0.76264	-0.28458	-0.25301	0.48909	-0.11932	-0.11932	0.57963	0.52329	-0.15575	-0.23660	-0.02838
AARONSON	-0.24745	0.28076	-0.09421	0.71061	-0.23108	0.63705	-0.28952	-0.05851	0.04256	-0.17126	-0.17126	0.22508	0.73015	-0.25094	-0.20541	-0.13535
ILYIN	-0.19550	-0.45774	0.28903	-0.45334	-0.17864	-0.41090	-0.22525	0.19969	-0.41948	0.84908	0.84908	-0.41088	-0.44333	0.86116	-0.20120	-0.22483
WU	0.98700	0.67303	0.16356	0.12940	0.98822	0.13456	0.95968	-0.03345	0.55925	-0.31300	-0.31300	0.40668	0.28661	-0.29119	0.86588	-0.08780
GILDEN	-0.35113	0.06582	-0.22183	0.72814	-0.34410	0.74516	-0.35349	-0.16318	-0.08359	0.17212	0.17212	-0.02116	0.41851	0.10756	-0.27773	0.46282

[a]Pearson correlation of respective rows (references) and columns (citations) of original data matrix.

[b]Data contain self-citations. Underlined (———) correlation coefficients represent individuals connected in the cosmopolitan coauthorship network. Wavy underlines (~~~) indicate high correlations (⩾ .5) between individuals who are not connected in the cosmopolitan coauthorship network.

system. The most that can be said is that Gilden, for instance, is like or not like the other 15 highly published coauthors within RT in his referencing and citing patterns. The quality or even visibility of one's work cannot be judged from such a closed system.

As we move to Tables 5.4 and 5.5 (away from the individuals who are marginal to the NCI research effort), there are high correlations in citation and referencing patterns between two individuals who are not directly connected in the coauthorship network. For example, the correlation between the citation patterns of Todaro and Reitz is .66, even though they did not coauthor an article in our set. Their referencing correlation, on the other hand, is only .23. More generally, all of the high correlations in citations and references which involve noncoauthorship relationships are only two steps removed from a direct one-step coauthorship relationship. What is implied by this is that high correlation similarity between two noncoauthoring individuals is due to a *mutual* coauthor of the two who contributes to their similarity in profiles. The degree of similarity between two individuals becomes an indicator of scientific "inbreeding" in this situation. One's citing and referencing patterns are accommodated by those with whom one authors articles. This extends to more than one step in the in-house network. Reitz, Wu, and Smith project similar referencing and citation patterns not only because they work on the same research topics but also because they work with Gallo. Lieber's high citation and referencing correlations with Parks and Scolnick are mediated by Todaro, Livingston, and also Aaronson.

What these data suggest is that such a series of overlapping spheres of influence gradually encompass a research group such as that found within the NCI, creating, in effect, typical citation and referencing profiles which lend unity to a research effort. Integrated centers of research within problem domains, perhaps laboratories, generate by their overlapping citation and referencing patterns a profile which delimits their efforts and helps define the boundaries of research questions. In particular, one would expect that numerous lesser researchers within the domain would exhibit a high correlation of their *referencing* patterns with this elite, but that their *citation* patterns would not be highly correlated at all. This accords with the refutation of the so-called Ortega hypothesis (Cole and Cole, 1972), but suggests that the social mechanism of the *large research laboratory* reinforces such citation patterns, rather than the elite characteristics of *individuals.* A social mechanism and not the elitist notion of innate ability or nurtured talent would seem to account for much of such concentration of citation behavior.

There remains one more intriguing perspective to consider regarding the person-to-person citation patterns within the cosmopolitan coauthorship network, namely, the asymmetrical correlation matrix (Table 5.6). The correlations entered in this matrix represent the relationship between the referencing vector of the individuals listed on the rows with the citation vector of the individuals in the columns. In sociometric terms, what is being compared is the relationship between choosing (referencing) and being chosen (citation behavior). The main diagonal of such an asymmetric correlation matrix may be thought of as an index of self-confirmation within the problem domain. It represents the degree that one's perception of the area (evaluated through referencing) coincides with others' perception of one's place within it (the way one is cited). The off-diagonal elements of the matrix can likewise be interpreted if the alter ego is placed outside of an individual and located in the hands of others, allowing the mirror of their citation structure to be compared with other referencing patterns.

It is possible, therefore, to subdivide the matrix in Table 5.6 into subsets of individuals whose chosen and choosing vectors have similar profiles (note those with correlations $\geqslant .5$). The groups that emerge are:

(1) Spiegelman-Schlom: Columbia University
(2) Gallo-Reitz-Wu-Smith: Laboratory of Tumor Cell Biology, NCI (Wu also at Litton Bionetics)
(3) Todaro-Lieber-Livingston: Viral Leukemia and Lymphoma Branch, NCI
(4) Parks-Aaronson-Scolnick: Viral Carcinogen Branch and Viral Leukemia and Lymphoma Branch, NCI
(5) Zhadnov-Ilyin-Bykovskii: Gamaleya Institute of Epidemiology and Microbiology, and D.I. Ivanovsky Institute of Virology, Moscow.

These groups seem to mirror the institutional and, particularly, the laboratory, structure of RT research. By capitalizing on a built-in autocorrelation of citations between individuals, we are able to decompose the network into those individuals whose referencing and citing behavior is congruent with the image of the domain held by others. The congruence found in Table 5.5 is such that one can even discern differences in the various branches of NCI. Autocorrelation analysis is an appropriate label to attach here because self (auto) correlation implies the functional unity created within laboratories through the vehicle of coauthorship and a commonality of referencing profiles (but see Tagliacozzo, 1977).

The analysis thus far yields a picture of the RT problem domain that amplifies the large laboratories (after the Temin and Baltimore discovery in 1970). The ability of these laboratories to produce research, and thus papers, was greatly aided by the tremendous resources of money and capable researchers. The laboratories were able to mobilize quickly since they had been in existence for some time as efficient ongoing research enterprises. As one editor aptly remarked after the Temin and Mitzutani and the Baltimore discoveries, "Spiegelman then set his machine to work and found the enzyme in a dozen or more other animal tumour viruses. Other followed suit and the enzyme was found in every RNA tumor virus examined" (Anonymous, 1971: 1616).[12] To "set Spiegelman's machine to work" accurately characterizes the phase of research that is portrayed by the in-house network. But it was not just Spiegelman; all of the big guns of the cancer war were trained upon RT and the newfound hope for unraveling the cancer mystery.

By concentrating first on the in-house coauthorship network within RT, we have observed the exploitation of research opportunities in large laboratories. In the postdiscovery period the advantages accruing to authors, in terms of coauthorship possibilities during such a period, become formidable. Those laboratories which are best equipped, staffed, and funded at the critical "take-off" moment—large governmental (e.g., NCI) and private (e.g., Flow Laboratories, Litton Bionetics) laboratories, plus established medical research centers (Institute of Cancer Research, Columbia)—are particularly amenable to expanding on the discoveries made elsewhere. This, of course, is not to suggest that such laboratories are always "exploitative" of smaller research facilities, but rather that they have the edge on smaller (in terms of manpower and dollars) facilities which cannot as readily channel their resources into an all-out mobilization. Nor is this to suggest that such large laboratories never make original discoveries of their own. Of course they do. But they also can more readily remain in the forefront of a problem area until its potentialities are sufficiently exhausted.

The crucial point is that by taking a macro view of the domain, by dealing only with the most published authors within RT, the analysis favors the large laboratory structures that are associated with, indeed are products of, the Big Science of cancer research. Based on such an analysis one might hastily conclude that the only or best kind of research to be supported by any mission-oriented cancer campaign should be located in large established laboratories. This may be true, our previous discussion (Chapter 3) notwithstanding, but the above macro-level analysis is insufficient to support such an argument. We still need a more "finely tuned" understanding of the social and cognitive factors which lend so much visibility to the large laboratories.

A TIME-DISAGGREGATED ANALYSIS OF THE COAUTHORSHIP STRUCTURE

The analysis of coauthorship on a microscopic level has already been introduced, namely the structure of Spiegelman's research group in 1972 and 1973 (Figure 5.5).[13] What shall be seen in this section is the dispersion and concentration of research in terms of work groups of coauthors; when groups are linked by coauthorship one can then ask how and why this linkage occurred. The continuity of this portion of the analysis with that of the cosmopolitan coauthorship analysis of the previous section should become evident. We confine our attention here to "annual" changes in patterns of coauthorship.

Of the 85 articles within the set for 1972, 79 (92%) have 2 or more authors with a total of 220 distinct authors involved in coauthorship relations. When the coauthor linkages are subjected to sociometric analysis,[14] it is discovered that 40 distinct disjoint subsets are formed. Of these 40 subsets, 5 are represented by more than 3 articles. These 5 subsets of coauthors account for 35 articles (41%) for the year. To establish continuity with the thrust of the previous section, only those coauthorship sets will be presented to augment understanding of the highly visible in-house structure. Thus, although presently only the coauthorship networks represented by 4 or more articles per year will be observed, this is not to suggest that the remaining groups are unimportant.[15] In the 1972 Spiegelman example (Figure 5.5), the network is formed by 10 articles and includes 24 authors dominated by Spiegelman at Columbia University and Moore at the Institute for Medical Research, Camden, New Jersey. The structure of coauthorships, however, definitely crystallizes around the leadership of Spiegelman.

Because most of the other one-laboratory networks are not as clearly defined as those of the Spiegelman group for 1972, the remaining four groups in 1972 will simply be described by noting the most prolific (co)authors. All are familiar names.

In addition to the Spiegelman-Moore network there is a Gallo network (not pictured) with 11 articles and 20 different coauthors. Gallo (11)[16] heads the list with his name included on every article. Again, as in the in-house coauthorship network, Gallo's group at the Laboratory of Tumor Cell Beiology (NCI) is in the central position surrounded by researchers who claim Litton Bionetics as their location. Thus, early on in the research on RT, the framework for contractual arrangements between these two laboratories was firmly established.

Two other coauthorship sets for 1972 also confirm relationships already established in the cosmopolitan network. The group composed of

Parks (5), Scolnick (4), Todaro (3), Aaronson (2), and Livingston (2) is identical to the one isolated earlier; in 1972 it wrote five articles. Another group mirroring the in-house network includes 13 Russian authors, led by Bykovskii and Zhadnov, who published five articles in 1972. This group, located at the Ivanovski Institute and the Gamaleya Institute in Moscow, was the first Russian contingent involved in RT research; it was also the one engaged in the NCI-orchestrated international study of virus particles in human cell lines which was cited earlier.

THE NETWORK PAIRING OF BALTIMORE AND TEMIN

The dyad that looms conspicuous by its absence from the in-house coauthorship network is the 1972 Baltimore-Temin group. The codiscoverers came together to author a review article on RT (Temin and Baltimore, 1972) and thus briefly unite their respective research teams in a coauthorship network (not pictured). The network is constructed by coauthorships on four articles, two articles by Baltimore's group, one article by Temin's group, and the Baltimore-Temin coauthored article. Baltimore and Temin are the only two who tie the groups together, the other five authors are mentioned only once in 1972. The striking thing about the discoverers in 1972 is their minor role in the early development of the RT literature. It is certainly surprising that Temin's total coauthor count for the 1972-1974 period is only four coauthors. Baltimore's coauthor count for the same period is considerably higher, 13. But when these are compared with Spiegelman's 40-plus coauthors, one suspects some radically different laboratory structures at work shaping the coauthorship networks.[17]

What one ideally would like to know is whether the collaboration of two individual researchers in different institutional settings increases their chances of developing creative ideas. But how could this be measured? We have already seen that internal self-citations within laboratories inflate the in-house citation structures to the point where one can virtually predict what laboratory a person works in by his citation profile. We must pursue our annual analysis further.

The Overall Network Structure 1972-1974

1972: DOMINATION BY LARGE LABORATORIES

In the five distinct subsets of authors for 1972 dwells a picture of the social structure of the problem domain as it existed in the early 1970s. The large laboratories quickly "get into the act" and publish numerous articles. Seemingly, they are much more qualified to divert both research personnel and funds to take advantage of new discoveries such as RT. If the war on cancer was to progress, then the large laboratories which were created to wage this war were the logical sites for the elucidation of RT.

There is no overarching coauthorship network, however, which would reflect interlaboratory cooperation in the "postpartum" period. The unity that existed was an intellectual unity: The problems had been specified by the discovery itself, although they were transparent to the researchers who had been working in neighboring areas for years. Each research group found it advantageous to withdraw, as it were, into its own laboratory, (re)formulate a program to extend the discovery, and work on its puzzles. Spiegelman, within weeks of the discovery, engaged his team in unraveling the techniques of the RT assay (Spiegelman et al., 1970).[18] It would appear that other researchers similarly intensified their research effort within their own laboratories during the early postdiscovery period. Something of the flavor of the early period of research is captured in *Nature's* commemoration of the first anniversary of the discovery:

> In the past year, reverse transcriptase—or RNA dependent DNA polymerase—has become the subject of a widening credibility gap, and those who have been dabbling with this enzyme have only themselves to blame for so rapid a change in atmosphere. During the first two or three months after the announcement of the discovery of reverse transcriptase, everyone was agog to hear the latest rumour of the latest one-shot experiment; and on such ephemeral foundations, castles of hot air, not to mention newsprint, arose alarmingly quickly. But as the number of groups mushroomed to play minor variations on too few original themes, scepticism about their sweeping conclusions has increased commensurately [Anonymous, 1971b: 161].

In the 1972 article set, the contagious excitement among the individual research groups described above is evident. Perhaps the hope that one's own research group would be responsible for discovering a cure for cancer, or at least a viral "common denominator," was motivating the researchers to act in such a frenzied fashion. Is it really surprising, then, that laboratories should exhibit such concentrated coauthorship patterns? Perhaps in a less active research front, graduate and postdoctoral students disperse before the research is published, thereby creating the impression of widespread interlaboratory cooperation. "Hot areas" may appear more laboratory-bound than they actually are simply because of little coauthorship *mobility*. Whatever the individual or social motivations were, the social structure changed noticeably in 1973.

1973: YEAR OF DIVERSITY

In 1973, out of 215 articles in the set, 173 (80%) have 2 or more authors. On these 173 coauthored articles there is a total of 460 authors represented who comprise 71 disjoint subsets. There are, however, only 5 subsets which published 4 or more articles within the year. Once again, the discussion will be confined to them.

In Figure 5.6 is displayed the coauthorship network for 1973 which encompasses the most authors (50) and articles (113); 43 authors function as mediator in this network and cluster in readily identifiable institutional groups in the graph. There is a clear grouping of Litton Bionetics (authors 1, 2, 5, 8) with the Viral Tumor and Carcinogenesis Branch (VTC) of NCI (6, 2, 12). The research of this Gallo cluster, as above noted, is essentially carried out in the same laboratory. A cluster which has not been previously encountered is composed of researchers (3, 4, 10, 11, 14) at the National Institute of Child Health and Human Development (NICHD). Also note on the left wing of the graph a contingent of Russian authors (18, 20, 22, 23, 24, 25, 26, 27, 30) that includes many of the same researchers at the Ivanovski Institute and the Gamaleya Institute in Moscow whom we discussed earlier. In fact, the article that unites this Russian group with the Americans is the Parks et al. (1973) article discussed under the in-house coauthorship network. It is once again Gilden's mediating role that ties the research of Flow Laboratories to that of the Russian group. But as we move to the lower right corner of the network, Gilden is also associated with researchers from the University of Southern California (41, 42, 43).[19] As we approach the center of this network of coauthors, the role of the Viral Leukemia and Lymphoma Branch and of the Viral Carcinogenesis Branch, headed by Todaro (15) and Huebner (33), respectively, comes into focus. Yet with the removal of Aaronson (17), for instance, the work of the NICHD researchers would form a subset by themselves. Individuals in large national laboratories, then, do seem to function as critical mediators of research to other large laboratories. The elimination of a few key individuals would surely cause the coauthorship network to fragment.

Of course, one must wonder about the structural significance of linkages based on single articles, as in the case of Gilden and the Russian researchers. If a linkage has appeared, no matter how weak (Granovetter, 1973), the potential for reestablishing the linkage of individuals or institutions in the future is greatly increased. We would hypothesize that it is precisely such linkages which expand the horizons of one's social resources beyond the strong bonds engendered by the laboratory situation. The in-house researchers, almost to a man, appear in this 1973 network as key

FIGURE 5.6 Reverse Transcriptase Coauthorship Network, 1973

1 Ting, R.C.Y., Litton Bionetics
2 Bhattacharyya, J., LTCB, NCI
3. Swan, D., NICHD
4. Packman, S., NICHD
5. Sarin, P.S., LTCB, NCI
6. Paran, M., LTCB, NCI
7. Wu, A.M., Litton Bionetics
8. Reitz, M.S., Litton Bionetics
9. Livingston, D.M., VLL, NCI
10. Aviv, H., LMG, NICHD
11. Leder, P., NICHD
12. Gallo, R., LTCB, NCI
13. Lieber, M.M., VLL, NCI
14. Ross, J., LMG, NICHD
15. Todaro, G., VLL, NCI
16. Benveniste, R.E., VLL, NCI
17. Aaronson, S.A., VC, NCI
18. Filatov, F.P. Ivanovsky Inst., USSR
19. Scolnick, E.M., VLL, NCI
20. Yershov, F.I., Gamaleya Inst. & Ivanovsky Inst., USSR
21. Parks, W.P., VC, NCI
22. Ilyin, K.V., Gamaleya Inst. & Ivanovsky Inst., USSR
23. Mazurenko, N.P., Gamaleya Inst. & Ivanovsky Inst., USSR
24. Bektenirov, T.A., Ivanovsky Inst.
25. Irlin, I.S., Ivanovsky Inst.
26. Uryvaev, L.V., Ivanovsky Inst.

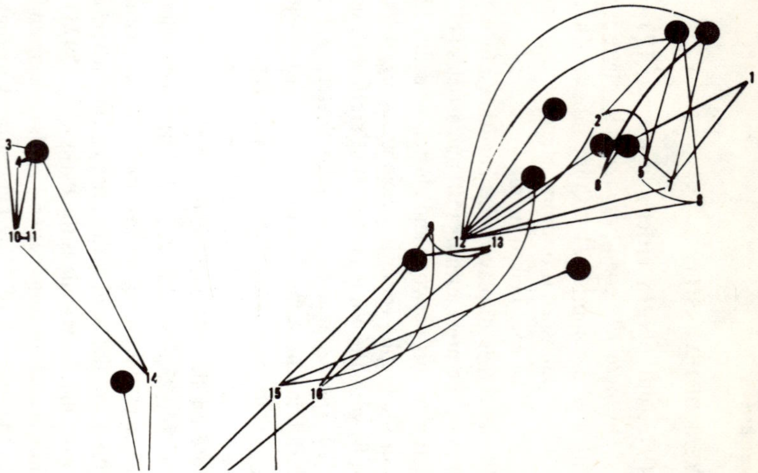

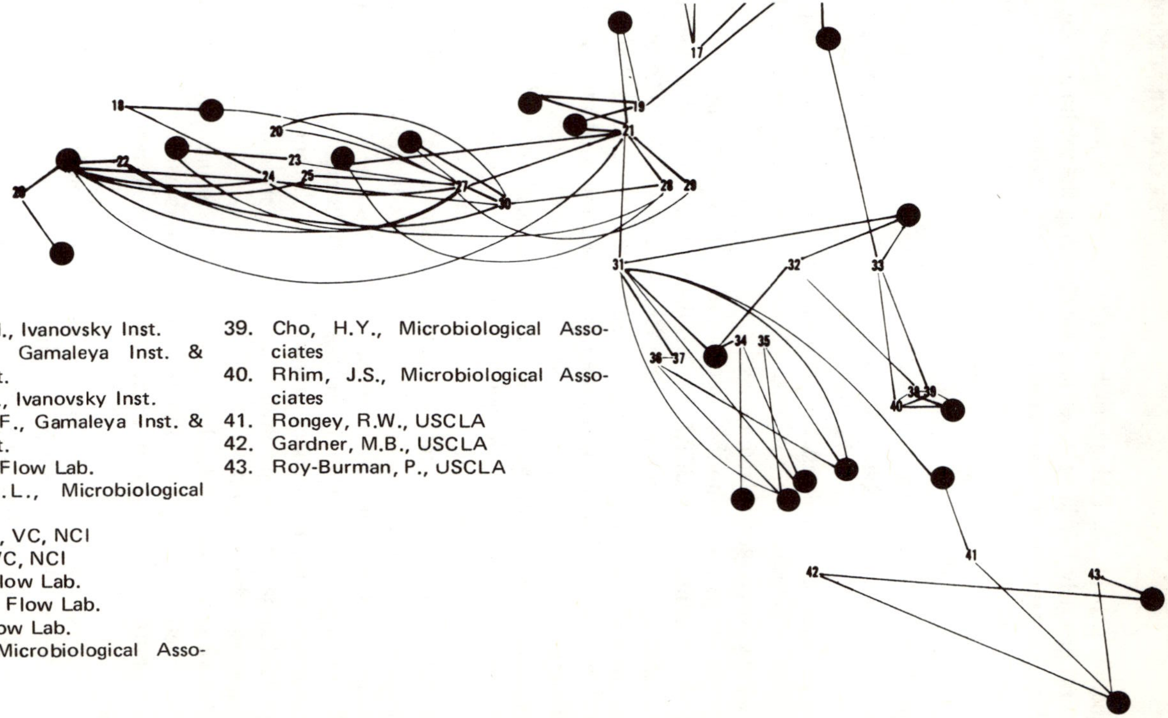

27. Zhdanov, V.M., Ivanovsky Inst.
28. Miller, G.G., Gamaleya Inst. & Ivanovsky Inst.
29. Solov'ev, V.D., Ivanovsky Inst.
30. Bykovskii, A.F., Gamaleya Inst. & Ivanovsky Inst.
31. Gilden, R.V., Flow Lab.
32. Vernon, M.L., Microbiological Associates
33. Huebner, R.J., VC, NCI
34. Sarma, P.S., VC, NCI
35. Long, C.W., Flow Lab.
36. Hatanaka, M., Flow Lab.
37. Okabe, H., Flow Lab.
38. Duh, F.G., Microbiological Associates
39. Cho, H.Y., Microbiological Associates
40. Rhim, J.S., Microbiological Associates
41. Rongey, R.W., USCLA
42. Gardner, M.B., USCLA
43. Roy-Burman, P., USCLA

mediating individuals. Perhaps such central individuals and laboratories perform precisely this integrative function, molding the relations within a problem domain into some semblance of social unity, particularly through the mediation by heads of laboratories. Men such as Huebner and Todaro appear both as critical links in coauthorship networks and also function as leading theorists.[20] If an "enforced" consensus on theories is being attained through contracts and coauthorship, then what appears as weak ties may actually be strong ties. If seemingly tenuous relations are "enforced" by contractual relations or by governmental exchange programs, then perhaps the "weakness" of a linkage in terms of coauthorship is merely a reflection of the "strength" of the authority structure within the sponsoring governmental laboratories.

In the largest coauthorship network for 1973, the only academic institution represented is UCLA. Yet it is the Spiegelman group defined by the academic research hospital setting (Figure 5.5) that in 1973 remains apart institutionally from the other coauthorship structures and attracts our attention. The sources of coauthors here are many: graduate students, postdoctoral students, visiting scholars, medical researchers, and so on. They form an abundant coauthorship pool and need not look to other laboratories. In some ways, though, this laboratory appears to be run like the government laboratories, that is, as head of the laboratory and the principal investigator on numerous grants, Spiegelman is often designated as a coauthor. Certainly the fact that Spiegelman is consistently associated with more coauthors than *any* other individual within the RT literature (in 1973 his name appeared on 12 articles with 30 different authors) minimally suggests that he oversees a very large research center. But it also suggests that he is vitally involved in an organizing effort that sustains an ongoing research program.

As indicated earlier, Spiegelman's group in 1973 seems fully mobilized for conducting RT research. But two other university-based groups had also mobilized by 1973, one at the Institute for Molecular Virology, St. Louis University School of Medicine, and the other at the University of California at San Francisco, Veterans Administration Hospital. The St. Louis group published five articles in the RT literature which included 14 different coauthors. Maurice Green's name appeared on each of these articles but only one other researcher, Grandgenett, appeared twice. Clearly, the laboratory structure crystallized around Green, with other researchers forming a more transient, perhaps typically academic, network of coauthors surrounding a postdoctoral mentor.[21]

The San Francisco group, on the other hand, has less concentration of individual focus. It published six articles on which 12 different authors were listed. Levinson (4) heads the list with the most coauthorships, followed by Bishop (3), Faras (3), Varmus (3), and Haase (2). The more diffuse nature of coauthorship within this group suggests that the collaboration was sustained more by common research *interests* than by the common *direction* of research found within Green's laboratory where all RT research focuses around one coauthor. Apparently, different organizational structures underlie the St. Louis and San Francisco efforts for 1973. What is unknown is whether these structures mirror authority/seniority patterns or are more the intellectual spoils of entrepreneurial victors.

The final research group that will be considered for 1973 is of special interest because of its international cast. It is created by the coauthorship of nine articles by 29 different U.S. and French authors. The list is headed by Haapala (6) and Fischinger (4) from the Viral Leukemia and Lymphoma Branch (VLL) of NCI, followed by Nomura (3) and Gerwin (3) from the same laboratory, Chermann (3) and Raynaud (3) from the Institut Pasteur (Garches, France), and Jasmin (3) from the Hospital Paul-Brousse (Villejiuf, France). Peebles (2) from the VLL and Sinoussi (2) from the Institut Pasteur complete the list of coauthors mentioned more than twice within this group. Exemplified by this collaboration is its focus on a very well-defined problem: the inhibition of tumor viruses with the heteropolyanion, silicotungstate. Such research is neither the stuff of Nobel prizes nor too mundane to quell interest. It functions on the level of difficult, fundamental, basic science requiring carefully executed research; it also seems to be eminently doable, but requiring technical skill and patience to execute. International cooperation is no doubt indicative of a level of problem specification within problem domains (see Crane, 1971), but precisely how the cognitive and the social interact on the international level beckons for more systematic study.

1974: YEAR OF EXPANSION

By 1974 the situation within RT coauthorship patterns once again reflected the changing and growing interest within the problem area. The international cooperative efforts, which were always tangential to and/or of broader interest than RT, disappear from the coauthorship networks. In all, there are 87 subsets of coauthors but only 8 of these coauthor networks have written 4 or more articles. The largest coauthorship network for 1974 (Figure 5.7) contains 123 researchers associated with 59 articles. From even a rapid scanning of this major coauthorship network, it can be seen that many of the individuals and groups already discussed as active in previous years are again present. Spiegelman's group, however, is tied into a larger network due to the Gallo-Spiegelman (1974) letter to

FIGURE 5.7 Reverse Transcriptase Coauthorship Network, 1974

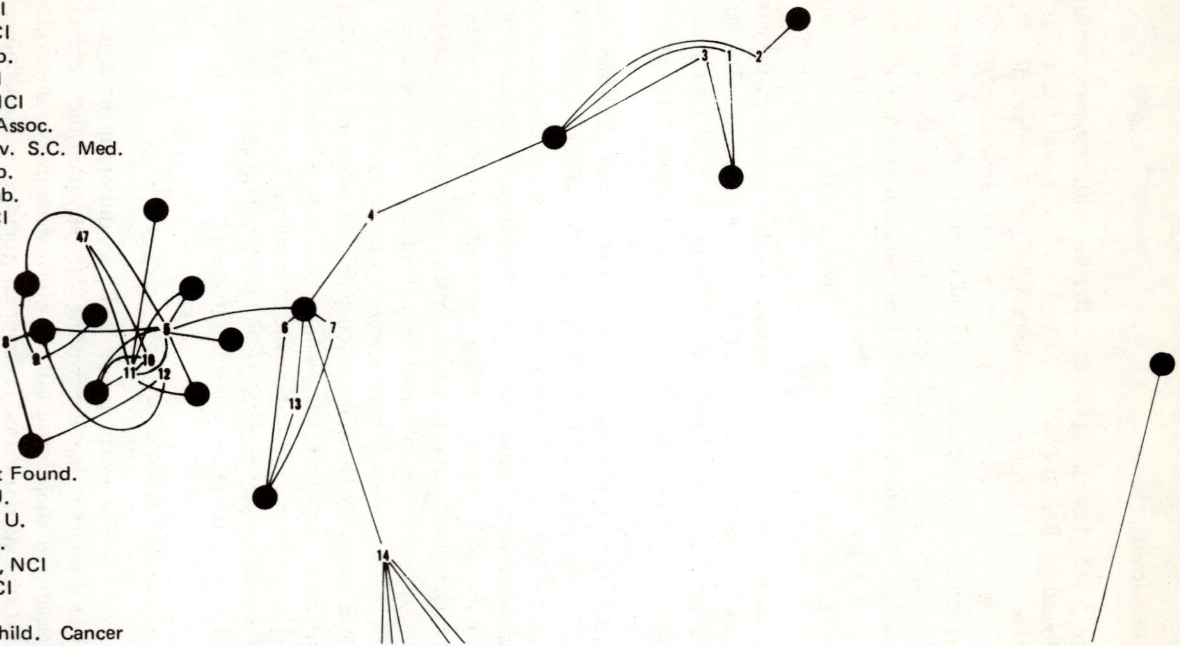

1. Mattern, C.F.T., LVD, NIAID
2. Fischinger, P.J., VLL, NCI
3. Gerwin, B.I., VLL, NCI
4. Peebles, P.T., VLL, NCI
5. Gilden, R.V., Flow Lab.
6. Fowler, A.K., VO, NCI
7. Strickland, J.E., VO, NCI
8. Rhim, J.S., Microbio. Assoc.
9. McAllister, R.M., Univ. S.C. Med.
10. Tsuchida, N., Flow Lab.
11. Hatanaka, M., Flow Lab.
12. Huebner, R.J., VC, NCI
13. Hellman, A., VO, NCI
14. Kalter, S.S., Southwest Found.
15. Burny, A., Columbia U.
16. Gulati, S.C., Columbia U.
17. Yaniv, A., Columbia U.
18. Benveniste, R.E., VLL, NCI
19. Lieber, M.M., VLL, NCI
20. Todaro, G., VLL, NCI
21. Livingston, D.M., Child. Cancer Res. Fdn. & VLL, NCI

22. Sherr, C.J., VLL, NCI
23. Spiegelman, S., Columbia U.
24. Gallagher, R., LTCB, NCI
25. Mondal, H., LTCB, NCI
26. Gallo, R.C., LTCB, NCI
27. Miller, N.R., LTCB, NCI & Litton Bionetics
28. Smith, R.G., LTCB, NCI
29. Hehlmann, R., Columbia U.
30. Schlom, J., Columbia U.
31. Gillespie, D.H., LTCB, NCI
32. Reitz, M.S., Litton Bionetics
33. Gambino, R., Columbia U.
34. Auld, D.S., Harvard Med. & P.B. Brigham Hosp.
35. Kacian, D., Columbia U.
36. Vallee, B.L., VLL, NCI
37. Paran, M., LTCB, NCI
38. Kawaguchi, H., Harvard Med. & P.B. Brigham Hosp.
39. Wu, A.M., Litton Bionetics
40. Abrell, J.W., Litton Bionetics
41. Sarin, P.S., LTCB, NCI
42. Ramirez, F., Columbia U.
43. Sarngadharan, M.G., LTCB, NCI & Litton Bionetics
44. Lewis, B.J., LTCB, NCI
45. Goldfeder, A. Cancer & Radiol. Lab. N.Y. City Dept. of Health
46. Bank, A., Columbia U.
47. Long, C., Flow Lab.

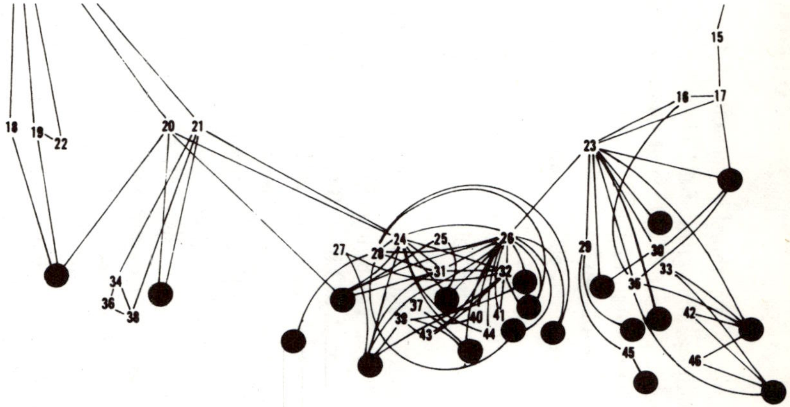

Nature discussed in the in-house coauthorship section. If that article/letter were deleted, then the Spiegelman group for 1974 would form, as in previous years, a research unit unto itself. Once again the dense group forming around Gallo and the research of the Laboratory of Tumor Cell Biology and Litton Bionetics is in full view.

Almost all of the individuals represented in Figure 5.7 are familiar from previous analysis. Those who bridge subgroups maintain their cosmopolitan responsibilities in 1974. Their linking function not only specifies the paths of research diffusion but also helps define migratory paths for researchers. In particular, an exchange pattern between government laboratories and their private affiliates seems to have definite repercussions on the recruitment of personnel. The expansion of the contractual arrangements with private laboratories such as Litton Bionetics can be seen in the shifting coauthorship patterns surrounding W. P. Parks. In 1972, he was predominantly publishing with individuals whose primary affiliation was NCI. In 1974, however, there is another group formed (8 articles, 16 authors) with Parks at the center. The group now includes Parks (4), Nuebauer (3), Rabin (3), Scolnick (3), Wallen (3), Ablashi (2), and Yang (2). Of this group, only Parks, Scolnick, and Yang are affiliated directly with the VLL of NCI. Yang is also connected with Litton Bionetics as are the remaining four authors, a fact indicative of the growing symbiotic relationship of Litton and the VLL of NCI during the 1972-1974 period.

These shifts no doubt reflect the policy shifts in cancer research discussed in Chapter 3, but they also signify a shift in the structure of this particular subgroup over time. In the case of 1972, Parks's name appeared on all five of the articles his group published in that year. The overlapping coauthorship network for 1974, however, contains eight articles but only four of these are attributable to Parks. This says, in effect, that although the group is larger, the centrality of Parks is maintained in the coauthor network for 1974 more by the interlocking laboratory structure than by authorship dominance. It is the organization of the research which is extended to incorporate other workers.

Two other U.S. groups of coauthors with 4 or more articles appear in 1974, namely, an MIT group and a University of California at San Francisco group. The MIT network is composed of 28 authors who are contributors on 12 articles. Nine authors from the MIT group have published two or more times, led by Verma (7) and Baltimore (6), and 5 others with 2 each. Such a distribution of coauthorships would seem to indicate a mentor-student relationship, the mentors Verma and Baltimore overseeing the research of numerous students.[22] One, the other, or both of these two central figures is on every article from this cluster. In contrast, the San Francisco group again seems to form a more diffuse coauthorship network. Although there are 16 authors in this group on 16 articles, there is a much higher percentage of authors with two or more authorships–50% for the San Francisco group versus 31% for the MIT group. The authors in the San Francisco group also seem to form a broader base for their coauthorship activities within their own group than is the case with the MIT network.

The remaining four coauthorship groups in 1974 all represent the work of non-U.S. laboratories. The Russian group anchored at the aforementioned institutes in Moscow has maintained a continuous interest in RT research. But the author signatories of this group by 1974 have swelled to 24 researchers listed on 10 articles. Zhadnov is the most central of individuals within this group appearing as author on all of the articles for this year. Bykovskii (6) and Ilyin (5) are the only other authors who have been continuously active in this research since 1972. Also of interest in the Russian research effort of 1974 is the appearance for the first time of another network of coauthors working at the Institute of Molecular Biology of the Russian Academy of Science and at the I. V. Kurchatov Institute of Atomic Energy, Moscow. This group in 1974 published 4 articles and included 14 authors. The largest share of this research concerns the successful synthesis of DNA complementary to pigeon globin messenger RNA using RT. Their claim, in other words, is to have synthesized a gene using messenger RNA from pigeons as the template for reverse transcription. Their extension of this research to the transcription of phage RNA shows that they are fundamentally involved in the genetic aspect of RT; this contrasts with the more cancer-oriented research of the other Russian coauthorship network.

By 1974 the Beatson Institute in Scotland, too, is contributing research on reverse transcription. Its 7 articles with 21 authors, centered around Paul with 6, suggest a large concentrated effort within the domain. Their research, as in the case of the new Russian group, centers on the uses of RT in understanding genetic defects; a *Nature* article on "The severe form of alpha thalassaemia caused by a haemoglobin gene deletion" is exemplary of the Beatson efforts.

RT in these newly appearing coauthorship networks has gradually found its way into areas which were not previously loci of concern. As the uses of RT proliferate, a broadening of research interests has resulted. Its new "reagent status" secure, RT can now be utilized in experimental contexts far removed from that of the viral research that stimulated it. Any further deductions from our broad structural analysis of coauthorship patterns, however, must await confirmation by more phenomenological, in situ, analysis (e.g., Woolgar and Latour, 1978).

A Career Profile of Reverse Transcriptase Researchers

The focus of this chapter hitherto has been the visible groups and clusters whose postdiscovery collaborative work on RT occupies a special place in the history of the domain. This history, however, has been a drama enlivened by several individual characters. The "characters" to which we refer are not only the most "public" of figures, the Nobel laureates Temin and Baltimore. Indeed, the cast includes the Spiegelmans, Greens, and a coterie of NCI and foreign researchers who have infused the history of RT with a personality and intensity all its own. We have not forgotten these scientists, just postponed analysis of them until now.

Our goal is to construct a set of biographical profiles which corresponds to the several categories of "structurally interesting" persons in the history of RT.[23] These profiles will "contextualize" the linkages among researchers, networks, and events by presenting backgrounds, tracing influences, and examining some idiosyncratic details that occupy the "backstage" of RT. Our analysis is also motivated by a sobering reality of science: Like other workers, scientists are constrained by their work environment. Yet too often, as Whitley (1977) correctly observes, scientists are treated like "free agents" subject to no local whim, indeed, engineering a career through an array of institutions which makes few demands but liberally dispenses the rewards of promotion, remuneration, local status, and so on. A more accurate portrayal–as the literature on creativity in work settings attests (e.g., Pelz and Andrews, 1976)–is that scientific work and its myriad expressions of productivity are fundamentally shaped–and comprised–by social, political, and logistical imperatives (see Hargens, 1975, for comparative data). The intellectual process, in other words, occurs in anything but a vacuum. It is collaborative, competitive, and part of a larger ongoing activity. The climate is established and maintained by the employing organization, and in accordance with *its* priorities and commitments.

If, in the course of work, scientists can subsume their goals under those of the organization, mutual goals may be achieved. Often, however, this is not the case. A coincidence of various means may never develop, and tensions may arise ranging from the sacrifice of personal goals to the obstruction or subversion of organizational goals. Such a range of "fit" between individual scientists and their organizational affiliations is apparent in the RT domain. For example, the glaring contrast in program focus, magnitude, and research style between NCI labs and academically based labs–even the more visible and well-funded of the latter–invites some assessment of the scientists involved in various team efforts, the constraints under which they labored, and the ways they adapted or became reconciled to the kind of scientific work they were compelled to do.

Of equal concern is the intellectual breadth of individuals and teams. For most, RT represented but one problem deserving two, perhaps three, years of investigation, among many problems to be explored along, say, the virology or epidemiology trail. Whence did the RT researchers come—in an intellectual sense? What was their graduate training? And where did they go after contributing to RT? Evidence on these queries begins to put RT in the wider perspective of cancer and biomedical research in general. It also suggests the demographic and ecological patterns which biomedical researchers create (see Duncan, 1959), both in response to their innermost intellectual cravings and to the unique attractions which certain labs, programs, and institutions hold. It is through analysis of scientists *in* organizations, therefore, that the RT case study assumes a more inferential meaning—about intellectual migrations, research productivity, career vagaries, and the institutionalization of scientific work.

THE CAST

The cast for biographical profiling are 58 RT researchers whose contributions to the domain were revealed above in several ways: prolific authorship or publication of highly (co)cited pre- or postdiscovery articles, membership in a visible NCI or academic lab team, and frequent acknowledgment as a reader, supplier of materials, and so on in RT articles. These criteria, of course, were used for selecting scientists as interview targets. Hence, our 15 interview subjects are among the 58; 26 others were sent letters soliciting a current curriculum vitae and 18 complied (a 69% response rate). In addition, dissertation abstracts were located for 31 North American Ph.D. holders in the *Comprehensive Dissertation Index*. The main source of biographical data, however, was *American Men and Women of Science* (12th and 13th editions). Indeed, 43 of 51 (or 84%) of the U.S.-based members of our purposive "structural" sample were listed in this directory, as testimony to their accomplishments and status relative to the scientific community at large (see Crane, 1965). To augment these data with information about overall research performance (not just publication in RT), we consulted the *Source Index* of the *Science Citation Index* and coded articles published into three periods: prediscovery, 1965-1969; postdiscovery domain development, 1970-1974; and domain transition (i.e., "current" applications of the enzyme), 1975-1976. Note that these periods refer to stages of RT activity, although the articles coded encompass *all* serial publications spanning the 12 years 1965-1976. In this way RT publication can be assessed vis-à-vis total research productivity.

As a further comparison, a second aggregate of scientists was defined as the complement of the structural sample: those who published in RT, published prior to the discovery, and were highly cited, or were often acknowledged in RT articles but had not gained the recognition of inclusion in *AMWS* and for whom no other biographic information could be found. For these 41 scientists, the identical publication data were coded from the *Source Index*. so that comparative analysis of research performance within and without RT between this heterogeneous "control group" and the purposive sample would be possible.

THE PROFILES: A PROVISIONAL CONSTRUCTION

No significant differences exist between the structural sample as a whole and its constituent subsamples in chronological or professional age. For all 58 scientists, their mean and median birth years are 1933 and 1936, respectively, while the mean year in which they received their highest degree is 1963 (median = 1966).[24] Thus, the principal researchers in RT were, on average, 34 to 37 years old (± 9 years) at the time of the discovery of the enzyme and had barely concluded a quarter of their projected 35-year postdoctoral career. For many, therefore, the advent of RT came during service in first professional positions, a "period effect" (Ryder, 1965) which we examine below in terms of subsequent research interests and productivity.

Although the period of transition from initial research interest to involvement in RT was brief for most of the cast, two kinds of migrations can be traced to reveal shifts in careers. One migration is intellectual (see Chubin, 1976, for a review), namely current field of (self-)identification compared to field of highest degree, as reported in *AMWS.* The striking finding on this professed migration or change of identification is that five years after the discovery of RT, 15 researchers (37.5%) regarded virology as their primary field identification; this includes 5 of the 12 M.D.'s. That 11 researchers would have gravitated to this field suggests a real intellectual attraction or "pull" effect.[25]

A second kind of migration, that between employment sectors (e.g., Crowley and Chubin, 1976), may also be indicative of shifts in career plans and goals. To examine this possibility, we constructed Table 5.7. Significantly, we observe virtually no intersectoral migration from the time of discovery to the peak period of domain growth. What is obscured on the diagonal is the amount of within-sector institutional migration. Other data (on median time employed by an institution) suggest that such movement is fairly common (an average of once every three years). Apparently, however, the work contexts distinguishing the three sectors—or the barriers

TABLE 5.7 Matrix of Employment of Reverse Transcriptase Researchers in Three Sectors, at Time of Discovery and During Peak Domain Growth

1969-71 SECTOR	1972-74 SECTOR: Academic/Medical School	Government	Private[a]	n
Academic/Medical	26	2	1	29
Government	–	6	-	6
Private	1	2	7	10
n	27	10	8	45

[a] Includes hospitals. Chi/square for academic vs. nonacademic = 29.88, 1 df, $p < .001$

which preclude entry and exit from them–are sufficient to retain research personnel. Several of our interviewees stated, in fact, that "academic researchers wouldn't work" in NCI labs[26] and, likewise, "NCI researchers can't afford to go back to academia, even to a well-endowed medical school." Clearly, the rewards differ in each setting, making a traversing of the boundaries separating academia from nonacademia a rare occurrence (only 4 cases in Table 5.7). What slippage does occur seems to stem from an M.D.'s desire to enter clinical practice or a scientist's wish to teach part-time instead of preparing contract proposals and researching full-time.

What the profiles presented thus far hint at are distinctive career trajectories for subsets of RT researchers. In general, these researchers are professionally young[27] and somewhat intellectually mobile. Many entered the RT domain through postdoctoral apprenticeship at large academic labs[28] or a shifting of research interest while at an NCI lab. The major referents for their work circa 1975, as measured by specialization and professional society membership, are tumor viorology and related microbiological and biochemical applications to cancer. Furthermore, their lack of mobility between employment sectors and the not-inconsiderable status attained in their positions by 1975[29] suggest that even the NCI *wunderkinder* have not forsaken the research role (see Zuckerman and Merton, 1972).[30] Indeed, most seem to be thriving in research, having made the adjustments necessary to capitalize upon local resources while satisfying administrative demands and, at a microscopic level, lending stability to the RT domain. To explore these impressions systematically, however, we must relate the emergent career paths to other research activities coterminous with the growth of the RT domain.

PRODUCTIVITY IN REVERSE TRANSCRIPTASE AND BEYOND

The measurement of research activity within the RT domain represents only a portion of the samples' overall productivity. The questions we now address center on changes over time in the proportion that is devoted to RT, and the correlation of productivity measures with various institutional and career-phase attributes. For this analysis, we compare four samples: the structural (n = 58), the control (n = 41), those scientists located only at NCI labs from 1970 to 1974 (n = 12), and the members of the visible in-house network (n = 16).[31]

As seen in Figure 5.8 the shape of the total article productivity distributions is almost identical for the four samples, though the level of effort in each period varies markedly with the most productive NCI sample outstripping the median output of the least productive control sample by ratios of 4:1, 2:1, and 4:1, respectively, in the three time periods.

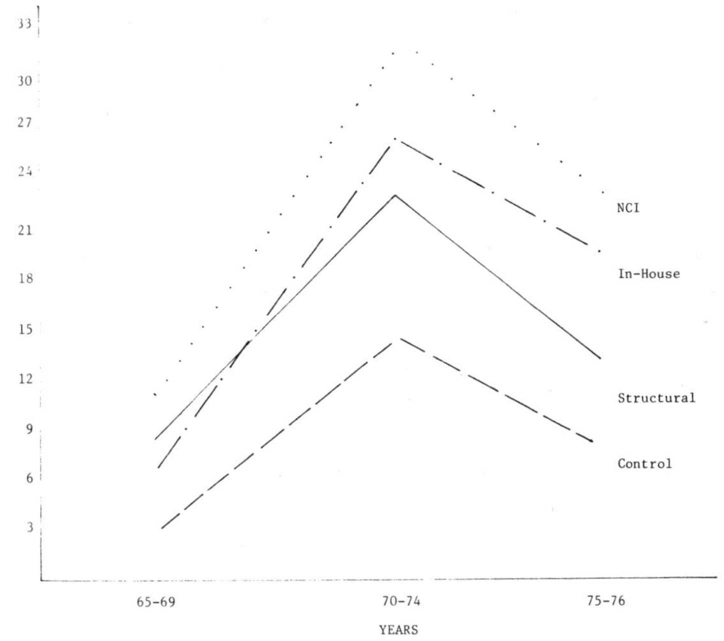

SOURCE: SCI, Source Index, Institute for Scientific Information (1965-77)

FIGURE 5.8 Total Article Productivity of RT Researchers in Three Periods

It is in Table 5.8, however, that the disparities in productivity both within the RT domain and relative to total article output are in full display. The first row of this table suggests that volume of productivity in the period preceding the discovery in 1970 is a poor predictor of RT productivity for all except the in-house sample. Conversely, the zero-order correlations for all except the control sample indicate that during the two postdiscovery periods, RT publication is significantly correlated with total publication output. Nevertheless, if median RT publications are divided by median articles for 1970-1974 (the interval basically covered by the RT effort and our article set), we see that the proportions for three of the samples hover around one-third. Only the in-house network devotes a majority of its effort to publication within the RT domain. This is not surprising, of course, since the productivity criterion for admission into this network was at least 10 articles, a threshold (recall from above) satisfied by only 23 scientists, a scant 2% of all the authors identified as publishing on RT. Admittedly, therefore, it is this criterion, in part, which

TABLE 5.8 Measures of Article Productivity Within the RT Domain Relative to Total Productivity, by Samples

	Structural (n=58)	Control (n=41)	NCI (n=12)	In-House (n=16)
Pearson r between RT articles and all articles in--				
1965-69	.153	.252	-.220	.478[a]
1970-74	.502[b]	.078	.496[a]	.600[a]
1975-76	.415[b]	.185	.703[b]	.524[a]
Median RT articles	6.9	4.4	12.5	16.5
Median RT articles ÷ all articles 1970-74	.288	.301	.385	.634

[a] $p < .05$

[b] $p < .005$

SOURCES: SCI Source Index and RT article file.

assures the high correlations for the in-house sample. The magnitude of those correlations reinforces the visibility accrued to these 16 by virtue of their *co*authoring together in the domain. Their median output of RT articles is more than that of the eminent structural sample, and even overshadows the voluminous contributions by NCI researchers.

What these data thus convey is the greater preoccupation with RT research by the in-house and NCI samples.[32] Both in an absolute and a relative sense, these researchers devoted a larger fraction of their effort to the problems raised by the discovery of the enzyme. The members of the structural sample concentrated the smallest proportion of their output (.288) in 1970-1974 on topics within the domain, a finding which prompts conjecture about the wider scope of their respective research programs and, in terms of their career patterns, the status they brought *with* them to the domain rather than that which they derived *from* it. For the members of the structural sample, as well as for the control aggregate, research on RT may well have represented more of a "passing interest" than a "going concern." We probe this next.

EXPLAINING PRODUCTIVITY: A DISCONTINUITY OF EFFORT

As a final attempt to determine the relationship of domain productivity to total research effort, we shall perform a series of linear (ordinary least-square) regression analyses. Inspection of the zero-order and partial correlations among demographic and ecological variables resulted in entering degree year into the equations (due to high collinearity, $r > .8$, with birth year), as well as two dummy variables—degree type (Ph.D. or M.D.) and academic/medical school only employment (1965-1976).[33]

In Table 5.9, the number of RT articles published by the structural and control samples is regressed separately on three career variables. Significantly, membership in the in-house network is a better predictor of within-domain productivity than 1965-1969 publications. In fact, the in-house variable—though in part a proxy for RT publication—accounts for 90% of the variance explained in each of the equations. The low magnitude of the zero-order and standardized regression coefficients for the structural sample is further evidence of discontinuity in research effort, namely, that the level of productivity by these 58 scientists prior to the discovery is a poor harbinger of productivity within the RT domain. But does the reverse obtain? Does RT productivity accurately predict the level of research output in 1975-1976? Or does a linear combination of other variables provide improved explanation?

To pursue these questions, the regression analyses summarized in Table 5.10 were performed. Proceeding from the most specific publication information—RT articles (see Table 5.10, Regression A) to the most recent 1970-1974 articles (Regression C)—we observe a three-fold increase in explained variance in the structural sample and a five-fold increase for the control. These data confirm the conventional wisdom that the best predictor of publication at t is publication at t - 1. But notice the significant β for membership in the in-house network for the structural sample under Regression B and the effect of location in an NCI lab for the control sample under B and C.[34] Work environment in the case of NCI researchers does contribute to their productivity level in 1975-1976. Academic/medical school employment—perhaps because it is less homogeneous in terms of size, resources, and work obligations—exhibits no explanatory power.

Once again, then, number of RT articles is far less predictive of subsequent overall productivity than earlier, that is, prediscovery, publication. This finding supports our earlier conjecture about the discontinuity in level of research effort. Contributions of the two samples to the unfolding microcosm of RT seem to be one aspect of ongoing programs that focus on, if our earlier characterization of *AMWS* specializations is correct, tumor virology and the cellular mechanisms underlying cancer.

CAREER PROFILES: RAMIFICATIONS AND LIMITATIONS

RT, as a research problem and domain of activity, derives coherence from the large laboratories which commit their resources and energies to it. This commitment is by no means exclusive; other research not depen-

TABLE 5.9 Regression of RT Productivity on Three Career Variables for the Structural and Control Samples

	STRUCTURAL		CONTROL	
	r	ß	r	ß
Total 1965-69 articles	.15[illegible]	.188	.252	.204[a]
Membership in in-house network	.675	.702[b]	.781	.723[b]
Location at NCI lab 1970-74	.355	.031	.462	.079
R^2	.436		.624	

[a]F-value $p < .05$

[b]F-value $p < .001$

dent on the enzyme appears to be maintained simultaneously (see Hagstrom, 1970). Hence, the connection of the domain to other research sites, even as seen through the productivity of the central RT scientists, labs, and networks, is of negligible assistance in identifying those other *particular* sites. One thing can be stated with certainty: Affiliation with an NCI lab promotes overall productivity. Regardless of whether this large laboratory effect inflates visibility in the biomedical literature,[35] as demonstrated earlier in this chapter, it undoubtedly furnishes the wherewithal and institutional support of readily available collaborators to seize upon and extend the discoveries made in smaller, modestly endowed and modestly staffed labs. This seems to be the legacy of Big Biology and perhaps the clearest benefit of mission-oriented research. As one of our interviewees declared, echoing an oft-heard sentiment, "The discovery of reverse transcriptase could not have been made in a large NCI lab because you just don't have time to think imaginatively."

If discovery is in the realm of basic unfettered science, then, in contrast, intramural NCI researchers are best equipped and poised to strike deeper at the targets hit by extramural researchers. We hasten to add, however, that most NCI scientists with whom we spoke confessed that their initial reaction to hearing of the discovery of RT was not surprise or shock but, "So what? Big deal!" Most claimed to be vaguely aware of the provirus hypothesis at the time but were utterly unconcerned with the repercussions that its confirmation would have for *their* own work.

One conclusion to be drawn from our career analysis is that specialization itself engenders the attraction of researchers to new problems.[36] Neither degree type nor professional youth predict where biologists will migrate in search of new problems or new angles on old problems. The

TABLE 5.10 Regression of 1975-1976 Article Productivity on Publication and Career Variables for the Structural and Control Samples

REGRESSION	STRUCTURAL		CONTROL	
A.	r	β	r	β
RT articles	.415	.433[a]	.185	.146
In-House Network	.225	-.091	.142	-.236[a]
NCI Location	.222	.194	.423	.486
Academic Employment	.020	.191	c	c
R^2	.198		.134	
B.				
1965-69 Articles	.694	.872[b]	.569	.620[b]
In-House Network	.225	.261[a]	.142	-.220
NCI Location	.222	-.078	.423	.580[b]
Academic Employment	-.020	.022	c	c
R^2	.542		.532	
C.				
1970-74 Articles	.804	.892[b]	.808	.764[b]
In-House Network	.255	-.051	.142	.013
NCI Location	.222	.047	.423	.304[a]
Academic Employment	.020	.111	c	c
R^2	.651		.726	

[a] F value $p < .05$

[a] F value $p < .001$

[c] No information for this sample.

traces of a problem domain that we detect in a concentration of literature must be extracted from the larger intellectual context in which it is enmeshed.[37] Ironically, what we extract is so intimately connected to so much that, upon separate analysis, the domain now isolated harbors few clues as to where to look *next.* For just as researchers become acclimated to a particular work environment, they are fickle in applying their energies to an assortment of problems; they preserve the setting for their research, while reordering their intellectual priorities.[38] Thus, when we examine a problem domain, we see a patchwork of fragmented individual, institutional, and perhaps even sectoral (e.g., government) research programs while the "missing" fragments of these programs attach to other literatures.

A domain captures a cross-section of the biomedical community—in terms of career trajectory, disciplinary background, and scientific role incumbency—that has converged sufficiently long on a problem to attract new resources, attention in the literature, funding from agencies, and personnel capable of shifting gears or sustaining multiple interests. This represents a fluidity of careers for some, a status change for others, a sudden wave of productivity, visibility, and prestige for many. A collective biography of the RT cast demonstrates the importance of careers, and their organizational exigencies, for the evolution of biomedical problem domains.

Conclusions

By analyzing the coauthorship structure of RT, we have placed in perspective the macro-social structure of this domain. Not only did the number of authors increase but also the number of important groups, U.S. and foreign, expanded. This expansion was stabilized by the continuity of large research groups. The unity of such large laboratories was apparently maintained by the central position of "cosmopolitan" researchers. These individuals are often major theoreticians and/or administrators of laboratories which have a contractual relationship with NCI.

It would also appear that the elite cosmopolitan coauthors not only unify the research programs of their laboratories but also exert an influence over the citation profiles of their respective group members. Although coauthorship consolidates individual-to-individual citation patterns, this very fact also allows one to demonstrate how laboratories present a uniform image to the larger biomedical research community. Individuals within laboratories "look alike" because of a repetition of citation patterns. It is difficult to differentiate an individual from a laboratory because intralaboratory coauthorship creates autocorrelation in the citation matrix. The individual becomes *part* of the *whole* through coauthorship.

It is true, as noted, that major theoretical forces within the problem domain, for example, Huebner, Todaro, and Gallo, are often central in the networks which represent the large federal laboratories. On the other hand, the discoverers of RT, Temin and Baltimore, seem conspicuously absent from the major coauthorship networks. Their research seems to be organized around different principles which are perhaps characteristic of their academic environment. The academic pool of potential coauthors seems to be modest compared to the manpower resources of the large NCI laboratories. Although the discovery of RT occurred in a social setting distinct from the highly visible research on the elucidation of the enzyme, we cannot determine from an analysis of coauthorship the "quality" of research in the academic versus the NCI sector of the domain. We can conclude that the dynamic differs in the two settings. It is also quite certain that the government research laboratories possess resources which shape the macro-social image of the research domain. Few would deny that funds can stimulate organizational development. The coauthorship algorithm is particularly amenable to analyzing the development of this macro-structure and, therefore, has focused our attention on this expression of Big Biology in the cancer war period.

Although the crescendo of organizational growth and proliferation within the biomedical community is deafening, it is impossible to conclude from analysis of collaboration patterns alone whether such organizational growth represents, in *pianissimo,* the moving force of progress in Big Biology. The issue is difficult to resolve because an independent criterion of the scientific merit and importance of research is needed to discover the significance of less visible organizational clusters. It is easier to argue that the elite, for example, Nobel laureates or the highly cited/cocited, only communicate with other elites (see Cole and Cole, 1972). It is less easy to argue, on either intuitive or empirical grounds, that the elite *need not communicate* with any but other members of the elite.

In addition, therefore, we undertook a collective biography of the RT elite. Our demographic profile reveals this set of biologists—those we interviewed and those we merely glimpsed at a distance—to be remarkably accomplished, insightful, and engaged in modally productive careers. Their coming together for a short time in a problem domain is just one in a succession of such confluences they will experience and help to foment. Yet we must be resigned to understanding mere segments of their intersecting professional lives spent in particular domains or abandon the confluence approach altogether and embrace a neater "cohort" design wherein the individual *sui generis,* and not the specialty or problem domain, commands the focus of analysis.

For by adopting a confluence approach, we have relegated the individual to a subordinate role as an agent of change and symbol of success in the historiography of the RT domain. By comparing two and sometimes three and four small aggregates of researchers whose career paths crossed within the RT domain, we have sampled a population which impinged upon, and became identified with, the specialization of RT. We know now, too, that it is indispensible to that historiography to track ideas through persons and organizations; idealized scientific objects alone—theories, methods, and apparatus—will not do. Such objects are manipulated and debated, socially transformed into structures that social analysts can then dissect and relate in time and space to a wider spectrum of esoteric artifacts and their specially trained producers.

Ours, finally, is a realistic approach to science in which the force of knowledge–within a domain and beyond–begets a demography and ecology of science which affect both the state of knowledge in biomedicine and the more idiosyncratic processes of scientific careers.[39] Thus, our methodological injunction persists: Large-sample unobtrusive sociological analysis of career patterns and small-sample intellectual and social history cannot stand alone in explaining migrations to and from problem domains. Motivations, intentions, and responses to organizational imperatives cannot be inferred from the operation of period effects on aggregates of scientific workers.

The subjectivity of career decisions must be probed with the subjects themselves,[40] ideally (but realistically) in the context of (1) their natural work environment and (2) the research program which dictates their manipulations of cognitive objects (see Whitley, 1977). This recourse to the living is why the problem domain is especially accessible; nonetheless, a domain is easy to reify and difficult to interpret apart from the *problem* which generated it. That is, RT is not the sole province of virology or molecular biology, because the problem is really "cancer" or "cellular transformation"–problems which require multiple-disciplinary perspectives and occupy correspondingly heterogeneous cadres of researchers. To divorce the problem from its attendant work force is to separate cognitive from social structure. And to separate these structures is to explain neither: A workerless science equals scienceless careers–an absurdity no social analyst can abide.

NOTES

1. Of this article set, 80% was retrieved from *Index Medicus*, while 22% of these articles were also found in *Biological Abstracts* and/or the *SCI Source Index*.

2. For a spirited exchange of views between advocates and detractors of this tool, see Griffith et al. (1977) and Edge (1977). The collected essays of Garfield (1977), as well as Narin (1976) and Moravcsik (1973), are also informative.

3. Some pertinent statistics to bear in mind while perusing Figures 5.2 and 5.3 include the following: The 656 articles were published in 162 journals. Yet 3 journals–*PNAS*, *Journal of Virology*, and *Virology*–account for one-fourth of the set. Of the journals, 12 capture 50% of the article set. As for citations, fewer than one-third of the 162 journals are represented by the articles in the set. Yet these 50 journals capture 90% of the articles *in* the set. In all, 306 RT articles (47%) are never

cited (through 1975) by other articles in the set, though some of this is due to "indexing lag." Mean citations per article, for example, decline from a high of 10.8 for 1971 articles to .67 in 1974. Finally, in the nearly 20,000 citations generated by the RT article set, over 1000 journals are represented with *PNAS* accounting for approximately 20% of the citations to articles both *in* and *out* of the set. *Nature (New Biology)* received 20% of the in-set citations, but only 5% out. *Journal of Virology* and *Science* are likewise cited twice as much within the set, 11% and 9%, respectively, than they are without. Both *Nature* and *Virology* are cited outside the set a greater proportion than within (by margins of 11% to 7% and 9% to 6%, respectively). The cancer journals, notably, *JNCI, International Journal of Cancer,* and *Cancer Research,* are less popular outlets in RT, accounting for only 5% to 7% of the citations. For a bibliometric analysis of the cancer literature, see Garfield (1974).

4. This aggregate of 23 prolific publishers constitutes 2.1% of the 1088 different authors of the 656 RT articles; of these 1088, fewer than half, however, published more than 1 RT article.

5. Of the article set, 12% (77/656) is accounted for by the coauthorships just among these 16 researchers.

6. This was indeed the result of a special NCI-supported collaboration (Gilden, 1978).

7. Gilden, former director of Flow Laboratories, has numerous grants over a million dollars; in 1973, for instance, he was the principal investigator of a grant for "The study of oncogenic potential of viruses" (9 N01 CP 33247-00), which carried a budget of $3.1 million (Department of Health, Education and Welfare, 1973). While a vice president of Flow Laboratories in 1976, he also chaired a Virus Cancer Program Scientific Review Committee whose stated purpose is to provide "advice to the Director, NCI, and the Director, Division of Cancer Cause and Prevention, or the Associate Director for Viral Oncology, on the scientific merit of proposals for contracts submitted to the Virus Cancer Program" (Department of Health, Education and Welfare, 1976: 132).

8. Furth says that, " 'One man' departments are those in which many investigators comprise a team working on one problem. For example, V. DuVigneaud's entire Department of Biochemistry at Cornell was devoted almost exclusively to the study of hormones of the posterior lobe of the pituitary" (1976: 873).

9. The answer is yes. This was confirmed by Schlom, Spiegelman's long-time collaborator, and by Spiegelman himself:

> It's very simple. I'm in view all the time. I am constantly available to any of my people who get into trouble or need something. . . . My feeling with postdocs is that they come generally to learn something from me. Hopefully, they will have something to contribute other than skillful hands, but the fact is that they are going to have the rest of their lives to think for themselves. If, during this period, I dominate their thinking because of the fact that I've been thinking about this damn thing for a long time, much longer than they, and I've made all the mistakes that they are going to make, and have already corrected them, and I don't want them to repeat it—it's very difficult under those circumstances for a guy to really show his ingenuity. Does he have it or not? I can usually tell, but he doesn't get much of an opportunity to really express it.

10. In Tables 5.4 to 5.6 the in-house coauthorship network is represented by the straight underlined correlation coefficients; other high ($\geqslant .5$) correlations are identified by wavy lines.

11. Recall that in 1976 Gilden moved to Fort Detrick's Frederick Cancer Center, a quasi-governmental facility that is ostensibly managed by Litton Bionetics.

12. This is consistent with Spiegelman's (1978) and Schlom's (1978) own descriptions of the former's operation.

13. To economize on the number of lines needed to express the coauthorship network in Figure 5.5, only those authors who published more than one article are listed by name; the remaining authors with whom they are linked are indicated by black dots. The authors linked on either side of a black dot are also, therefore, directly linked together on the same articles. The function of mediators between coauthorship groups is stressed by this mode of graphing linkages.

14. Alba's computer program SOCK (see Alba and Gutmann, 1972) was utilized to discover the disjoint subsets of coauthors within the data and to scale the sets in two dimensions. Figures 5.5, 5.6, and 5.7 were scaled using Alba's algorithm (see Appendix C for further details).

15. If time and resources permitted, it would be advisable to analyze the remaining authorship groups. Such an analysis would address the question of how, for example, lesser published authors contribute to the evolution of the problem domain.

16. The number of articles attributable to the individual authors is noted in parentheses after the author's name.

17. We are again reminded that the social structure of a research area can drastically influence interpretations of findings on relationships such as coauthorship. A caveat must always accompany coauthorship analysis: The analyst is not simply studying the social structure of a freely formed research area. Thus the large laboratory spurred by the sizable investment in cancer research has created very dense coauthorship surrounding government and private cancer research laboratories in the Northeast. If our methods isolate such concentrations, and we interpret them as "hot-spots" where more money should be invested, then we cannot help but fulfill our own sociological prophecy. The fact that the discoverers of RT were from relatively small laboratories should itself cast doubt on any facile policy pronouncements based on the social relationships discovered via coauthorship.

18. This "introversion" accounts for the separation until 1974 of this group, as depicted in Figure 5.5, from the major coauthorship network.

19. Gilden's doctoral work was done at UCLA (Ph.D. in zoology, 1962) so this association could be due to his West Coast connection.

20. Several of our NCI interview subjects, however, denied the "programmatic" status of the oncogene hypothesis.

21. One such postdoctorate and now research associate in Green's lab spoke with ambivalence about the diversity of projects which Green encourages. Unlike Spiegelman's centralized approach, Green tends to be laissez-faire, except during periods such as that following the discovery of RT: "when you have post-doctoral and graduate students, it's an awful lot of fun. When you're all working at night . . . round the clock. I didn't come home for three months" (Green, 1978).

22. Actually, Verma, now at the Salk Institute in San Diego, was completing a postdoctorate under Baltimore that began in 1971.

23. What we propose to do is a collective biography (for a review, see Pyenson, 1977) that delineates career patterns of the RT cast, particularly its stratification and mobility as an *intellectual* force rather than as a labor force (for the latter, see Harmon, 1965; Hargens, 1969).

24. If we consider Ph.D.'s only (n = 37 or 64%), or those with M.D.'s (n = 16), or both the Ph.D. and M.D. (n = 5), no deviations obtain. Furthermore, of the 55 scientists for whom Ph.D./M.D. institution information was secured, 15 were trained in 12 schools located in 10 different foreign countries. Ten of these foreign-trained scientists took postdoctoral positions in visible U.S. labs, for example, Spiegelman's, and most of these found permanent jobs in academic departments and private institutes, for example, Sloan-Kettering and the Salk Institute. Among the 40 American-trained scientists, 30 different institutions granted the M.D. or Ph.D. with only the University of Illinois (4) and Washington University (St. Louis; 3) awarding three or more such degrees. The doctoral fields most represented–irrespective of national origin–are biochemistry and microbiology.

25. This is supported, indeed amplified, by the specializations and research interests listed at the end of the *AMWS* biographies. Although the number and terminology of these responses are open-ended, a coding of keywords reveals that three-fourths of the biographies contain "viruses"; one-fourth mention "RNA viruses" in particular. Other variants include "viral oncogenesis," "oncornaviruses," "tumor viruses," and "replication of viruses."

Still another dimension of professional identification is society/association membership. With multiple responses possible, one-half of the researchers listed affiliation with the American Society for Microbiology, a third with the American Association for Cancer Research, and less than a fifth with the American Society for Biological Chemistry or the American Chemical Society.

26. The most celebrated exception to this dictum would be Schlom's experience. A Rutgers Ph.D., Schlom did predoctoral research at NCI, was invited by then-NCI director Rauscher (himself a Rutgers Ph.D. in virology) and John Moloney to join Spiegelman when he moved from Illinois to Columbia (in search of a medical school and clinical climate). Spiegelman invited Schlom and a productive four-year collaboration ensued, whereupon Rauscher "called" Schlom back to NCI to chair the Breast Cancer Virus Segment of the Tumor Virus Detection Section in the Laboratory of Viral Carcinogenesis. Like Aaronson, Gallo, Scolnick, Todaro, and Parks (who has since left NCI to practice pediatrics), Schlom "grew up" in NCI. All are young men in their late 30s who now hold key administrative positions while remaining "at the bench."

27. The only "elder statesmen" of the domain are Spiegelman and Huebner, both in their 60s, and Green, who is only 53.

28. This is consistent with Crane's (1972) findings on the attraction of young scientists to visible senior researchers in mathematics and sociology specialties, but underscores the import of studying the *postdoctoral* mentor-student relationship (see Zuckerman, 1977, and Mullins, 1973, for evidence on the predoctoral version of this relationship).

29. Among the mail respondents, 14 report (median) advisory service on two editorial boards of major journals such as *Journal of Virology, Cancer Research, Cell,* and *Journal of Molecular Biology*. In all, the honorific-functional role of gatekeeper was being executed for 21 different journals.

30. As one of the *wunderkinder* with whom we spoke put it:

> In an institute of NIH like NCI, to get really top-flight scientists to become administrators at these high levels, you really have to be fairly dedicated . . . because in most universities you can make a lot more money as you move up towards the deans and, you know, presidents; and in institutes like Sloan-Kettering or McArdle or some of these other places, as you move up, that

doesn't mean you move out of your lab relationships. In a government situation, beyond the level that I'm at now, which is lab chief, if you move higher than that, you're involved in sort of distributing money to the world. You really can't, I don't think, compete at that point. You have to be above the battle, so it isn't that easy to fill these higher positions.

31. Note that whereas the first two samples are mutually exclusive, the latter two are subsets which cut across the combined membership (n = 99) of the former. Specifically, one half of the in-house network membership were NCI employees from 1970 to 1974.

32. Interestingly, if only first-authored articles are considered (a measure Zuckerman, 1968, has shown to indicate *junior* status, i.e., its frequency wanes with increased professional age), three-fourths of the NCI sample's median output in the 1965-1969 period qualifies, a proportion almost twice that of the structural sample. In the postdiscovery period, these proportions decline to a similar level of one-third, but the median *number* of the first-authored articles by NCI researchers is 11.8 as compared with 10.5 for the in-house sample and 8.5 for the structural sample. In short, youth and the visibility achieved via first authorship in collaborative publication need not go hand in hand.

33. In the equations predicting RT productivity, none of these variables had more than a miniscule effect (though "academic only" employment does appear in the regressions reported below). In addition, type of degree is inconsequential for predicting productivity. Apparently, a research M.D. and a Ph.D. are comparable, though the orientation and focus of their respective researches (even within a problem domain) may differ. Our suggestion that a medical-clinical model may be guiding the work of M.D.'s more than basic Ph.D. scientists was pooh-poohed unanimously by our interviewees. Distinguishing orientations is not that clean or simple.

34. A similar effect was revealed in the equation using 1970-1974 articles as the primary independent variable for predicting 1975-1976 productivity of the in-house sample (R^2 = .763).

35. Due to the suspected confounding of individuals by laboratory citation profiles, we did not use citations as a variable in the previous regression analyses.

36. A quote from one of our subjects ably summarizes the attraction phenomenon: "You know, at some point in your life, you become fairly wedded to a given area. You've done well, you know it. But the young guy . . . coming out of school . . . if there is money, he'd be a fool not to look at it."

37. As one of our interviewees put it: "All you have to do is read the *Proceedings of the National Academy of Sciences* and find several good areas which are being minimally explored, which you can do experiments on, and which will be contributory." And yet another claimed: "You ask anybody in what section of *PNAS* their paper was published, and they probably will not be able to tell you–whether it was microbiology or biochemistry or genetics. I mean, they don't know."

38. Consider some of our interviewees' comments:

> I guess I consciously decided after the discovery of RT that I wanted to take that as an opportunity to get deeply involved in studying RNA tumor viruses and the whole problem of cancer. And being a lab scientist, I thought it most appropriate to let the experiments take me.
>
> I've heard of people who were disappointed because they didn't get the Nobel prize. When they . . . started working on RT problems after the discovery,

> they then thought that they should somehow be prized. I just thought that was silly.
>
> Any small investigator would be crazy to start working on RT [after the discovery] . . . knowing that he was going to have to compete with these huge laboratories [e.g., Spiegelman's, Gallo's, Todaro's].
>
> The guys who got the Nobel prize for this thing are the ones who have issued by executive fear . . . that RNA tumor viruses have nothing to do with human cancer. Right? This has been taken very seriously by the guys who dole out the money. And so young people who just don't have the security required to stick with their convictions are just not applying for money [to do] research on a human disease. . . . It makes life difficult in the sense that I don't get any intellectual and experimental support in the community. . . . That means everything has to be done in one place . . . and is slowed down enormously. So instead of getting help and cross-fertilization in terms of ideas and data coming out of the laboratories, that's just dried up.

39. For example, one of our subjects, a veteran academic researcher, said on NCI employment:

> If you are at NIH . . . you have some security in that you have a laboratory and a stable source of money. However, you have a problem: You can't expand your laboratory and bring more people in, so you have to go and get some other building someplace run by somebody else under a contract, [and] . . . you're going to have to do all the administration. In addition, at NCI you get paid less . . . and furthermore you're given tasks. The tasks are that if you have these contracts, you have to go out, and as part of your obligation, write reports about these contracts, defend those contracts, evaluate them, present them to other study sections; so there is a lot of scientific administrative work that goes along with it. It's sort of a mixed blessing being at NCI.

The minority viewpoint is that of a prominent lab chief:

> I came from an academic setting, and if I ever left NCI, I would go back to an academic setting. I consider myself a reasonably good scientist in standing with the academic community, but I am told that actually their perception—the academicians' perception—of the way government does business in fact is not the way that the government does business.

This relates to another lament we frequently heard concering Civil Service: It affords the lab workers a measure of security that can haunt the lab chief. Because civil servants can't be fired, only minor realignment of such personnel is allowed. As one NCI chief assured us, "If one wanted to get rid of someone who was obviously incompetent, one would have to give up science for a year and make it a full-time desire."

40. A flurry of biographical and autobiographical accounts has recently appeared which traces the evolution of personal research programs against the backdrop of intellectual and social histories of disciplines. These memoirs, taken together, offer new opportunities for weighing the forces which shaped scientific careers and ostensibly altered the face of those disciplines as well (see Bernstein, 1978; Kuhn, 1977; Merton, 1977; Toulmin, 1977).

CHAPTER 6

CITATION AND COCITATION STRUCTURES

> The recognition of the existence of the enzyme reverse transcriptase may well have been delayed by failure to properly interpret data available by 1967. It would indeed be ironic if full exploitation of reverse transcriptase were now delayed by a too intense focus on this enzyme at the expense of other entities. In particular a rational approach to molecular inhibition of either viral infection or cellular oncogenesis surely requires understanding of the comparison and function of other cellular polymerases. In this connection . . . recall that replication of oncornaviruses and cellular transformation by these agents appear to require *cell division* as well as DNA synthesis. Understanding of the activity of reverse transcriptase and of other cellular polymerases may well proceed apace. Such a broad based approach may best yield understanding of the modes of division of normal and malignant cells and provide significant clues to the control of these processes.
>
> O'Connor (1973: 1177)

Introduction

The coauthorship relation has been shown to distinguish laboratory research groups for further inspection and that, upon inspection, there emerged a relatively coherent body of RT researchers. The analysis of coauthorship could be carried out satisfactorily with visual representations of the networks; the key individuals and institutional units clustered nicely due to the nature of the relation. However, in this chapter a different type of relationship is at issue and it will require another mode of analysis.

Cocitation analysis allows the set of RT articles to suggest which research articles are most relevant to the advancement of the problem domain. Thus the individual and institutional constraints which operate on coauthorship–heightening laboratory self-citation while both inflating and blurring the contributions of some researchers—are reduced. Here the clustering of articles will represent more of an intellectual cohesiveness than a social relationship. The problem of meaningful clustering of articles in a cocitation matrix can be solved, however, by the use of eigenstructure analysis (consult Appendix C) which is also interpretable in network terms. This technique will be applied to cocitation matrices to help expose what is now beyond simple visual inspection.

The Cosmopolitan Cocitation Network: A Prelude to Analysis

In Appendix D is assembled a list of 66 articles from the article set which have been cited 25 times or more. This list has been ordered according to its date of *submission* for publication, thus constituting a research chronology. Also included are the authors' locations and the funding information given in each article. The identification numbers are consecutive and match the eigenvectors given in Table 6.1 and the scaling in Figure 6.1.[1] The total number of citations received (CT), the total number of cocitations (CC), and the weight received by the article on the first eigenvector (WT) are also recorded for each article. It is this set of highly visible articles that will be analyzed with the cocitation algorithm.

The cocitation algorithm is equivalent to the everyday expression of "being mentioned in the same breath" with someone else. It is a way of associating articles through an analysis of how they are mentioned together by the referencing articles within the RT problem domain. By allowing the choosing articles to occur throughout the time span of the domain, 1970-1975, the analysis favors early articles that have had a longer period within which to be cited.[2] The analysis will be based on the articles that received 25 or more citations (1.5 standard deviations above the mean citation rate) from other articles in the RT set. For reasons presented below, we shall refer to these 66 highly cocited articles as the "cosmopolitan" network.

Through the analysis of the cosmopolitan cocitation network, we will discern how the shift from individuals to articles as the main focal point of analysis alters our perception of the problem domain. Do the important articles come from the in-house authors and laboratories or do the heavily cited articles offer evidence of other structures shaping the development of RT research?

Before we proceed with a formal analysis of the cosmopolitan cocitation network, however, there are some characteristics of the list of 66

(text continued on p. 201)

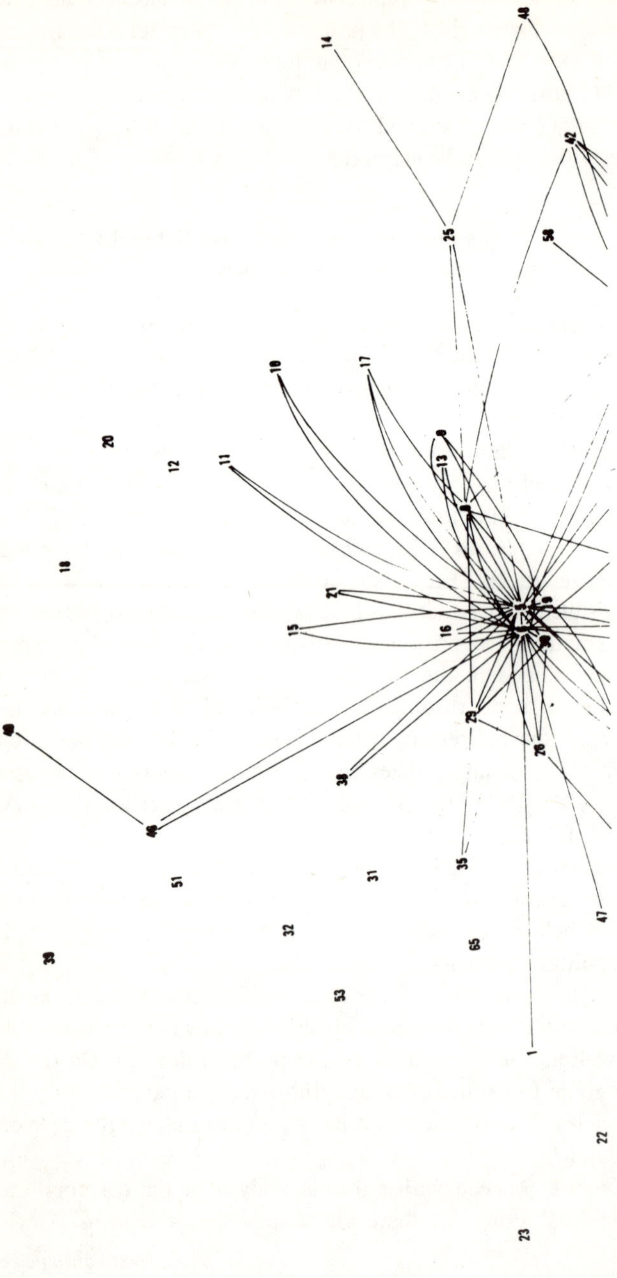
14
48
42
25
58
10
17
20
12
11
8
13
18
21
15
16
9
29
26
40
38
46
35
51
31
47
32
65
39
53
1
22
23

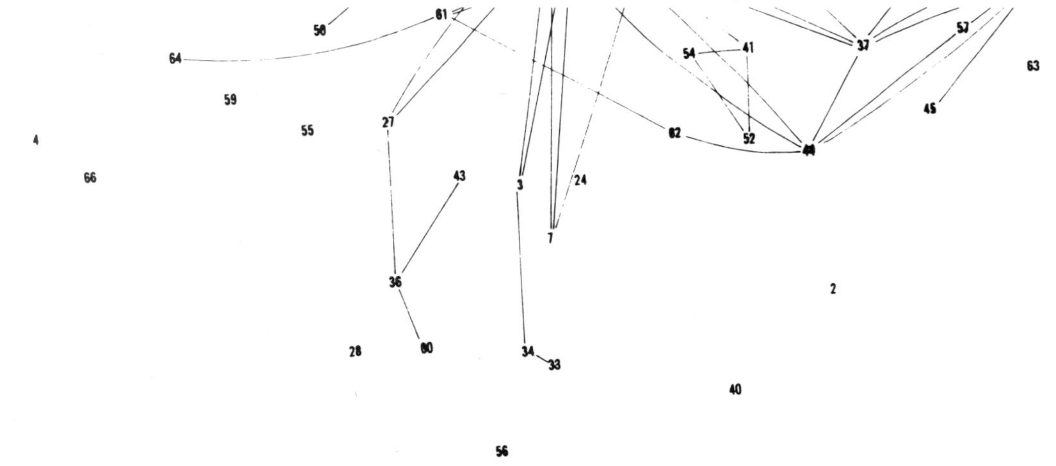

[a]For each eigenvector, the major clusters discussed in the text are noted by two symbols (* and #). These symbols are assigned independently for each vector and no similarity across vectors is implied by use of the same symbol. Because eigenvectors give relative solutions to a set of equations they are accurate only to within a sign change; in other words, the signs in any column could be reversed. All vectors are orthonormal.

FIGURE 6.1 Cocitation Network for Most Highly Cited ($\geqslant$ 25) Articles by the RT Article Set[a]

TABLE 6.1 Eigenvectors of Cocitation Network for Most Highly Cited (⩾ 25) Reverse Transcriptase Articles[a]

Article ID	1st Eigenvector	2nd Eigenvector	3rd Eigenvector	4th Eigenvector
1	0.0934	-0.1371 #	0.0078	0.0254
2	0.0664	0.0142	0.0100	0.0390
3	0.1109	-0.0864	-0.1361	0.2366 *
4	0.0332	-0.0273	0.0890	-0.0247
5	0.3845 *	0.0231	0.2514 *	0.0729
6	0.3897 *	0.0106	0.2461 *	0.0605
7	0.1048	-0.0188	0.1234 *	0.0256
8	0.2373 *	0.1968 *	0.2191 *	0.0476
9	0.1392 *	0.1099	0.0981	-0.0159
10	0.0911	0.0365	0.1093 *	0.0539
11	0.0948	-0.0068	0.1502 *	0.0955
12	0.0760	0.0128	0.0780	0.0137
13	0.1330 *	0.0031	0.1218 *	0.0888
14	0.0643	0.1366 *	0.0821	0.0922
15	0.1001	-0.0623	0.0646	0.1111
16	0.1177	-0.0293	0.0347	0.0355
17	0.1056	0.0531	0.1089 *	0.0917
18	0.0717	-0.0071	0.1052 *	-0.0088
19	0.1868 *	-0.0316	0.0408	-0.0687
20	0.0748	-0.0020	0.0996	0.0400
21	0.1217	-0.0459	0.1047 *	0.0952
22	0.0616	-0.0388	-0.0587	-0.0483
23	0.0378	-0.0237	-0.0187	-0.0481
24	0.0950	-0.0849	-0.0179	0.2041 *
25	0.1039	0.1802 *	0.0181	0.0793
26	0.1866 *	-0.1816 #	-0.0321	-0.1467 #
27	0.1232	-0.1843 #	-0.1025	0.0835
28	0.0669	-0.0777	-0.1265	0.1528 *
29	0.1716 *	-0.1094	0.0927	-0.1496 #
30	0.1892 *	-0.1311 #	-0.0459	-0.1066
31	0.0850	-0.0673	0.0257	-0.0167
32	0.0758	-0.0509	0.0241	-0.1053
33	0.0781	-0.0920	-0.2136 #	0.2792 *
34	0.0822	-0.0957	-0.2235 #	0.2899 *
35	0.1116	-0.1222 #	0.0116	-0.1550 #
36	0.0862	-0.1376 #	-0.1689 #	0.2331 *
37	0.1283	0.2767 *	-0.1271	0.0181
38	0.1070	-0.0590	-0.0088	-0.1871 #
39	0.0407	-0.0351	0.0160	-0.0553
40	0.0638	-0.0053	-0.0741	0.1527 *
41	0.1153	0.0780	-0.1475	-0.0190
42	0.0960	0.3118 *	-0.1182	-0.0345
43	0.1079	-0.1312 #	-0.1760 #	0.1738 *
44	0.1170	0.2353 *	-0.2010 #	-0.0499
45	0.0998	0.2571 *	-0.1388	0.0075
46	0.0806	-0.0440	0.0975	-0.1189
47	0.1014	-0.1316 #	-0.1098	-0.1339 #
48	0.0700	0.2452 *	-0.0897	-0.0210
49	0.0484	-0.0194	0.0526	-0.0497
50	0.1106	-0.1462 #	-0.1775 #	-0.1888 #
51	0.0758	-0.0291	0.0349	-0.1357 #
52	0.0992	0.0401	-0.1334	-0.0056
53	0.0740	-0.0707	0.0299	-0.1186
54	0.1092	0.0123	-0.1386	0.0098
55	0.0888	-0.0724	-0.0954	-0.0792
56	0.0638	-0.0503	-0.1233	0.1900 *
57	0.1011	0.2809 *	-0.1391	-0.0515
58	0.0891	0.2272 *	-0.1347	-0.0507
59	0.0774	-0.0810	-0.0778	-0.0986
60	0.0735	-0.0909	-0.1819 #	0.1911 *
61	0.1359 *	-0.0641	-0.1934 #	-0.2622 #
62	0.1095	0.1236	-0.2172 #	-0.1917 #
63	0.0659	0.1942 *	-0.1372	-0.0348
64	0.0935	-0.1466 #	-0.1527 #	-0.2196 #
65	0.0849	-0.1092	-0.0302	-0.1004
66	0.0577	-0.1094	-0.1253	-0.1228
Eigenvalues	533.4	137.2	105.2	73.0

a. For each eigenvector, the major clusters discussed in the text are noted by two symbols (* and #). These symbols are assigned independently for each vector and no similarity across vectors is implied by use of the same symbol. Because eigenvectors give relative solutions to a set of equations they are accurate only to within a sign change; in other words, the signs in any column could be reversed. All vectors are orthonormal.

articles which warrant comment.[3] For instance, the first article on the list (Lowry et al.) appears to confirm the hypothesis (see Garfield, 1972) that suggests that the most highly cited articles in science are methodological in content. Such methodological prerequisites seem to obtain in biomedicine in an operational fashion, that is, methods articles help to define researchable questions and propose what apparatus, procedure, or material is needed for experimentation. This differs from the view that methodology is somehow distinct from theory and must be "imported" into an area from "outside" (see Griffith et al., 1974). In other words, "protein measurement with the Folin phenol reagent" appears to form some of the conceptual prerequisites for the emergence of the domain of RT research. It illuminated some questions, albeit from a historical distance, that were deemed researchable within the problem domain. Techniques were not merely a "means" imported to realize some research end. Methodology, in short, should be thought of less in an instrumental context than in the substantive, problem context of research.

This argument, initially presented in Chapter 1, needs to be reiterated here because the results of citation analysis are easily misconstrued.[4] When the discussion, later in this chapter, turns to an analysis of the highly cited articles that predated the discovery of RT, the temptation might be to label the electron microscopes and other techniques as instruments rather than as the substantive operations of research which they represent. But methodological articles need to be interpreted in their substantive capacity as problem "facilitators" which circumscribe and, at the same time, promote research in a domain. Numerous articles in our set make reference to the fact that "Protein concentrations were determined using the procedure of Lowry et al." (ID 1); our immediate question is, "How did this article help shape the domain?"

Likewise, the Huebner and Todaro article (ID 3), "Oncogenes of RNA tumor viruses as determinants of cancer," should not be seen as merely a theoretical one, speculating on the mechanism of RNA tumor viruses. It functions as a statement of an orientation to cancer, as a prelude to further discoveries such as that of the enzyme RT itself. It is a confluence point, a compactor of ideas, an attractor of funds, and a means of focusing past research onto a narrowing set of problems. In short, it is a complex of ideas and social forces that could aid in forming a problem domain. It is interesting to note how Huebner and Todaro summarize the background research for their oncogene theory (which we reviewed fully in Chapter 4):

> The viruses [dealt with by the oncogene theory] belong to the group of C-type RNA viruses first demonstrated to be oncogenic in chick-

> ens by Ellerman and Bang and by Rous about 60 years ago and in mice by Gross in 1951. Since that time, but especially in the last few years, morphologically and functionally similar C-type viruses have also been isolated from hamsters and cats and have been seen, though infrequently, by electron microscopy in several other species, including man. While the complete infectious form of the virus is rarely observed under natural conditions, in certain inbred mouse strains with high leukemia incidence, such as AKR and C58, and some lines of chickens, overt virus is commonly observed and is demonstrable even prior to birth. In low or moderate leukemia-incidence mouse strains, overt expression is generally absent early in life but appears in certain tissues later at a time when there is also an increased incidence of tumors. Whether infectious virus and/or tumor become expressed is determined largely by host genetic factors, but expression can be influenced by environmental factors such as radiation and exposure to carcinogens. While full viral expression can occur, we postulate that more frequently there is only partial expression, with perhaps the only gene of the virus expressed being that responsible for transforming the cell into a tumor cell (the oncogene) [1969: 1087].

In this statement prefacing their theory, Huebner and Todaro call upon the research that has been discussed in Chapter 1. They also make reference to the work of W. Bernhard on specifying the type of viruses known as C-type viruses. Bernhard's (1960) article "The detection and study of tumor viruses with the electron microscope" might appear to be methodological. But it turns out to be much, much more. It is indeed substantive and helps shape the emerging problem domain. The work of the French cytologist-virologist Bernhard with the electron microscope becomes another cumulative stepping-stone for Huebner and Todaro. They utilize such previous research to focus on a new area. They, as it were, "see through a glass darkly" only what in the future (after the discovery of RT) would seem to come into view. The various theories discussed earlier seem to fulfill a similar function for the ongoing life of the RT domain.

In comparing the function of the Lowry et al. (ID 1) and the Huebner and Todaro (ID 3) articles, it is vital to note how they rank in terms of citations and number of cocitations relative to the other 64 articles. In citations the Huebner and Todaro article (with 55) ranks 12th; in cocitation it ranks 18th. In the case of the Lowry et al. article the contrast is even more striking; it ranks 7th with 71 citations, but places in the 40th position with 343 cocitations. What this suggests is that the citation of these two important early works is diffuse and not as highly concentrated in articles which reference the other 64 articles. Indeed, the reasons for referencing these articles may differ from the reasons for citing others within the domain.[5] Perhaps away from the center of the domain (defined in terms of high citations) there is more need to cite these articles in a very specific fashion, but in the research center it is enough to say that the Folin phenol reagent method was used or that what is under consideration is the oncogene theory of cancer. There is perhaps, too, a tendency for certain tools and analyses that relate to an ever-widening research community of discourse to cumulate and enter into scientific common knowledge, becoming simply the "assumptions" for further research. But there is also the possibility, if not the stricture, that citation counts should not be extrapolated beyond the structural networks in which they occur. It is to this structure that the following decomposition of network patterns applies.

The Eigenstructure of Cocitations

After the multidimensional scaling of the 66 articles found in Table 6.1 and Figure 6.1 was completed (stress = .29), we graphed the articles that were cited together (cocited) 20 or more times by the *entire* RT article set. This permits the problem domain to project how it "saw" the relations of the various highly cited articles. First and foremost the graph conveys that the two most central articles within the set of 66 are the two discovery articles written by Baltimore (ID 5) and Temin and Mizutani (ID 6). The hub of the problem domain in network terms is clearly these two discovery articles, but certainly hovering nearby are Goodman and Spiegelman's article on "RNA dependent DNA polymerase of human acute leukaemic cells" (ID 19).

What is lacking at this juncture is a formal network criterion for analyzing the structure of the cocitation matrix which was used to generate this visual representation of the problem domain. Fortunately, algorithms similar to those used in multidimensional scaling, namely, eigenvector routines (see Appendix C), can help detect the structure of the network and interpret the picture in Figure 6.1. Because the cocitation matrix is a symmetric real matrix, with the same units of measurement in every cell, we can compute the eigenvectors and discern the connectivity structures of the network.

Returning to Table 6.1, the first four eigenvectors reveal what one might call the eigenstructure of the network. These vectors rank and cluster the various articles in terms of their structural position within the network. It is the task of the analyst, then, to study these various dimensions of the network and assess their meaning. Note that the first vector contains only one clustering of the articles, whereas the remaining vectors contain two clusters each, surrounding the high positive and low negative poles of the vector. Thus in studying the vectors, we have the opportunity to identify seven different clusterings of the cocitation network. These clusters must reflect the results of networking, that is, linkages generated by the cocitation relationship.[6]

THE FIRST VECTOR: DISCOVERY AND CHARACTERIZATION OF THE ENZYME

The first vector in Table 6.1 is not difficult to interpret for it mirrors the centrality found via the multidimensional scaling analysis (see Figure 6.1). The articles in order of their importance on this vector are, in Appendix D, ID numbers 6, 5, 8, 30, 19, 26, 29, 9, 61, and 13. This is essentially the tight center cluster discussed above that dominates the cocitation structure. It is the discovery cluster, the seminal cluster around which the problem domain took shape; it is also the isolation and purification cluster of the network. This vector spans several years of research in RT–evidence that the cocitation of these various works encompasses an evolving research program. The isolation and purification work should not be viewed apart from the attempts to decipher the function of the enzyme and its capacity to allow RNA viral replication. All of the articles in this cluster are empirical research articles suggesting the "dominance of the experiment" in the RT literature. It would be difficult to classify any of the articles in this cluster as "purely" theoretical.

Significantly, the set of important scientists discussed in the previous chapter intersects with the authors of these cosmopolitan cocited articles. Besides the discoverers Baltimore and Temin, we once again see the importance of men such as Spiegelman, Gallo, and Green. It is with incredible speed that these researchers jumped into the problem area after the discovery had been announced. What can be seen by simply looking at the submission dates (recorded to the left of the articles in Appendix D) is that after the discovery articles were received at the beginning (Baltimore) and the middle (Temin and Mizutani) of June and published within a matter of weeks, the publishing lag lengthens into months. This is despite the rapidity with which other researchers submitted their manuscripts. Perhaps the novelty of the discovery and the unclaimed priority rights had begun to fade.

It is incorrect to think, however, that these postdiscovery researchers were converging on the area in an exploitative fashion. It would, indeed, seem just as logical to say that the discoverer Baltimore had jumped the fence of his work with vesicular stomatitis virus to apply analogically some of his research skill (for a discussion, see his Nobel address, Baltimore, 1976b). It would seem that the time was ripe for an empirical reversal of Watson's "Central Dogma" of DNA replication; the quest for the enzyme, indeed, the need for the discovery of such an enzyme, was becoming apparent to virologists. The discoverers correctly formulated the problem and allowed the rapid successive discovery and analysis of the DNA polymerase in other viruses. Thus Spiegelman et al. (ID 8) follow immediately, discovering the polymerase in feline leukemia virus; and so the process continued until the area was inundated by reports on the various viral sources of the enzyme.[7]

On the first eigenvector the institutional progression is from McArdle Laboratory for Cancer Research (ID 6), to the Department of Biology at MIT (ID 5), to the Institute of Cancer Research, Columbia (ID 8, 30), to the Human Tumor Cell Biology Branch of NCI and Litton Bionetics (ID 19), back to MIT (ID 26) and Columbia (ID 29), then to the Institute for Molecular Virology, St. Louis University School of Medicine (ID 9), and finally back to Columbia (ID 13), Litton Bionetics, and the Laboratory of Tumor Cell Biology, NCI (ID 61). What is especially revealing here is the secondary status on this vector which Green's laboratory at St. Louis occupies. As we shall see, this status carries dual significance for our analysis, clarifying the gulf between intellectual history and the methodological lessons derived from citation manipulation.

Green et al. (ID 7), within weeks of the submission of the discovery articles, had submitted their own article on RNA-dependent DNA polymerase in murine sarcoma viruses, but this article seems to qualify as an also-ran. In it Green et al. cite the Baltimore and the Temin and Mizutani discovery and state that they have received a preprint of Spiegelman's work on feline leukemia virus. But more appears to be going on here than first meets the eye: Baltimore begins his discovery article with the sentence, "DNA seems to have a critical role in the multiplication and transforming ability of RNA tumour viruses" (ID 5) and cites Green's forthcoming article "Oncogenic viruses." Green's group (Rokutanda et al.; ID 9) begins its article "Formation of viral RNA-DNA hybrid molecules by the DNA polymerase of sarcoma-leukemia viruses" with the statement, "We have postulated that the RNA tumour viruses possess a DNA polymerase dependent on viral RNA [here Green's review of "Oncogenic viruses" is referenced], and several laboratories have recently reported that leukaemia and sarcoma viruses of the mouse, chicken and cat incorporate radioactive deoxyribonucleotides into an acid-insoluble form" (1970: 1026). What can be inferred is that Green, more directly than *anyone else,*[8] had postulated the existence of the DNA polymerase within the protein capsid and others had demonstrated it in a series of animal viruses (see Green and Gerard, 1974). But the scientific credits (in terms of citation counts) did not swing in any overwhelming fashion toward Green's work. In fact, he receives very little credit (10 citations) from articles within the set.

It is by weighing the evidence in Table 6.1 and its accompanying scenario that one grows circumspect about the uncritical usage of citation structures, whether in the form of simple citation or cocitation counts or in networks. For as was surmised in the previous chapter, one can attribute much of the similarity of citation profiles to extensive in-group citation. This behavior would appear to muddle the cocitation picture, too. If certain groups emerge as high publishers in a research domain and cite their own earlier work more heavily than an idealized "nonaffiliated researcher," then these articles emerge as highly cited works and, moreover, as densely connected through cocitations. In other words, *there develops a tendency in cocitation analysis to pick off the large laboratories and research groups, just as the central individuals within such laboratories were made more visible in the in-house coauthorship network.* The extent of such exertions of influence on network structures is rather difficult to determine. At present, we must tread lightly on the implications of cocitation analysis until the parameters that boost visibility and usage, much of which seem artifactual, are better known.[9] As our analysis enhances understanding of the underlying relationships implied by the cocitation network, one must remember that the institutional structures out of which the ideas arise may actually be distorting our perceptions of scientific development.

Thus, the first eigenvector in Table 6.1 represents the discovery and characterization (isolation, purification) of RT. This interpretation is visually reinforced by the starlike pattern surrounding the discovery articles presented in Figure 6.1. The remaining three vectors make more interpretive demands than the first, but the cognitive consistency of the clusterings can be appreciated by just reading the article titles. For each of the remaining three vectors, two substantive clusters will be briefly discussed.

THE SECOND VECTOR: REVERSE TRANSCRIPTASE AND BREAST CANCER RESEARCH

In Figure 6.1, we observe on the right side of the graph a group of interconnected articles. Glancing at the second vector of Table 6.2, we notice that the high positive (*) numbers[10] represent 11 articles contained in Appendix D. The predominant subject matter of this subset is mammary carcinoma, a subject which has a checkered tradition in viral cell transformation. Long since Bittner's work in the 1930s on the transmission of mouse mammary carcinomas, the factor responsible for the propagation of this carcinoma was not known. The great advance came when Moore et al. (ID 14) fractionated the milk from 212 carefully selected women from Philadelphia and Bombay (selected on the basis of history of mammary carcinomas in the family) and began examining these samples with an electron microscope. They found that

> Particles with the same morphological characteristics as those that cause breast cancer in mice (B particles) were found in the milk of all three groups, but the incidences in the groups were vastly different. B particles were found in the milk of seven (5%) of the American women with no history of the disease in their families; they were found in the milk of six (60%) of the Americans with a history of the disease in their families; eighteen (39%) of the Parsi women were found to contain the particles in their milk [Moore et al., 1970: 611].

This discovery of particles physically identical to those found in mouse mammary tumor virus research accounts for the spurt of research found in this second vector. One can at least surmise this by going to the citations in the critical article within the cluster (ID 42) and noting that the research of Moore et al. is treated as the major impetus for ensuing breast cancer research. It should also be emphasized that the original Moore et al. article did not deal at all with RT, but immediately stimulated research in that direction. Before long, Schlom, Spiegelman, and Moore (ID 48) were to investigate whether the particles Moore's group discovered did contain an RT. Their discovery of the enzyme in these particles similar to known RNA tumor viruses was itself already cited (as a manuscript in preparation) in the central article of this cluster (ID 42). In some sense, therefore, the key Spiegelman et al. article reviews and summarizes the earlier discovery articles in the domain.[11]

What is so striking in this cluster is, once again, the dominance of one laboratory, namely, the Columbia laboratory of Spiegelman. Whether it accurately portrays the concentration in the field of viral induction of mammary cancer remains an open question. It could be, once again, that large research groups can so self-cite their work (within a laboratory) that cocitation clusters emerge whenever they tackle a problem.

The other cluster (#) which is isolated by the second vector involves 10 articles that are somewhat more difficult to classify. Scrutiny of Figure 6.1 reveals that this set of articles is not as highly connected as the previous one. If we were to attach labels to this set, we would probably identify it as the separation, purification, and specification cluster. The Lowry et al. (ID 1) article appears in this cluster along with discussions of the nature of synthetic versus natural polymerases. This cluster represents what is so typical of the biological orientation to methodology: a means of understanding and an embodiment of the understanding process as well—operational, concrete, substantive methodology. The flavor of this orientation can be found in the central article in this cluster (Ross et al.; ID 27) and is worth extensive quotation:

> The virions of RNA tumour viruses contain enzyme(s) capable of synthesizing DNA from viral RNA and from synthetic RNA-RNA or RNA-DNA templates. Synthetic RNA-DNA templates provide a very sensitive method for the detection of enzyme activity, and so a search for such activity was made in tumour cells. Although DNA polymerase activity was detected in neoplastic cells using synthetic RNA-RNA and RNA-DNA templates, similar activity has been found in normal cells as well. Thus, the presence of polymerase activity *per se* could not be used as an accurate indicator either of neoplasia or of the presence of a covert RNA tumour virus. It was critical, then, to determine the relationship, if any, between the viral enzyme and the enzymes found in normal, non-tumorigenic cells and in virus-transformed, tumorigenic cells [1971: 163].

The careful wrapping of methodological questions in substantive understanding is perhaps one of the most difficult aspects of the biological sciences for the social scientist to comprehend. The careful weighing and comparing of evidence from synthetic templates of RNA-DNA providing the leverage for discerning the physical properties of viral versus normal enzymes should not be cast aside as a mere difference of experimental design or methodological technique. It is a peculiar form of understanding, part of the structure of rationality within the biological sciences, that needs to be fathomed if one is to understand its social implications. The cluster formed around the problem of the "separation of murine cellular and murine leukaemia virus DNA polymerases" is a good example of substantive methodology within biomedical research.

Again, as in earlier clusters, it is highly instructure to note the institutions involved in the research contained in the "methodological" cluster. This cluster moves into the heart of the federal, in-house NCI research effort. It is the intellectual territory of the Viral Leukemia and Lymphoma Branch along with the Laboratory of Tumor Cell Biology, both of NCI. The work of MIT's Department of Biology along with the private facilities of Litton Bionetics and the Roche Institute is also represented. It is clear that this is not Spiegelman's main interest at Columbia. The domain is somewhat removed from the clinical interactions that seem to specify the aforementioned research on mammary carcinomas, moving toward the "pure" research wing of RT research.

THE THIRD VECTOR: VIROLOGY AND LEUKEMIA

On the third eigenvector still other orientations to the RT domain emerge. One of the clusters (positive) represents a viral component and the other (negative) relates to a leukemia portion of the highly cited literature. After the discovery of mouse, chicken, and cat viral RT, the work continues on other RNA tumor viruses, for example, visna virus, and gradually involves research on inhibitors of DNA polymerase activity, for example, streptovaricins (ID 20). This cluster of virology articles is virtually entirely at home in the academic sector of RT research and suggests that traditional departmental and disciplinary structures may be more accommodating to this type of biological research than, say, to the other areas which are dominated by NCI (separation and purification).

This contrasts with the leukemia cluster found on the third vector where the research indicates large government laboratory concentration and more mission-oriented research, for example, contracts with Litton Bionetics. Hints of such developments can be seen as one traces the locations of the research in this cluster of articles concentrated around ID 34. It is interesting that this Lowy et al. article comes from the Laboratory of Viral Diseases at the National Institute of Allergy and Infectious Diseases; it received support from the Etiology Area of the NCI and became a cornerstone for in vitro studies of leukemia virus. Essentially, the methodology allowed the artificial activation of leukemia viruses in tissue culture cell lines. But the methodological "how" and the substantive "why" never seem to be far apart in cancer research of this sort. For instance, in Aaronson et al. (ID 33), the "Induction of murine C-type viruses from clonal lines of virus-free BALB/3T3 cells" becomes both a method for studying cancer and a contribution to viral and chemical carcinogenesis.

What is being witnessed in this cluster is the advent of new orientations toward leukemia research stimulated by the discovery of RT. For in this cluster the work in RT becomes a means of assaying C-type viral activity within cells. Even the Baxt et al. (ID 62) article is more than a declaration that "human leukaemic cells contain reverse transcriptase associated with a high molecular weight virus-related RNA." They realize that,

> To pursue further the aetiological implications of these [earlier] findings for human cancer, it is necessary to perform experiments designed to answer the following questions concerning the virus-related RNA: (1) How large is the RNA being detected in human tumours? and (2) Is it associated with a reverse transcriptase of Temin and Mizutani and Baltimore? Finally, if a large RNA molecule is found in association with a reverse transcriptase, it is further necessary to determine whether the DNA synthesized by the two in concert is complementary to a relevant "oncogenic" RNA (that is, RNA homologous to that of an RNA tumour virus) [Baxt et al., 1972: 72].

It is such a synthesis of knowledge that one might call it the prototype of the growth of biomedical science. The Baxt et al. (1972) attempt to utilize, for example, the Rauscher murine leukemia virus as a model to purify the DNA-polymerase and see whether it will transcribe a known RNA molecule (e.g., avian myeloblastosis virus, ID 61) is typical of the indirect tactics needed for the analysis. Thus, the leukemia research found within this cluster shows how the intellectual web of research coheres in problem specification and how the confluence of ideas into this network creates an integral research front.

THE FOURTH VECTOR: THE ONCOGENE PLUS

The manner in which research interests cluster and in which the unity of a domain is created can be seen in the clusters in the fourth eigenvector. Although the clustering of articles along institutional lines in this vector is exemplified by the (1) Viral Leukemia and Lymphoma Branch of NCI and (2) the Laboratory of Tumor Cell Biology and Litton Bionetics, we see that certain distinct problem concerns dominate their respective programs.

The first cluster that relates leukemia research to the larger cancer effort also manifests the unity of the research program of Todaro and Huebner.

Articles 3 and 56 are two elegantly argued statements of Todaro and Huebner's "oncogene hypothesis." As demonstrated earlier, the first of these two articles attempted to integrate the historical work of Bertrand, Ellerman and Bang, Rous, and Gross into a coherent statement of the cause of cancer: "The new hypothesis predicts that both spontaneous cancers and cancers induced by chemical and physical agents will be the result of expression of the oncogene(s) of covert C-type RNA virus" (Huebner and Todaro, 1969: 1088; ID 3). What followed was a rehearsal of the evidence in support of their synthesis, and within the span of a few years they were able to give a cogent and convincing review ("new evidence," ID 56) of how current research has supported their work. This cluster reads like the bibliography of a polemic for the oncogene hypothesis. Lowy's (ID 34) and Aaronson's (ID 33) work, which has been encountered before, now become cornerstones for the oncogene theory; for if one can induce murine C-type viruses from clonal lines of virus-free BALB/3T3 cells, then one must explain whence the viruses came. Their "spontaneous" appearance is seen as having originated from the genetic, vertically transmitted potential that all cells possess.[12]

Of the 10 (*) articles in this fourth vector, only 2 are not cited in Huebner and Todaro's oncogene article. One was on the "C-type virus in tumor tissue of a woolly monkey with fibrosarcoma," from the School of Veterinary Medicine, University of California at Davis, and the other, coauthored by Todaro which appeared a few months after the oncogene article. The other studies represented in the cluster on antibodies, immunology, and "C-type virus released from cultured human rhabdomyosarcoma cells" (ID 40) are primary supports for the synthesis proposed by Huebner and Todaro.

Observing such a cluster and seeing that it has isolated not only a group of authors with the same institutional affiliation, that is, the Viral Leukemia and Lymphoma Branch of NCI, but an intellectual unity as well, we are particularly satisfied. The technique seems to have isolated not just individuals but a research program; it has captured not just related empirical research but also the theoretical unity that motivates it. At the same time, we recognize that the other clusters, while not as intuitively pleasing perhaps, have efficiently isolated intense areas of research which are equally vital for the ongoing research effort. The caveat, therefore, is that one should not be enticed to study only those cluster complexes comprehensible to the sociologist; it is the scientist's usage which is of prime interest. The rationality of a problem domain may not be intuitively obvious, as in the next cluster discussed, but may nevertheless represent vital pieces of the puzzle of scientific growth.

Certainly the other (#) cluster that is found on the fourth vector represents the type of group that strains interpretation. It is not neat; its theoretical unity is not readily accessible in a program statement. It would appear to be institutionally connected with the Laboratory of Tumor Cell Biology of NCI and with the associated Litton Bionetics Research Laboratories. Perhaps the company of these articles is, to a large extent, an artifact of the laboratory structure, that is, large laboratories publish much and self-cite the work of the same laboratory. But even if this were the case, one should be able to discern the rationale for the particular research within the cluster.

CONCLUSIONS FROM THE EIGENSTRUCTURE ANALYSIS OF COSMOPOLITAN COCITATIONS AND THE UNFINISHED AGENDA

Thus far in the analysis of the cosmopolitan cocitation network, much has been learned about the institutional structure and intellectual orientations within RT. It has become clear that the focus of the domain, as predicted, has been elaboration of the work of Baltimore and of Temin and Mizutani. It has also become apparent that the large laboratories exert a formidable influence in the cocitation network. By taking into account not only the citation or cocitation counts but also the eigenstructure, we have been able to display the important network clusters within the cocitation matrix. By taking into account network properties, the secondary structures indicate the parameters of confluence onto the problem domain, that is, how ideas come together and how scientists focus their research interests. Such an analysis also illustrates how research areas emerge and split off again, to wit, the oncogene hypothesis reaches out to make virology part of genetics.

The analysis of the cosmopolitan cocitation network notwithstanding, it is still not clear how the confluences as inferred from the chronology of important articles actually *created* the domain. In other words, a fairly detailed picture of the postdiscovery era of the domain has been painted, but the structural themes (intellectual, social, and so on) which converged to *create* the domain have yet to be probed. How did the science which exploded out of the discovery articles come to be? What we have been analyzing is, for the most part, articles from within the domain proper. To finish the agenda, what we must now ask is, "What were the prerequisites, in terms of important articles and arguments, for the discovery of reverse transcriptase and the creation of the new research problems?" To pursue this analysis, a set of articles which are highly cited (10 or more citations) and *predate* the discovery era of RT research have been selected. What articles, in other words, do the authors of the RT literature deem important in the prediscovery era?[13] Granted, the question runs counter to the stream of the historical unfolding of the domain. But this is intentional; it permits better exposure of the undergirding of the domain and dramatizes the nature of developments which begat explosive growth in the postdiscovery period.

Prediscovery Cocitation Analysis

Analysis of the research on which the discovery articles were erected could be performed on the references within the discovery articles or on some larger slice of the "precursor" literature. Neither method has been chosen because what is of interest is not what led the *discoverers,* as it were, to the Nobel prize, but rather what preceded the development of the *entire* problem domain. By allowing the entire set to choose articles from this prediscovery period, one can discover the structure of the literature which supports the domain as a whole. The analysis, in other words, is aimed at explaining problem domain creation and subsequent research pathways.

Once again the analysis proceeds from a cocitation matrix which relates the prediscovery articles to one another through their simultaneous appearance on the reference list of a given article in the set of 54 reproduced in Appendix E. The articles in this appendix, as in Appendix D, are arranged by order of their submission dates to journals, though all were published before June 1970. Each was cited 10 or more times, cocited at least 20 times, and scaled in the manner of the previous analysis. The total number of citations (CT), the total number of cocitations (CC), and the weight received by the article on the first eigenvector (WT) are again recorded for each article.

First, it is instructive to identify those articles which are most highly cited in this period. Notably, the "Folin phenol reagent measurement of protein" heads the list of most highly cited articles followed by the first oncogene hypothesis article by Huebner and Todaro. These are followed by articles on vesicular stomatitis virus (Baltimore's chief interest prior to his ground-breaking research on RT), Rous sarcoma virus, DNA sequences, and the enzymology of DNA. The highly cited articles during this prediscovery period manifest some of the prerequisites (in retrospect) for discovering RT.

But surprisingly, an assay based on the Folin phenol reagent comes to the forefront as a key article within the RT domain. Even though it is well known that this is the single most cited article in all of biology, it still seems unusual that in the microcosm we are studying it would command such status. To us, this illustrates the far-reaching tentacles of scientific development—when some basic protein assays discovered by Wu and developed by Folin in the 1920s, later perfected by Lowry et al. (1951) in the 1950s, recur in the most sophisticated of molecular biology research. Why, for instance, has the technique not been lost for citation analysis through eponymy, for example, the Wu-Folin protein assay? We would conjecture that there is ample complexity in the assay to assure that the article will be referred to for reasons of economy and the sheer simplicity of the method.[14]

Whatever the specific reasons for the high citation counts of this particular article, in areas where protein analysis is routine (as in studies involving molecular biology of DNA or RNA), the Lowry et al. article should represent for us a compelling argument for the cumulative growth of science. The diffusion throughout biology of such assays demonstrates the ease with which such research spans the problems of a large segment of biological science. Other assays, such as the RT assay itself, may have a more limited scope for its diffusion, but it, too, is continually enlarging its area of "relevance." As problems get redefined with the accumulation of knowledge, relevance looms and the interweaving of biological knowledge enhances the growth process. The Lowry et al. work stands as a symbol of such historically important discoveries that make themselves felt long after other articles have been forgotten or thoroughly absorbed by a specialty or field. Because it is vitally relevant to all areas of biology, much the same as Darwinian theory or the discovery of DNA was/is, it continues to assume an integrating role for biological researchers much beyond its seemingly modest content.[15]

Of immediate interest is the ordering of cocitations that does not match the ordering of the articles by citations. Lowry's article is not nearly as highly cocited as one would expect from its citations; it does not appear in the reference lists along with the other highly cited articles as frequently as one might expect. What is happening is that by implementing a new criterion of importance, namely, association with other articles that are highly cited, the Lowry article suffers in the ranking process. This emphasizes that its relevance for this new system of relations is surpassed by articles more central to the inchoative RT research. The Lowry et al. article is, in other words, more randomly distributed across the problem domain. It is now the oncogene hypothesis of Huebner and Todaro (ID

(text continued on p. 218)

TABLE 6.2 Eigenvectors of Cocitation Network for Most Highly Cited (⩾ 10) Prediscovery Articles[a]

Article ID	1st Eigenvector	2nd Eigenvector	3rd Eigenvector	4th Eigenvector
1	0.0659	-0.1676 #	0.2880 *	0.0917
2	0.1341	0.0911	0.1545	-0.5022 #
3	0.1093	-0.0970	0.0854	0.0472
4	0.1812	-0.1243	0.0276	0.0610
5	0.0717	-0.0281	0.0026	-0.2128 #
6	0.0534	-0.1192	0.1780	0.0520
7	0.0451	0.0037	0.0128	-0.1491 #
8	0.0600	0.0353	-0.0043	0.0050
9	0.1620	0.0512	-0.1476	0.0292
10	0.1195	-0.0066	-0.1622 #	0.0330
11	0.2466 *	-0.0300	-0.0872	0.0170
12	0.2217	-0.0330	-0.1561 #	0.0348
13	0.1683	-0.0533	-0.1816 #	0.0114
14	0.0767	-0.0222	-0.0664	-0.1150 #
15	0.0907	0.2186 *	0.0724	0.1230 *
16	0.0460	0.0013	-0.0363	-0.0550
17	0.2111	-0.0053	-0.0989	0.0223
18	0.1191	0.0137	-0.0034	-0.0271
19	0.0892	0.2540 *	0.0982	0.1065 *
20	0.0983	0.3456 *	0.2060	0.0154
21	0.1113	0.2517 *	0.1314	0.0542
22	0.1780	-0.2216 #	0.1790	0.0643
23	0.1726	0.0324	-0.1437	0.0781
24	0.3051 *	-0.1171	-0.0358	-0.0220
25	0.0443	0.1674	0.1178	-0.0169
26	0.1016	-0.0129	-0.0722	-0.0615
27	0.0401	-0.0030	0.0563	-0.4023 #
28	0.2253 *	-0.1061	-0.1447	-0.0122
29	0.1505	-0.1963 #	0.1305	0.0439
30	0.1592	-0.0160	0.0456	0.0115
31	0.0391	0.0148	-0.0101	-0.1509 #
32	0.0742	0.2046 *	0.0983	0.0845
33	0.0568	0.0812	0.0186	-0.0867
34	0.1074	0.2237 *	0.0719	0.1100 *
35	0.0700	-0.2240 #	0.3927 *	0.0975
36	0.0123	0.0102	0.0111	-0.1147 #
37	0.1989	-0.1030	-0.0728	-0.0854
38	0.0921	0.1891 *	0.0590	0.0335
39	0.0598	0.2013 *	0.1200	-0.0098
40	0.0748	-0.1982 #	0.3251 *	0.0940
41	0.0200	0.0134	0.0501	-0.3415 #
42	0.3450 *	0.1508	-0.0901	0.0865
43	0.0288	0.0286	0.0036	-0.0746
44	0.0476	0.0006	-0.0538	-0.0560
45	0.1308	0.0296	0.0363	0.0084
46	0.0869	-0.1614 #	0.2968 *	-0.0132
47	0.1924	-0.1011	-0.1535	0.0488
48	0.0572	0.0354	0.0794	-0.4437 *
49	0.1962	-0.0855	0.0108	0.0526
50	0.0584	-0.0759 #	0.2175 *	-0.0334
51	0.1073	0.1874 *	0.0985	0.0022
52	0.1226	0.2928 *	0.1358	0.0850
53	0.1546	-0.0752	-0.1512	-0.0245
54	0.0668	-0.0177	-0.0644	-0.0034
Eigenvalues	63.2	28.6	22.0	18.0

a. For each eigenvector, the major clusters discussed in the text are noted by two symbols (* and #). These symbols are assigned independently for each vector and no similarity across vectors is implied by the use of the same symbol. Because eigenvectors give relative solutions to a set of equations they are accurate only to within a sign change; in other words, the signs in any column could be reversed. All vectors are orthonormal.

FIGURE 6.2 Cocitation Network for Most Highly Cited (⩾ 10) Prediscovery Articles[a]

[a]For each eigenvector, the major clusters discussed in the text are noted by two symbols (* and #). These symbols are assigned independently for each vector and no similarity across vectors is implied by the use of the same symbol. Because eigenvectors give relative solutions to a set of equations they are accurate only to within a sign change; in other words, the signs in any column could be reversed. All vectors are orthonormal.

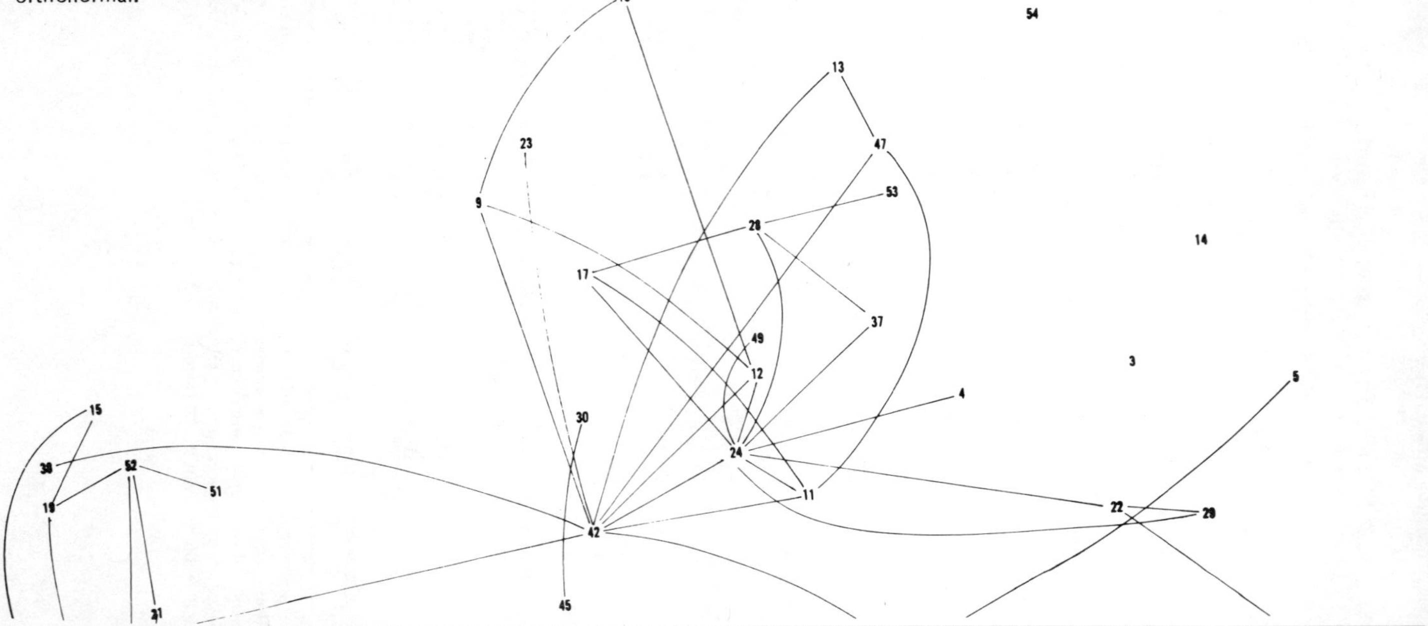

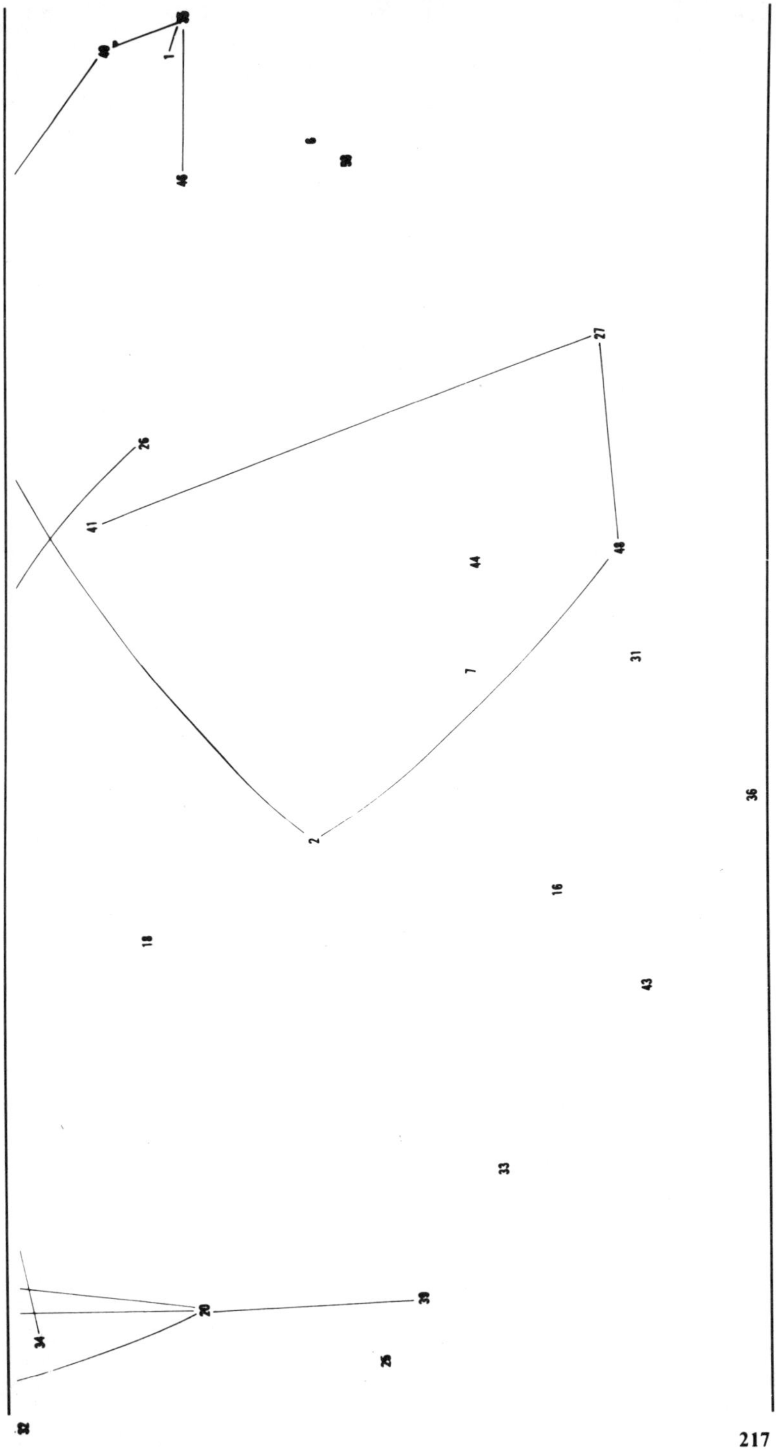
1
46
27
26
41
48
44
7
31
2
36
16
18
43
33
39
20
34
25

42) and the work of Duesberg on the "physical properties of Rous sarcoma virus RNA" (ID 24) that move onto center stage. Perhaps the structural milieux of problem domains so consolidate discrete events, for example, individual citations, that unless the structure of consolidation is understood, importance cannot be determined. Importance here refers to relevance of research to other ongoing research; it is the relevance structure in scientific growth and progress that must be uncovered.

The clusters of articles (derived from an eigenvector analysis) in this prediscovery period represent the delineation of such spheres of relevance within the emerging problem domain of RT. Because the cocitation matrix for this early period is not dense, that is, there are many zeroes in the cocitation matrix, we will not proceed on a vector-by-vector basis, but rather summarize the findings contained in Table 6.2 and Figure 6.2.

On the first vector, two distinctive styles of thinking are represented in the citations themselves. Baltimore and Temin both seem to base their discovery on Temin's provirus theory (see Temin, 1976). Although in different laboratories during the prediscovery period, they were both experimenting with actinomycin D and found that it inhibited the production of certain RNA viruses. They did not need the most central article on the first eigenvector, the Huebner and Todaro "oncogene theory," to make their discovery. But if this is the case, then what is the function of the Huebner and Todaro article within RT research? Is it used predominantly as a foil for the statement of other views—Temin and Baltimore cite the oncogene theory although they disagree with it—or is it the unifying force for the whole problem domain?

The second vector divides the research on murine leukemia viruses from that on mammary tumor viruses. The former (*) cluster is dominated by the development and utilization of tissue cultures whose experimental control would facilitate the discovery of RT. The second (#) cluster overlaps considerably with the first (*) in the third vector. Their commonality is research on mammary carcinomas and includes Bittner's classic (ID 1) statement on the transmission of mouse mammary tumors. But most vital in this cluster for the advancement of RT research is the electron microscopy study of "type B particles in human milk" (ID 35). Moore et al. were doing for human milk virions what Bernhard (as reviewed earlier) had done for tumor viruses. Their meticulously designed experiment became a building block for further research and thinking about the causes of human mammary cancer. If the time seemed ripe for the discovery of the mechanisms of RNA virus propagation, there also was developing a renewed research sensibility to the issue of human cancer. Excitement for a war on cancer was mounting. And with the increasing evidence of the presence of RNA viruses in human milk homologous to that found in mouse tumors, all that was needed was another Bittner to complete the etiological research.

The second cluster in the third vector conveys the feeling of "imminent" discovery—about six years early. The provirus hypothesis, which Temin had propounded a year earlier (Temin, 1963; 1976) was beginning to yield experimental dividends. He was ready to present evidence which confirmed his prediction, "by showing that labeled RNA from RSV has homology with DNA from RSV-infected cells, but not with DNA from parallel uninfected cells" (Temin, 1964a: 323).[16]

But others, notably Bader (ID 10), were also experimenting in the early 1960s with inhibitors (Bromodeoxyuridine and actinomycin D) which would not allow DNA synthesis. Bader, for instance, was able to suppress with actinomycin D the propagation of Rous sarcoma virus in chick embryo cells, but could not suppress propagation of vesticular stomatitis virus using the same inhibitor. Recall that it was Baltimore's later work with the enzymatic relations within the vesicular stomatitis virus that gave him the clue to the discovery by analogy of RT. Bader and Temin were already, independently, unraveling the mysteries of viral propagation, paying no heed to Watson's contention that "RNA never acts as a template for DNA" (1970: 330); rather, they were following the experimental leads of the virology research front.

In vector four, the development of tissue culture assays appears once again. This cluster (*) intersects with the earlier one, but does pick off the articles which were specifically concerned with the development of virus titration, neutralization, and purification assays. What is curious is that these three articles are all written by the Hartley-Rowe research group, which was located at the National Institute of Allergy and Infectious Diseases. Of all the research represented in the highly cited prediscovery set, the tissue culture research in vectors two and four seems to be most concentrated within government research laboratories.

It is appropriate that the other (#) cluster in the fourth vector deals with the problem of enzyme detection. In 1968, when Shatkin and Sipe (ID 27) demonstrated that the enzyme necessary for the reovirus replication was contained in the virus itself and not synthesized in the host cell, the research agenda for other RNA viruses was established. The Baltimore et al. (ID 48) demonstration that the virions of vesicular stomatitis virus also contain an RNA polymerase was one of the penultimate steps in the prediscovery process. One needed only to combine the information known about DNA polymerases with that of RNA viruses to discover the DNA polymerase of a class of cancer-causing RNA viruses.

Conclusions

O'Connor's caution which was quoted at the outset of this chapter has now taken on new meaning. As the discussion of the prediscovery process and the cosmopolitan structure has unfolded, some of the necessary components of the problem domain have become clearer. Once one is able to obtain a perspective on the domain through the use of cocitation analysis, the fabric from which the domain is woven by the various research efforts, and the concentration of diverse research styles and subject areas, becomes visible. The danger is that discoveries such as RT, which can catch the public eye (e.g., through the Nobel Prize), will be perceived as remote from the ongoing process of science and consequently viewed as extraordinary events, that is, outside the "normal" structures of scientific progress. The sociological and philosophical publics, on the other hand, can compound the same distortion by emphasizing that science only progresses through a series of radical breaks from the past. The judgment that a paradigm shift occurred in the case of RT, negating Watson's (1970) statement of the Central Dogma of DNA-RNA synthesis, would be gratuitous. Indeed, the discovery of the enzyme consummated a continuous cumulation of experimental evidence in support of the provirus hypothesis.

What this chapter underscores is the continuity of research that both preceded the discovery and followed in its wake. Such an evolutionary process is more subtle than the resolution of crises we have been taught to perceive and the research successes we tend to celebrate. We have been socialized into accepting a certain scientific *event,* rather than a research *process,* as worthy of attention and reward. By emphasizing the fact that RT research continues programs on viral and chemical transformation, we are not thereby implying that the scientists involved in unraveling the mysteries of the transformation process are not great men. We are suggesting, however, that the meaning of "greatness" must be critically assessed in terms of its social and cognitive prerequisites within a research setting.

Some of these prerequisites, of course, reflect the policy effects of the massive funding mandated by the National Cancer Act of 1971. The exact effect of the funding process is difficult to ascertain, but when it should be clearly in force is during the postdiscovery period of RT research. The concentration of research during this period in large governmental and private laboratories (e.g., Litton Bionetics, Flow Laboratories) can be seen in the cocitation analysis which reveals their dominance in the literature of the domain. But how does one know what the research would have been like if the funding had not materialized? Would the confluence patterns have been "better," "more advantageous," or "earlier?" Most arguments pertaining to the effects of funding, we fear, will remain mired in the perennial difficulty of asking hypothetical questions of history.

On another plane, continuity which emerges from a discussion of the cocitation analyses illuminates the pitfalls of discussing social structure divorced from the cognitive, rational dimension of a problem domain. We social scientists need not pretend to understand this fundamental aspect of any problem domain in all of its ramifications. But more than a cursory knowledge of the problems attacked by the "inside" researchers seems mandatory *or the social dimensions of the problem domain will remain impenetrable.*

If there is any *mysterium* left in the simultaneous discovery of RT, it fades in the shadow of the seeming historical "teleology" of the confluence process. How is it that so many different efforts from the remote past (e.g., Bittner, 1936) and from widely separate fields (as the sociologist might see fit to define them) can prepare the way for present biological discoveries? The answer seems to lie both in the process of confluence and in the objects of analysis themselves; the biological organism and its structure set the parameters of knowledge confluence. The structure of the scientific process mirrors to some extent the "engineering" of the physical world. Thus the study of science must consider knowledge structures that science proposes and which the scientist, in myriad ways, disposes. When social scientists deny scientific reason a material role in their analysis, they face the prospect of fashioning ideologies and perpetuating myths about scientific processes.

This is not to insist that only the scientist active in a specialty can uncover the research structure of particular problem domains. Our analytical tools for understanding the growth of knowledge often differ from the perspectives of active researchers. For instance, O'Connor contends that the discovery of RT was delayed "by a failure to properly interpret data available by 1967" (1973: 1177).[17] But like prematurity, it would appear that the relevance of data controls their interpretation. What one needs to know is how information comes to be seen as relevant to nurturing its development through the production of knowledge claims, and not how the active researcher imagines it *could* have been.

Nevertheless, for the active researcher, imagination is coupled with high social stakes. How (or whether) one acquires a sense of relevance or timing of one's research may determine who anticipates and who replicates the work of whom. Remember that Watson, the Nobel laureate, and central dogmatist of molecular biology, too, was not aware of the importance of the virological research being conducted in the early 1960s. If relevance is the social catalyst of knowledge and reward, then Spiegelman's (1970) remark that the real goal of the war on cancer is to help cure leukemia and not to spend a weekend in Stockholm expresses the tension that exists between knowledge and social reward. There is no need to deny either aspect of this reality in order to develop a theory of scientific growth. Indeed, that is what a sociology of knowledge specialization is all about.

NOTES

1. All eigenvectors reported in this chapter have been computed using subroutine EIGRS provided by the International Mathematical and Statistical Libraries (1975). The multidimensional scaling routine used for Figures 6.1 and 6.2 was the "Torgerson Multidimensional Scaling Program" (TORSCA; see Green and Carmone, 1970).

2. Specifically, the mean citations per article decline monotonically from 1971 to 1974 (10.8, 9.0, 3.3, .7). With the three-fold increase in the RT literature from 1972 to 1973, the number of article "targets" for citation has expanded to reduce the probability that a *particular* article will be cited. Admittedly, this assumes more randomness in citation than may be the case. For now we recognize that the more recent citation means are depressed by our truncation of the RT article set in 1975 (see Chapter 5, Note 3).

3. Articles in Appendix D and Table 6.1 will be referred to by their respective identification numbers.

4. A common confusion which we shall not address here is the inferential leap made, on the basis of citation counts to articles, about the "quality" of authors. Even highly cited and venerated scholars produce—for whatever reason—poorly cited articles. Articles, after all, are discrete events. Yet the advantage of high status and visibility (which bears on citation behavior) accumulates (Merton, 1968) to suggest that the quality of product, like its producer, never wavers. To the contrary, and to use Merton's phrase, we would argue that that attribution of quality involves a "misallocation of credit."

5. See Kaplan (1965) for an early statement of citation "etiquette" and Mulkay (1974a) for an update.

6. This is true, even though the linkages do not appear on the graph in Figure 6.1. The criteria for placing the linkages on the graph were arbitrary—20 or more cocitations are needed—with the remainder of the linkages implied when the eigenstructure is studied. In fact, more linkages could have been included in the graph but then one would not be able to interpret the linkages amid all the confusion of the lines. We could also have attempted to interpret more vectors but, as will be seen, the more vectors one considers, the less highly connected becomes the network. This indicates that we would be interpreting less and less strongly connected units within the network. As a rule, this is the case and, therefore, analysis must terminate at the

point at which minor network structures are encountered which seem uninterpretable. Yet there are no formal criteria that signal termination of analysis.

7. Spiegelman (1978) is adamant in calling "unjustifiable"

> the way *Nature* blew this thing [the discovery] up into violation of the Central Dogma. That's just a lot of nonsense. None of the molecular biologists involved . . . ever looked upon that as an impossible reaction. . . . John Tooze, who was then one of the writing editors for *Nature,* he of course knew of our work on hybridization . . . and he said, "If you want, we'll hold up the Baltimore-Temin papers until yours is ready and we can publish all three in the same issue." And I said, "No, they made the discovery and this really confirms and extends it, true"–because I had the key piece of information–but frankly, if I had made the discovery I would not have published until I had done the hybridization.

8. As recounted in Chapter 4, Green based his prediction of a protein capsid in the virus on the then-unpublished data of NCI microbiologist Bader whose inhibitor research paralleled that of Temin since 1965.

9. Meadows and O'Connor, in their research on pulsar literature, lend support to our argument. They argue:

> In the initial stages of a new growth area only a few scientific groups are likely to participate in the research. Hence, to begin with, the literature available for citing by any group will be to a significant extent that group's own work. As time passes and more scientists are attracted into a new area, the proportion of the literature due to any given group of authors must decrease. Thus, the self-citation rate should be above average at first, decreasing gradually to the normal level for the field [1971: 97].

But if such is the case, then cocitations cannot be taken at face value as indicative of the intellectual state of a field, specialty, or problem domain. Cocitation clusters may simply be isolating the early institutional contexts of scientific development, that is, the most "coherent groups" (Griffith and Mullins, 1972) and, later, the most visible "invisible colleges."

10. We will refer to positive (*) and negative (#) numbers on the eigenvector tables only to facilitate identification. Of course, because eigenvectors give relative solutions to a set of equations, they are accurate only to within a sign change. In other words the signs could all be reversed within an eigenvector and not change the relative position of any element.

11. Of course, by using as choosing (referencing) articles only those found within the RT set, there is necessarily a de-emphasis on articles which do not deal directly with the enzyme. This also precludes viewing how the precise confluence occurred, for example, from the electron microscopy of Moore to the reverse transcription analysis of Spiegelman's group.

12. Recall the Rorschach-like qualities of the oncogene theory reviewed in Chapter 4: It elicited a range of interpretation by our interviewees.

13. By posing this question, we are adopting the posture that citation is a measure of intellectual indebtedness or utility and that the etiquette of selective referencing follows accordingly. Citation proponents (e.g., Weinstock, 1971) concede that the motivations which prompt citation are many; as critics and skeptical users of citation data, we hereby express our concern over the signal-to-noise ratio in the measure and proceed with fingers crossed.

14. If this line of thought were pursued, one might be able to develop a minimax theorem for maximizing one's citation count.

15. It has often been argued that the Darwinian and DNA discoveries are exemplary of the Kuhnian (Kuhn, 1962) concept of a paradigmatic revolution (see Greene, 1971; Ruse, 1970, 1971a, 1971b). Certainly those attracted to such views would find it difficult to consider Lowry's work of the same ground-breaking caliber. But if one's criteria shift to the structure of relevance within specialties and disciplines and take into account the ability of a discovery to facilitate further research and ideas, then certainly Lowry et al. can justifiably be mentioned in the same breath with Crick and Watson. When the theory of relevance changes, so must the theory of greatness.

16. As we have seen, however, this evidence was disputed and dismissed by most, then resisted until the multiple independent discovery of the RNA-directed DNA polymerase occurred.

17. Many of our interviewees echoed this sentiment, adding that everything is "easy" and "obvious" in retrospect. Hindsight is a great humbler, as some of the RT researchers wistfully acknowledged.

EPILOGUE: THE PLACE OF KNOWLEDGE IN SCIENTIFIC GROWTH

> Proponents of the "autonomy" of biology have called attention to many features of their science which do exist, and which mark differences between it and the physical sciences. Thus, for example, biology does characteristically deal with that subject matter in a more "concrete" way (in its "richness" and "fullness") than does physics. Yet these differences have tended to be misunderstood. . . . I have argued that these differences arise fundamentally from the fact that biology deals with entities and interactions whose character makes difficult (not "impossible") the application of techniques which are employed easily and fruitfully in physics. Employment of those techniques is, however, not logically precluded in biology, since ingenuity, factual discoveries, mathematical innovations, and refinement of problems can all make useful application of them feasible. Thus, when properly understood, these differences do not justify the extravagant conclusions that have often been drawn from them, regarding, for example, the "uniqueness" of biological subject matter, the "essentially historical "character of its explanations, and, in general, the irreducibility of biology to physics.
>
> Shapere (1969a: 15)

Introduction

The preceding six chapters represent not merely the unfolding of a research journey, but the development of a framework for conceptualizing growth and change in biomedical science. By tapping biologists' concerns—as expressed in print and in informal conversations—about the social and intellectual structures of their research, we have wrought from a case study a view which diverges from more traditional views of scientific growth. Unlike analysts who have studied the *bigness* of modern science on a macroscopic level (e.g., Weinberg, 1961; Price, 1975; Holton, 1962; Menard, 1971), we followed the path distinguished by less aggregated units and analysts (e.g., Price, 1963; Crane, 1972; Griffith and Mullins, 1972). Hence, we focused on cell transformation research (in Part I) and a rationale for narrowing our scope further to the subspecialty level of the problem domain of RT (in Part II). In many respects, we found that the latter path was not very well-trodden. For even the critics of the (exponential-logistic) curve-fitting approach (notably Rose, 1967; Gilbert and Woolgar, 1974; Studer, 1977a) write as though the growth of scientific knowledge is synonymous with the growth of research communities that produce that knowledge. Here at the micro-level, the sociology of communication networks has replaced what Barnes (1977) aptly calls "the potency of ideas and knowledge" as the key to scientific development.

Where, then, has *knowledge* gone? Have we subtly substituted the problems of the network approach (e.g., scientific growth as a process of information transmission among technical specialists) for the question of how novel ideas (discoveries, new syntheses, and so on) are conceived and modified, shared, negotiated, and recognized? Have we so methodologized the objects of science that we are content to measure them as products and structures, bundles of cultural artifacts? This is surely an implicit assertion of this study. Now we make the assertion explicit: *The place of knowledge has been lost in the study of scientific growth. The centrality of ideas as a prime mover or rationale for research activity has been denied.* With this denial comes not only an intellectual or disciplinary division of labor but also a substitution of products for process, a "phrenology" of science[1] instead of a penetrating gaze inside the "black box" of science (Whitley, 1972).

If knowledge explains the social phenomena we take as indicative of scientific growth, then it is mandatory to approach the products and structures of a scientific community through the cognitive content of its esoteric objects and through the cognitive orientations of those who produce, make claims about and ultimately certify that content as new or obsolete knowledge. Thus, schematically, the knowledge process is seen as an independent variable that interacts with the environing (i.e., wider societal or sociocultural) context to determine the form of scientific growth. Social forms are the visible measurable results or traces of the knowledge process. To describe these forms or structures of or within a scientific community is to report a number of "runs, hits, and errors." But these results may bear little resemblance to the sequence of events and processes leading to the "final" tally. Here the analogy crumbles. The point of baseball is to score; the "scores" of interest to us must be directly implicated in the continuing growth or deterioration of science.

In our analysis of the RT domain, we have (1) sought to restore knowledge to a central place in the study of scientific growth; (2) focused on the content of biomedical research, particularly that of cell transformation and cancer virology, as a guide to measuring change in social forms or structures; and (3) entertained the possibility that observed social patterns may defy generalization across all science or for all time. (After all, we have dwelled on the history of a *single* research domain in the *modern* era of *biomedicine.*) These three objectives are by no means independent. They virtually restate the same proposition: Blanket explanations of scientific growth are unfounded because sciences differ in their cognitive objects, technical (or evidential) norms, and resultant knowledge claims—in short, their rationality.

Rationality refers to the process of scientific argumentation, peculiar logic, or "ways of knowing" which characterizes a domain and, perhaps, whole regions of science. As used throughout our study, rationality is no mere appendage to the scientific "organism"; it is the heart of scientific process (see Laudan, 1977). Further, rationality is the feature of a science which enhances *our understanding* of scientific growth; it is the basis for the accumulation and obsolescence—the progress—of knowledge. If one does not *begin* with an appreciation and understanding of the scientific argumentation process in a domain, one's end product will be an interpretation of a social aggregate which incidentally happens to do science. The reason for its *communitas* will be lacking; it will be *denied.* But if "the characteristic of scientific action is the predominance of cognitive orientation" (Boehme, 1975: 214), then it is both pretentious and intellectually untenable for the sociologist to *replace* rationality with "explanatory" variables that are social, psychological, political, or economic in nature or origin (see Boehme, 1977).

There are difficulties, of course, in maintaining this view (which Bhaskar, 1975, calls "transcendental realism").[2] Contemporary sociology and philosophy, for example, have found common grounds for merging the cognitive with the social aspects of science (see Scheffler, 1967, and below), thereby, vitiating the need to understand the argumentation process of new knowledge—especially as a potential generator of structures in science. In what follows we shall employ evidence from our case study to (1) review various formulations and analyses of scientific growth and (2) extend a "confluence theory" of knowledge growth in which lines of research are seen as converging on specific problems to create "problems domains." A domain, we reiterate, is an intellectual entity, a nexus of research interests at a subspecialty, noninstitutional(ized) level, formed by multidisciplinary confluences for relatively brief durations (seldom exceeding five years). We maintain that unless processes of confluence are captured, the sociologist will resort to viewing paradigm communities and theory groups as the primary units of science and scientific growth since these units coincide with the group structures sociologists are trained to perceive and examine.

In contrast, confluence theory suggests it is not the development of such groups—their unity and differentiation—which underlies scientific growth, but rather the ability of diverse lines of research to converge and mingle within a cognitive region on a specific problem set.[3] Ironically, this ability can be contorted, stymied, or obstructed altogether by institutionalized policies (e.g., the war on cancer), which earmark funds for targeted research programs (e.g., NCI's Virus Cancer Program) at the expense of others. The effect is to impose on scientific rationality an "idealistic" mode of organization which, though successful in *other* sciences, is alien to that particular region (e.g., biomedicine) or unit (e.g., the lab or team) of science. It is these kinds of constraints that render a case study of a biomedical problem domain instructive far beyond its seemingly modest limits of generalization (Chubin, 1978b: Introduction). For not only can we refine a confluence theory of scientific growth but we can also relate that theory to the ongoing debates over (1) relativism and realism in science studies, (2) the role of micro-level studies in the construction and evaluation of science policy, and, finally, (3) the conceptualization, measurement, and meaning of scientific growth.[4]

Relativism and Realism in the Sociology of Science

It is easy to view the problems of realism and relativism as essentially philosophical questions that are beyond the scope of sociological methodology.[5] Analysts of scientific growth—whether they admit it or not—can ill-afford the luxury of disciplinary parochialism, however. If the sociologist's all-encompassing views of society do lead to a social relativism, it is the philosopher's comprehensive view of theorizing within science that has paved the way to that relativism (see Laudan, 1977; Doppelt, 1977). Specifically, the distinction between observational and theoretical terms (see Shapere, 1969b, 1974), which philosophers have routinely made in the past, is now being seen more and more from the perspective of theory. If, as in the case of Kuhn (1962), all observational terms are seen as theory-dependent, then scientific statements become relative to the theoretical context in which they occur. In such a situation, reference to objects in the real world can become incommensurable with other statements which make use of the same terms but in a different theoretical context.

In this philosophical framework, the scientific world is decomposed into theory groups, research communities, and specialties with their own scientific identities—a philosophical affinity with the sociology of science that Kuhn (1970, 1974) explicitly recognizes. It would appear that much of this affinity can be traced to a common mode of theorizing about science and society. Indeed, the Kuhnian terminology is quite attractive to the sociologist because it couches scientific progress in terms of religious and organizational metaphors; the theory-dependent view of science and the social relativism of sociology come to occupy common ground. Therefore, it should not be surprising to find more than one critic of Kuhn (e.g., Scheffler, 1967; Brush, 1974) suggesting that by sociologizing science, Kuhn has undermined the very belief in reality upon which science is based.

Because of the entrenchment within sociology and philosophy of a relativistic mode of viewing science, it is incumbent upon the analyst to understand how this view delimits analyses of science. An attempted reformulation would be of value merely as a heuristic device, but in the following we shall argue that by approaching the analysis of science from a realistic perspective—à la Bhaskar (1975) and Shapere (1974)—the sociologist can do greater justice to understanding the structure of scientific growth. The full importance of such a shift in analytical procedure cannot be fully appreciated, of course, until sufficient research has been completed.[6]

For us, a more realistic evaluation of scientific growth is encompassed in the conceptualization and study of problem domains. In the present context of the philosophy-sociology of science interface, Shapere's discussion of "scientific theories and their domains" is most instructive:

> The concept of a domain is intended to replace the old "observational-theoretical" distinction as a fundamental conceptual tool for illuminating the nature of science. "That which is to be accounted for" includes, especially at sophisticated stages of scientific development (and thus at those stages where characteristically scientific

reasoning is most apparent and predominant), elements from both the traditional "observational" and "theoretical" categories [1974: 528].

The distinction between theoretical terms and observational terms has resulted in the absorption of all references to entities. The concept of a domain refocuses the issue for Shapere emphasizing that

> The items of a domain are generally problematic not in isolation but rather through being *related* to other such items in a body about which the problem exists: scientific research is in such cases generated by items in association with one another, rather than by "facts" in isolation from one another. Philosophers of science, working within a tradition according to which all "facts" are "atomic," have been blinded to this primary source of scientific problems [1974: 530].

By shifting philosophical interest to the problem content of science rather than to isolated facts being assimilated into theories, Shapere is able to view the shifts in the structure of relevant research. Shapere's discussion of the development of the periodic table of chemical elements clearly displays how the domain of relevance expands within a region of science. As ideas developed regarding the nature of particles, their atomic weight, and their possible structures,

> Expectation increased in strength until it reached the status of a *demand,* reinforced by the following considerations: (a) more and more other areas revealed themselves as domains in which an atomistic explanation was expected (for example, the case of chemical spectroscopy . . .); (b) atomistic explanations became more and more successful (statistical mechanics) or at least more and more promising (Kelvin's vortex atom was applied in a great many areas) in other domains; and (c) reasons accumulated, . . . for suspecting the domain under consideration (the chemical elements related through the periodic table) to be itself related, as part of a larger-domain, to others, including ones in which atomistic explanations were either expected, demanded, or actually provided [Shapere, 1974: 540].

By focusing on the domain of research, therefore, we visualize the confluences which make scientific progress possible. In the case of the periodic table, developments in other areas had raised expectations; there was an anticipation of discovery. Likewise, we found review articles in RT attempting to capture the expectations of the domain; they foreshadow the convergence of lines of research and what must be done to accomplish certain theoretical and research tasks. Thus, adumbrations of the sphere of relevance seem to be present even before discoveries occur and tell us something about problem selection or "demand" for answers.[7]

Shapere's analysis of the structure of domains within chemistry and physics is so very instructive because it suggests that a confluence theory may have wider applicability than we originally suspected. Shapere's (1969a) analysis of biology shows that his views extend to this region of science as well; his views also demonstrate no attempt to defend the uniqueness of various regions on any grounds *except* the objects which they study. Hence, any similarity of domain structures must be credited to either the stage in the growth of knowledge or the nature of the observed objects within a science. The point of comparison between domains does not rest upon similarities of theoretical formulations or social structure which have emerged, but rather in the structuring processes within the domain itself. The region-specific confluence processes associated with various lines of inquiry within a domain should provide the *eventual* basis for comparative research within science studies. (Emboldened by our case study, we prefer to restrict generalizability to biomedical problem domains.)

By now it may appear that the differences between domains must reside ultimately in the nature of the object under investigation. In this light, Smart has precipitated a most interesting debate by trying "to show that the important analogy is not between biology and the physical sciences, but between biology and the technologies, such as electronics" (1963: 52):

> If it is asked whether biology can be made an exact science the answer is "No more and no less than technology." If by an "exact science" is meant one with strict laws and unitary theories of its own, then the search for an exact biological science is a wild-goose chase. We do not have laws and theories of electronics or chemical engineering, and engineers do not worry about the lack. They see that their subjects get scientific exactness from the application of the sciences of physics and chemistry. No one wishes to axiomatize electronics. Why should Woodger have wished to axiomatize genetics? There are no real laws of biology for the very same reason that there are no special "laws of engineering" [Smart, 1963: 57].

The view of biological laws which Smart espouses is, of course, debatable (see Ruse, 1973; Schaffner, 1969), but the essential point of his argument is that the real world of biology involves organizational principles which differentiate it from the physical and chemical sciences. Because the object is different, the science is different.[8] If this is true, then one should expect the confluence patterns within biomedicine to differ from those in other regions of science. That most theories within the sociology of science have been erected with the natural sciences as a "paragon" should engender questions, if Smart is correct, concerning the relevance of traditional sociological analysis to biology (see Martins, 1972). If sociology is to account effectively for the "object world" of biological thought, it must acknowledge the idiosyncratic relationships between the organization of biological entities and biological thought.

EVIDENTIAL NORMS AND BIOLOGICAL PROBLEM DOMAINS

Our survey of the intellectual foci within RT research (Chapter 4) illustrated that the systemic properties of the object world, for example, viral-cellular interactions, played a vital role in directing research. For example, Temin's criticism of the oncogene theory suggested that it was essentially epigenetic, and therefore unnecessary, given the genetic structure of cells. Similarly, the evidential norms Baltimore stated represented a method of "capturing" certain systemic properties within the problem domain. If the discovery of RT did not prove the DNA provirus hypothesis, it was because other possibilities could exist within the systemic structure of the cell. RT might be present but not needed by the RNA virus. Hill and Hillova may have consummated the systemic analysis, but the biological system "provided" a definition of the relevant lines of research which were needed for scientific advancement. Was it the object world or the theoretical structures of paradigm groups which ultimately focused research and gave extant theoretical models of the region a relevance or meaningful baseline for comparison within one of its domains?

Consider further this relationship between cognitive regions and problem domains: in the case of RT, the evidential norms undergirding the developmental process of virology yielded several insights. First, it can be argued that such norms illuminate a course of research events. Without such norms the biologist would not know when research results were fortuitous; the normal process provides the background for interpreting "irregularities" (not "anomalies") in the progress of research.

Second, such norms allow for a variety of theoretical perspectives to coexist within a problem domain. They allow communication across seemingly "incommensurable" paradigms (Kuhn, 1962) by asserting the existence of a test criterion. Because the test criterion must reflect biological reality, it will often, as in the case of the provirus hypothesis, implicate other relevant research problems of a region, for example, in embryology, bacteriology, or molecular biology.

Third, the founding of research strategies upon evidential norms allows researchers to put knowledge claims in perspective. Temin's lamentation, "My hypothesis was essentially ignored," can be interpreted in terms of its evidential maturity. Temin's theory was not *premature*—prematurity is a judgment that can be made only after the fact of scientific progress (see Chapter 1)—it was *immature.* To use an analogy, to throw out the Central Dogma would have been like discarding the Newtonian system when the orbit of Uranus was seen to deviate from the expected path. At this juncture in the developmental process, it was much more rational to attempt to search for a Neptune which would account for the discrepancy, rather than to dispose of a profitable working hypothesis (see Richter, 1972). In other words, there is often *good reason* for the "resistance by scientists to scientific discovery" (see Barber, 1961; Barnes, 1972). In the case of the provirus hypothesis, acceptance would have required a scientific decision which could potentially undermine a very fruitful line of research.[9] To argue convincingly for the provirus hypothesis, one would need the freedom provided by evidential norms *outside* of molecular biology, for example, in enzymology, virology, or oncology. Indeed, Baltimore (1976b) states that he "approached the problem of the virus' effect on intracellular RNA synthesis as a question in enzymology," later describing his RT research as a "foray into tumor virology." "Luckily," he observes, "I had no experience in the field and so no axe to grind." By shifting the context of analysis under the rubric of enzymology, the rules of the game (for him and, soon thereafter, for others) had shifted. As an enzyme, RNA-directed DNA polymerase could be intrinsically interesting. But after the enzyme was discovered, virologists resisted claims that the DNA provirus hypothesis had been *confirmed.* Not so. For the evidence for the existence of an enzyme was not the same as the evidence required to explain the genetic system of a virus. The knowledge claims made by researchers find meaning only against the background of a set of evidential norms. And sometimes by shifting one's focus to a "neighboring" set of norms, that is, current in another domain, one can solve, as Baltimore did, a question that had previously seemed intractable.

The relevance of evidential norms to the exploration and/or potential solution of problems in a domain resides in the "openness" of a cognitive region. Within biology, evidential norms may be defined "regionally" and can be readily brought to bear on a neighboring domain. In other words, evidential norms seem to constitute a class of Mulkay's (1969) "cognitive and technical norms," perhaps as norms "in action" applied to a particular problem. Their application, to use Mulkay's (1976) subsequent normative terminology, is part of the "evaluative repertoire" of scientists. Just as certain vocabularies are invoked to persuade nonscientific audiences of the value of esoteric research, *other* vocabularies are invoked to convince one's fellow researchers that the evidence specific to a region, for example, from a neighboring discipline or domain, has relevance, indeed may represent key information for the problem at hand and its domain.[10] Evidential norms thus embed the object world of biological thought; by mirroring biological reality in evidential norms, biomedicine itself reflects what comes to be perceived, as seen in preceding chapters, as a distinctively "biological" mode of cognitive organization.[11] But the expression of this rationality or process of argumentation differs with the audience to be addressed, that is, the rhetorical vocabulary is adapted for nonscientists, nondisciplinarians, or inhabitants of neighboring domains as the situation demands.

SEPARATION OF THE INTELLECTUAL AND SOCIAL ASPECTS OF SCIENCE: A RECONNAISSANCE

Social adaptations to scientific reality raise anew a theoretical issue that derives from the relativism-realism debate: the possibility or desirability of separating empirically the intellectual from the social aspects of science. In the foregoing, we have stipulated (redundantly) that the object world of biomedicine constrains the research process—its problems, logic of inquiry, and the configuration of practitioners who converge thereon. Thus, we have affirmed that the intellectual (content) must be used to inform analyses of the social (structure) in science. To do so, the analyst must examine *processes* by which content is negotiated by scientists—in terms of their beliefs, interests, allegiances, and positions (both within and outside of science).

Our response to the separation issue is forthright: Separation is both *im*possible and *un*desirable. This is not to say, however, that these two aspects of science can be treated as one; they should not. Too often, such treatments ignore content and measure structure,[12] concluding that scientific "progress," "development," or "growth" has occurred. In reality, neither aspect nor the interplay of both has been illuminated. Rather, the growth of knowledge has gone *un*measured, with scientific progress an artifact of measurement (for the policy implications of such artifacts, see Cole and Cole, 1972; Turner and Chubin, 1976; and below).

Allocating guilt or alleging ideological commitment by self-interested analysts to the belief that science *is* developing is not our purpose; a recasting of the separation issue *is*. Indeed, those who envision science as a relatively autonomous social system (e.g., Storer, 1966, 1974) and those who consider it essentially a politically determined system (e.g., Ravetz, 1971; Blume, 1974, 1977) seem to present incompatible views on it. Furthermore, it is questionable whether *either* of these two approaches addresses the issue of cognition and society. The manner in which sociologists formulate the issue is more reminiscent of an ethical issue—Who has the right to exercise moral authority over science?—than of a problem of discovery through sociological research. As Bendix states,

> In an era of mounting scarcities (or what comes to the same, our awareness of mounting scarcities), the old assumptions become less and less serviceable. As long as the private pursuit of knowledge yielded public benefits, the question of priorities could be ignored and the pluralism of seeking knowledge wherever it might lead enjoyed. But when priorities become pressing, choices must be made and these encroach sooner or later upon the bastions of academic freedom. The old equation of progress and knowledge is in jeopardy and the road ahead is lost in the twilight [1975: 358].

Thus, whatever one may argue about the early development of science and its social determination, one is faced with the *new* reality of the politics and economics of science. Those who maintain that science is autonomous would point to the distinctive institutional norms and social structures present within the scientific community; those who are intent on defending the political nature of science can find enough examples of deviance and anomaly to "prove" their point. But both views are, in fact, concerned with the social, not the cognitive. It is the autonomous research community versus the socially and politically determined research community which becomes, for us anyway, a surrogate issue. This issue has been defined in terms of the social control of *social* systems, not in terms of the relationship of social controls to a *cognitive* system. Bendix and others are concerned with the shifting social acceptance and control of science rather than with the interactions of knowledge and social structure (see Studer and Chubin, 1977). Once again, both views *assume* a relationship between cognition and social structure but fail to formulate the question so that the relationship itself can be brought under scrutiny (see Mendelsohn et al., 1979).

In Chapter 3 of the RT case study, the political context of the U.S. war on cancer was discussed, including scientists' commentary on this massive research effort. What emerged from that discussion was that a federally endorsed organizational structure *could* overwhelm scientists' testimony concerning the rationality of biological research. The confluences liberated by the evidential norms found within biomedicine seemed (often unwittingly) to be jeopardized by a linear, mission-oriented approach to problem solving. The political issues were indeed epistemological issues for the scientists. But most of the biologists who voiced opposition to the new funding policies were not powerless members of a faceless mass of scientists; they were individuals with much responsibility, eminence, and clout within their respective research communities. What is significant, moreover, is that even with direct political involvement of the biomedical community, the main issues were still discussed (with aplomb) in terms of the discovery process and the evolution of research programs in biomedicine. It was the problem of progress—cure, prevention, and control—that was at issue. The demands of the logic-in-use of the biologists were on display within the context of politics but, at the same time, the biologist-witnesses enjoyed an autonomy accorded experts (see Nelkin, 1975b) which was conducive to criticism of the political process when it impinged upon established prerogatives. Among those prerogatives was *not* the earmarking of funds for cancer research—that was a foregone conclusion—but the making of a policy which would disburse those funds in an intellectually responsible way. Yes, there was rhetoric, but rhetoric asserting cognitive autonomy in the midst of an overriding social (political) determination.

The cynical view is that, assured of a booty (if not a blank check) to conduct cancer research for the foreseeable future, the scientists could well afford to mouth a pious vocabulary. Instead, the targeting of cancer research as the paramount research priority raised a specter of success, a climate of expectation, and visibility that the biomedical community refused to endorse. They had spoken as scientists, not as organization men. They were to be allies of the federal bureaucracy in the war on cancer; the Cancer Act of 1971 was the legislative declaration of that war. Science was being called to battle with a strategy that the scientists insisted could not win, at least not in the urgent time frame that the political process had mandated. The object world is at the beck and call of no government, however. We learned that for some of those pushed, or led, into battle, the evidential norms *had* been violated and research reduced to contract drudgery. Yet for others, no change in work tempo had occurred; the research challenge was as exhilarating as ever; the coincidence of mission and norms, timely.

What about progress–the burden of the war, the promise to win? How does one measure this one albeit special dimension of scientific growth? We have no cures, but a growing archive of literature. Through a politically abetted multiplicity of effort, competition has intensified, expediting discovery, if not directly producing it (Merton, 1961; Gaston, 1973). So the timetable for apprehending scientific reality, that is, producing new claims to knowledge of it, *can* be nudged ahead, even if the justification for doing so is dubious.

To restate the crux of our argument, the analytical separation of the cognitive and the social in science can inform our inferences about the growth of knowledge only insofar as social structure is neither accorded primacy over nor substituted for intellectual content. There is, however, a reciprocity of content and structure that must be captured in the measurement of process. Whitley for instance, emphasizes that he does

> not intend a separation of the cognitive from the social where scientists' cognitive activity is seen as unconnected to their social actions. On the contrary, I am concerned with the different modes of connection between these aspects. Scientists are social beings and science is a social activity. In distinguishing cognitive institutionalization from social institutionalization, I am suggesting it is fruitful to analyze differences in the extent of coherence and cohesion between intellectual products, their mode of production, and the social circumstances surrounding their production, evaluation and revision [1974: 71].

The basic analytical separation in Whitley's view between cognitive and social institutionalization resembles the concern of the biomedical community for the imposition of organizational structures on the rationality of their science. If Whitley's views and those of the anti-cancer war biologists are correct, then social analyses of scientific growth qua research activity would have to undergo substantial revision.

Recall that the conventional view of scientific growth features a "stage" process. Crane (1972) argues, for instance, that the logistic *growth* of science proceeds through four basic stages; Mullins (1973) likewise postulates that there are four stages to network *development:* normal, network, cluster, and specialty; and Clark (1972) suggests five stages of scientific *institutionalization:* the solitary scientist, amateur science, emerging academic science, established science, and Big Science. All of these developmental schema, and the others reviewed by Edge and Mulkay (1976), prescribe that the growth of specialties and disciplines follows a certain *social* order. Thus, despite the fact that networks are being referred to, a linear pattern of development is posited. The correlation of social and intellectual characteristics—in form and content—is assumed to be high. But Whitley observes:

> I see no reason to suggest that monistic, highly institutionalized specialties are any more "mature" or "scientific" than others. There is no inevitable tendency towards higher institutionalization in all specialties and it would be unduly restrictive to insist on a linear model of cognitive development leading to greater consensus and "normality" in all situations. *The cognitive and social conditions under which specialty cognitive institutionalization takes place are problematic and await investigation* [1972: 86; italics added].

In other words, what needs investigation is *assumed* to be true by most analysts because the knowledge component of science has become identified with its social component. Knowledge growth has been subsumed under scientific growth; the formalization of policy governing the institutionalization of structures that produce knowledge sanctions the measurement of those structures as *indicative* of scientific growth. But the epistemological requirements for the production of knowledge and the formation of problem domains go unmeasured. What underlies institutional manifestations of growth is assumed to exist in one-to-one correspondence with those structural manifestations. Whither knowledge? Whither the preinstitutionalized, ephemeral biological problem domains? Has scientific growth been so equated with institutionalized forms that knowledge, rationality, and evidential norms—the object world—are rendered impotent, incidental epiphenomena to social forms? We think so.

Even Whitley's concern with institutionalization belies his sensitivity to the inversion of the cognitive and the social. By beginning with the "problem situation," Whitley does seem to have recognized the problem of domain formation, that is, the need to analyze a less visible and coherent form of cognitive organization:

> It is doubtful if such highly socially and cognitively institutionalized specialties are representative of all activities we term "scientific." By whatever criteria that honorific title is bestowed, it seems possible that the statistical norm of specialty structure may prove rather less institutionalized than, say, solid state physics or inorganic chemistry.

> The difficulty that biologists, in particular, have in naming their specialty attests to the ambiguity of cognitive and social structures in this field and may well occur in others. *Here, a multiplicity of models, techniques and contradictory results is to be expected and controversy about relatively fundamental points endemic* [Whitley, 1972: 80; italics added].

Surely the task must be to analyze the "multiplicity of models" and discover why results often seem to be "contradictory" in the biological sciences (see Mullins, 1968). What is needed is case specifics and not premature generalizations about (1) similarities that scientific domains share (e.g., Griffith and Mullins, 1972; Law, 1973); (2) the inferiority of biological organization relative to more mature sciences (e.g., Allison and Stewart, 1974); or (3) the more-than-adequate measurement of scientific growth through "the literature explosion" and the innovative citation indicators thus begotten (e.g., Garfield et al., 1977). The task of ascertaining the growth of knowledge is far more challenging (Gilbert, 1978). Few analysts have yet to recognize the challenge, much less cope with it; we think, realistically, we have begun to do so.

A Confluence Theory: Genesis and Evidence

If a realistic epistemology has guided our study of a contemporary biomedical problem domain, the genesis of this approach can be traced to a corpus of evidence within the history of biology. This evidence is by no means confined to cancer virology or even viral genetics; hence, it lends credence to an inchoative confluence theory of problem domain formation and the subsequent growth of knowledge within and beyond such domains. A partial recounting of this evidence, we believe, should precede further claims that confluence is a pervasive process of innovation in biology and not just a configuration of serendipitous events related to RT.[13]

We begin by quoting Teich's observation that

> Proneness to specialization and tendency to overcome it have been a marked feature of scientific history. But perhaps never before did so many specialists, at least in Britain and the U.S.A., with varied scientific background think about and work side by side on common problems as during the Second World War. Through these experiences the value of cross-fertilization of ideas and techniques was confirmed [1975: 273].

What Teich makes clear is that "common problems" have helped define the convergence of ideas from different socially defined specialties. World War II was the social occasion for convergence, but the structure of the argumentation process within science is what made such cross-fertilization fruitful. Similarly, the "intellectual migrations" to which Olby (1974b) refers are the multiple paths to the double helix, that is, the product of a successful cross-fertilization of relevant lines of inquiry.[14]

Attempts to exploit (and refute) Kuhn's (1962) classic analysis of the scientific community in understanding the impact of Darwin (Greene, 1971; Ruse, 1970, 1971a) and *modern* molecular biology (Ruse, 1971a, 1971b) have also proved illuminating of the process in question. Although Greene is circumspect about the applicability of Kuhn's framework to the work of Darwin, the philosopher Ruse asserts that Darwin indeed manifests all the characteristics of Kuhn's paradigm shift:

> The Darwinian revolution stands, to some extent, *outside the bounds of reason.* Reason, like games, requires rules. Since the argument was not conducted within rules, but was about rules, reason in a strict sense was not applicable here. One had rather to choose one's side by something akin to a "*leap of faith*" [1971a: 20; italics added].

When it comes to the advent of molecular biology, however, Ruse claims:

> The reason for the change came not from the fact that classical biology became riddled with anomaly, or unwieldy through the addition of *ad hoc* hypotheses expressly added to eliminate anomaly, and that biologists were thus driven to embrace molecular biology, but from the fact that biological investigation had *led to the study of smaller and smaller phenomena and that eventually it seemed pointless to explain these phenomena by purely biological concepts,* when there were already at hand scientific theories specifically designed to account for phenomena of the same order of magnitude, albeit nonorganic phenomena. . . . Hence I would suggest that the cause of the molecular revolution was a function of the merits of molecular biology, rather than a failure of classical biology. Thus here also, Kuhn's thesis does not find support [1971a: 36; italics added].

This is why Ruse sees the relationship between classical and molecular biology as one of "reduction" (or "informal reduction") even though, strictly speaking, he sees the relationship between the two biologies as one of replacement (Ruse, 1971b).

Yet the flaw in Ruse's analysis is exposed if one entertains a theory of the intertwining of the biological rationality with biological reality. Certainly Darwin's and also Crick and Watson's contributions are not denigrated if the paths of research which brought them to their discoveries are carefully traced. This does not imply a fixation on "precursoritis" (Shapere, 1966) as opposed to a revolutionary view of science; it simply argues that for the discoveries of Darwin and of Watson and Crick to be *recognized as discoveries,* lines of research must have confirmed the essential "truth" of their findings (see Bourdieu, 1975). By insisting that significant discoveries consistently lie "outside the bounds of reason," or by simply affirming that older points of view seemed "pointless," one eliminates the "good reasons" (see Shapere, 1974) which scientists can give for scientific change. It is, in fact, the same type of reasoning process which places in high esteem so-called premature discoveries within science. For if a theory such as that proposed by Temin in 1964 (the DNA provirus hypothesis) later proves tenable, then Temin can be viewed as "ahead of his time." But such prematurity is misunderstood if the broader domain which focuses the reasoning process is not taken into account. If prematurity is meaningful at all it must be understood in the context of anticipation which various lines of research have created and which seem to *demand* answers. Again Shapere captures the spirit of the process:

> One might even speak here of a general principle of non-rejection of theories: that when a discrepancy is found between the predictions of the theory and the results of observation or experiment, do not reject the theory as fundamentally incorrect before examining areas of the theory in which simplifications have been made which might be responsible for the discrepancy [1974: 167].

On this basis there was good reason to "detain" Temin's DNA provirus hypothesis until the implications of the Central Dogma were allowed to play out.

The crucial point is that if one understands the reason why "scientific revolutions" may be perceived retrospectively in science, then one can suggest *alternatives* to paradigm shifts, leaps of faith, and other discontinuities as explanations of the development of science. The fact that lines of research converge and create a context for recognizing discoveries when they do occur suggests a framework for rethinking scientific growth. Smart's contention that the biological world resembles an engineered product suggests some of the impediments to explaining the development of biological science.[15] The intertwining of various lines of research establishes a research strategy which "tacks" (to use a nautical metaphor) along various courses of understanding in order to arrive at the "destination" of biological progress.

The destinations of confluences, whether they demarcate prospective sites of scientific progress or not, are problem domains. Other analysts have conceptualized this "end product" as a repository of innovation and hypothesized the necessity of certain antecedent conditions. Among the more popular conditions to dominate studies of scientific innovation is "hybridization" (Ben-David, 1960; Ben-David and Collins, 1966). Though the focus of these studies has been trained upon social roles and institutionalization of disciplines, the spirit of the hybridization concept is most pertinent to a theory of confluence.

Mendelsohn, for example, has reinterpreted Ben-David's theory of role hybridization:

> As I look back at the history of biology, I might be led to ask where have major conceptual changes in the biological sciences come from, not in every field but in several important ones? They come very often from what I would call role hybrids—people who crossed from one field of science into another. What they seem to bring with them is the search for different types of clues and indeed a tradition of using different explanatory models and different modes of thought. *Their expectation of what might be considered an acceptable explanatory model is different from the expectations of the men whom they joined in their new area of research* [Mendelsohn, 1969: 136; italics added].

It is the role hybrid's "explanatory model" which "is different" because different evidential norms have been associated with the line of research from which he came. In Mendelsohn's view, it would appear that sometimes *lines of inquiry* crystallize in individuals ("look at Lavoisier, who in the eighteenth century brought to his analysis of respiration the insight and all of the tools of chemistry [Mendelsohn, 1969: 136])," consequently transplanting ways of thought which create major conceptual shifts. From this perspective, good reasons can be given for the efficacy of the underlying social process. The new view of the world actually accords with the object of scientific investigation; a new set of rules has been applied to the investigation of a problem and its explanatory power has proven effective in explaining a scientific reality.

Demarcating the hybridized science and its attendant intellectual roles and role incumbents, however, is *not* the issue. As Edge and Mulkay conclude:

> The three factors that Ben-David and Collins regard as particularly important in bringing about the differentiation of experimental psychology from philosophy, namely, the existence of a blocked career ladder in physiology, the difference in scientific repute between physiology and philosophy, and the activities of a group of migrants and converts who were committed to remodelling the latter discipline along the lines of the former, were *all absent* in radio astronomy. In addition there were two factors in the development of radio astronomy that fostered integration with the established discipline: namely, a considerable *cognitive overlap between the two groupings* and a *continuous and fruitful exchange* of information [1976: 368; italics added].

The emphases of Edge and Mulkay strike us as more than a *non* replication of findings; they represent a view of the real world as constraining scientists—in the fullest Durkheimian sense—to gravitate toward a mutual problem site, setting respective lines of inquiry on a confluence course. Assuming for a moment that hybrid sciences, such as astrophysics and biochemistry (the earliest of this genre, according to Ihde, 1969), need *not* be institutionalized disciplines, the following characterization could pass as a statement of confluence:

> Hybrid sciences have their origins in a unique stimulus. Certainly, the questions characterizing a hybrid science are in the air even if they are not being openly asked. The stimulus without the incipient questions would fall on sterile ground. The questions, however, are of very little significance as long as a reasonable mode of attack is not available [Ihde, 1969: 195].

It is the potential significance of cognitive tools that define them as relevant to a problem domain, triggering both the perception of a fruitful application in the minds of certain scientists and subsequently the confluence process (through intellectual mobility) itself. Consider an example from the history of cell transformation. Certainly Griffith's (1928) research on the transformation of pneumococcal types developed from a tradition of research in bacteriology and epidemiology, but it set in motion a very potent line of inquiry by calling into question research being conducted by Avery's group at the Rockefeller Institute. Griffith, throughout his career, seemed to be occupied with essentially epidemiological questions, and Avery's group maintained its interest in the transforming principle. Other lines of research also converged to create a new context for the specification of researchable questions. But when lines of inquiry converged and knowledge did advance, a new context for research advancement was created and not (necessarily) role hybrids. The normal convergence of knowledge of the real world with which scientists must deal, therefore, defines as rational and relevant the incorporation of divergent lines of research results into other lines of inquiry.[16] Perhaps this process crystallized around "great men" in the early stages of scientific development (Ben-David, 1971); we might better regard this, however, more as a historical "necessity" at the inception of science than the sine qua non of scientific growth today.

Another condition hypothesized as a necessary antecedent to growth in science is what Edge and Mulkay (1976) have called "marginal innovation" and "mobility." Indeed, these were the only noninstitutional factors common to the growth of the six specialties and disciplines they reviewed in *Astronomy Transformed.* That marginality and mobility are implicit in hybridization is no coincidence. The "marginal man," according to Park's definition, is "a cultural hybrid . . . living and sharing intimately in the cultural life and traditions of two distinct peoples" (1928: 892). As pointed out elsewhere (Chubin, 1976), the analogy is far from perfect; it is sufficiently heuristic, however, to extend the confluence theory.

As Kuhn (1962) intimated, and Schon (1963) and Mulkay (1974b) demonstrated, innovations in a science often come from outside its perceived boundaries. What is crucial, of course, is the *perception* that a novel idea and its bearer are marginal to a particular domain. Such perceptions of centrality or peripherality are hopelessly relativistic, regardless of the perspective one adopts. For example, if the significant intellectual unit is deemed to be a region rather than a problem domain, the definitions of marginality and mobility become far more restrictive, hence reducing the number of mobile cases observed.

We are dealing, however, with a more subtle phenomenon. Remember, novel ideas are transmitted all the time via the literature and the spoken word. More socially decisive is the transition of a *scientist* from one research area, network, or discipline to another. The movement of one with specialized expertise to a destination wherein his "cognitive baggage" is unpacked and his tools wielded in the solution or exploitation of a problem would label this scientist a migrant. Or would it? Hufbauer (1978) recently undertook an examination of the migration concept in the context of the stellar-energy problem, 1919-1938. Based on a dozen minibiographies, he concluded that the movement between physics and astronomy in this era qualifies the protagonist scientists as "interlopers" more frequently than as migrants. This status distinction is not merely semantic. For if the *career* mobility of researchers is traced, a truer picture of sequential change in intellectual activity emerges (see Garvey and Tomita, 1972; Gieryn, 1978). Whereas the interloper may dabble, the migrant will persist; the intellectual handiwork of both, however, will alter the state of the domain. It is because domains, like other scientific units, are *not* static that definitions of marginality and migration are constantly subject to change. After all, even if the coming together of researchers was marginal, they, in effect, formed a "center" (Shils, 1961) where formerly none existed.[17] As an intellectual process, it is the coming together of scientists (and not just their writings)[18] that renders a confluence theory not only plausible but also genuinely explicational.

Thus, the genesis of confluence are the cognitive norms of a (problem-defining) region[19] and the evidential norms which specify strategies of problem exploitation and solution. In this regard, it is telling that when management experts (Carrese and Baker, 1967) were called upon to organize the Special Virus Leukemia Program in 1965, they availed themselves of the *scientist's* understanding of the anticipated needs for various lines of research and took organizational cues from them (Carrese, 1978). The convergence technique which Carrese had developed effectively summarizes, on the one hand, the ability of scientists to anticipate the confluence of various research traditions; the degree to which such a program does *not* work, on the other hand, displays for us the time span over which anticipations can realistically operate. Perhaps one of the greatest differences between the physical sciences and the biological sciences may reduce to anticipations over time of their respective research needs, biology requiring a shorter span for anticipations than would the physical sciences (see Boehme et al., 1973). What we have already seen, for instance, is that even when Baltimore (1971) was anticipating the need for a direct proof of the DNA intermediary of RNA viruses, another line of research concerned with the uptake of DNA in cells (Hill and Hillova, 1974) was "prepared" to make a contribution. No Ben-Davidian role hybridization or quantum leap of insight was needed in this case because other researchers had been working on a similar problem (in a different context) for some time. It was the confluence of lines of research onto a problem site that solved the problem, and researchers in these areas continued to pursue their research according to a set of problem-solving evidential norms.

Genesis, however, is not maintenance. Indeed, we would be remiss not to consider briefly here the role of the external sociopolitical context in intensifying, perhaps expediting, the confluence process. Even prior to passage of the 1971 Cancer Act, NIH and NCI had earmarked money in programs like Virus (Leukemia) Cancer, and Cancer Chemotherapy. To deny the allure of research funds would be unpardonably naive. Yet the mercenary shadow cast across the so-called cancer establishment is too cynical; it does a disservice to both the establishment *and* its critics. Why? First, there is a question of capability: much biological research cannot even remotely be marketed under the cancer rubric. Second, even self-serving and rationalizing scientists prefer not to work on problems they find unchallenging or dull. How many will forsake their true research interests for funding to study such problems? Third, and perhaps most decisive, plentiful funding attracts plentiful competition (aside from the responsibility of working in the glare of the media focused on the cancer war). Competition, we know (Gaston, 1973; Hagstrom, 1974; Sullivan, 1975), carries the risk of anticipation, along with the vainglory of priority struggles (Merton, 1957). Indeed, Mulkay and Edge note that

> Individual researchers are concerned and encouraged to select problems which are not too close to those of other group members, so research groups tend to avoid areas where work by other groups is well advanced. The adoption of such a policy of avoiding duplication, and thereby avoiding competition, has been one important factor promoting differentiation between the two main British radio astronomy groups [1973: 38].

In this example of research choice, researchers minimize competition by differentiating their research from that of their prospective competitors: "Thus the tendency to avoid competition leads groups to move quickly into new fields, such as quasars and pulsars, which appear important and where no group has established an outstanding lead" (Mulkay and Edge, 1973: 41). Once the competitive situation has been resolved through negotiation, researchers must learn to live with their decisions.

"Living with one's decisions," as our interviewees (NCI and non-NCI personnel alike) assured us, is a real burden, particularly since many of them were "drafted" to fight (armed with big research budgets) an ill-conceived war for which, years earlier, they had "enlisted." Though some of the postdiscovery literature and personnel growth in RT can be attributed to cancer wartime migration (i.e., the inducement of prospective funding), the initial confluences (1970-1973) *were* intellectually motivated.

Our data, with auxiliary support from the biological and other case studies cited above, imbue a confluence theory with a modicum of explanatory power. This power originated in the object reality which biologists perceive and to which they react by changing the focus—slightly or radically—of their research, their perspective on problems within their cognitive region, and, finally, their own location in various domains.[20] The collective result of such change is a growth in knowledge signalled by such factors as hybridization, marginal innovation, the intellectual migration of the innovators, and the formation of "transient specialties" (to use Edge and Mulkay's term again).

The upshot of the theory, therefore, is to restore scientific rationality—in the present case, biomedical rationality—to its rightful place as a *generator* of research collaboration, competition, and community (network) structure. Any active researcher, pursuing leads from within his domain of inquiry and aware that key discoveries can occur outside of his immediate realm of interest, could surely perceive what new paths through the biological maze are potentially relevant. The RT protagonists' commentary eloquently testified to that. What demands analysis in the future is (1) *how* scientists construct their views of relevant research, that is, how argumentation "finds its way around" the cognitive regions that envelop problem domains, and (2) how science policy can seize upon such knowledge to identify viable research missions and then satisfy the intellectual prerequisites for "success" of the mission. The chief ramification of confluence, in sum, is an alternative approach to conceptualizing and studying scientific growth, particularly its congruence with scientific reality and the environing social (organizational) forms of science policy.

Scientific Growth and Science Policy: Conclusions From a Biomedical Case Study

Near the end of Part I of this study and again in the introduction to this chapter, we suggested that the uncritical fusion of the social and cognitive aspects of science endows analysis with an ideological flavor. It is ideological not merely due to the ascendance of scientists' vested interests in the research they undertake and the rewards they pursue (Gouldner, 1976); it is also ideological because connections between scientific rationality and social structure are no longer seen as problematic (see Krohn, 1977). A realistic account of science must recognize the operation of ideology, for within it the relationship of science and its organization finds meaning. Thus, too, the relationship of scientific growth or progress and science policy finds meaning. For the sociologist to attempt analysis of this relationship uncritically, without first reflecting on these questions of ideology, is to embrace a normative perspective that substitutes the social for the cognitive and forecloses the possibility of yielding policy-relevant knowledge claims about growth *or* progress.

The question of foremost import is this: Does the distinctive rationality or mode of organizing knowledge in biomedicine, as we have claimed, have consequences for the social structure of researchers and research programs in this region of science? Because science possesses a distinctive relationship to its social milieu, as Richter has argued,

> allowances must be made for aspects of science which are unique; in particular, for the special relationship between science and nature which limits the range of possible relationships between science and society [1972: 130].

To carry this realistic view a step further, must biological rationality be mirrored in its social organization and research structures? Or does this rationality possess a certain "robustness" which allows it to be expressed in various contexts, indeed, in spite of federal efforts to optimize its scientific output through the imposition of idealistic policies which nonetheless "worked" in other sciences, for example, the interwar period? If the rationality or cognitive norms within biology, for instance, is more reticulate than that found within physics (see Arber, 1954), what does this mean to the social analyst of science and the science policy maker? It means that to study the progress of biological research is to ask how robust is its development within differing cultural and social structural contexts.

What departures from, or adaptations of, the idealistic science-society "partnership" have we witnessed in the case of RT? By reconstructing the micro-level processes of problem domain formation and elaboration, we have traced the internal history of cell transformation to the "inevitable" simultaneous multiple discovery of an enzyme. The implications of this discovery for linking RNA viruses to (the prevention and treatment of) human cancer subjected this domain to the external political mission of the conquest of cancer. The question, then, is whether the organizational imperatives of Big Biology, activated by legislative mandate and represented by large governmental and private laboratories, actually *do justice* to the research effort within the problem domain. Do these imperatives optimize or impede? Do they hamper the ability of biologists perceived as outside the contemporary "bounds of reason" to bring the research foci of their problem domains to a new site? In short, can confluences occur?

To pose these questions allows those interested in shaping policy to entertain the question: How *should* biomedical research be organized? Should it be organized in a manner which differs from physics or chemistry?[21] Is it "incorrectly" (inefficiently) organized at the present time? Such normative questions are intrinsic to the dialogue on "contextual knowledge" (Johnston, 1976) that supersedes "the crude internalist/externalist dichotomy" in analyses of science. To be policy relevant, sociologists must enter this dialogue.[22] We have even suggested how: by not "investing" in any one representation of science. By seeking a middle ground between scientist-insiders' claims to expert knowledge and social analyst-outsiders' claims of neutrality, keywords, review articles, bibliometric networks, and retrospective oral accounts can *all* be scrutinized as representations of the socially mediated object world of science. As we have suggested in Part II of this study, there are no facile answers to questions concerning the relationships among these various representations. The generation of inconsistent views of a problem domain, however, becomes a policy tool; analyses of a domain's various dimensions throw into relief the biases (or eccentricities) of method, data, and theory.[23] Thus, the promise exists of a sociology of science that can extract from representations clues as to how, when, and where a science can be stimulated to "surrender" new knowledge. It is in this knowledge of *process* that an understanding of structure and growth in science will be found.

To cite a final example, the reason Miescher's work on DNA in the 19th century was infertile and Crick and Watson's work was fertile cannot be explained if environmental mechanisms are not recast to include the intellectual content of science. No one would deny that the increased effectiveness of an idea has socially interesting aspects, but to proffer purely social explanations, as if the principal *cause* of the growth of science *were social,* is to contort the problem of scientific change and, at best, to do violence to the many dimensions of scientific growth. By simply equating scientific growth with burgeoning literatures and communities of specialists, the analysis of scientific progress is withdrawn from the context of argumentation and evaluation which ultimately must arbitrate the effectiveness of ideas.

A responsible sociology of science will abet the formulation of responsible science policy only by addressing the complex reality with tools it has already yielded. Evidential norms and confluence are tools extracted from a case study of viruses and cancer. A study of the RT problem domain warrants no change in biomedical research policy; rather, it compels consideration of *alternative* policies—and the realistic promise of new knowledge.

NOTES

1. This marvelous word was applied to citation analysis by Ian Mitroff in a conversation with D.E.C. years ago; its application, it occurs to us as surveyors of the science studies terrain, is even wider than was initially intended.

2. In Bhaskar's words,

> Science is a process in motion, continually on the move from manifest behaviour to essential nature, from the description of things identified at any one level of reality to the construction and testing of possible explanations and thus the discovery of the mechanisms responsible for them. This process necessitates the construction of both new concepts and new tools (or the ressurrection or refinement of old ones). The aim of science is the discovery of the mechanism of the production of phenomena in nature; and it proceeds by way of a dialectic of taxonomic (or descriptive) and explanatory knowledge, in which the conflicing principles of empiricism and rationalism can be reconciled, a dialectic which has no foreseeable end.

An endless dialectic, of course, is no reconciliation at all. Since we subscribe to *this* view, we could be perceived (and rightly so) as endorsing a *weak* version of what has been popularized as "the strong program in the sociology of knowledge."

3. In a private conversation with D.E.C., Thaddeus Trenn has described local interinstitutional programs in West Germany which bring together diverse specialists to exchange views and plan research on selected topics. These *Sonderforschungsbereich* contrast with unplanned, noninstitutionalized confluences which form cosmopolitan (national and international) problem domains.

4. For an alternate (but similar) statement of this latter debate, see Lemaine et al.'s (1976) discussion of the rate, direction, and content of scientific development.

5. Sociologists, it should be noted, have been thrust down the road to relativism before, only to have rejected such an epistemology at the last possible moment (see Phillips, 1974). Recently, however, Elkana (1978) came to the rescue, as it were, claiming that "the two positions (realism and relativism) are not inconsistent. This polarization is not only unnecessary but dangerously misleading, and the solution to the apparent inconsistency is simply to hold them both simultaneously. This is what I mean by *two-tier-thinking*." Our response to this *fait accompli* of logic emerges as the Epilogue unfolds (but see especially Note 16).

6. Rather than beg the question of what is "sufficient research," we offer a provisional answer that we expound on below. Interestingly, our "answer" differs from that of Edge and Mulkay who, after comparing the sociological implications of their meticulous analysis of radio astronomy with previous studies of scientific innovation, caution that:

> Satisfactory answers cannot be provided by case studies alone. They can be achieved only by means of systematic comparison on a scale that, owing to the scarcity of suitable empirical material, is at present impossible [1976: 389].

To the contrary, comparative analyses are precisely the reason why the bulk of Edge and Mulkay's findings diverge from those in the sociological literature. That literature has paid little heed to the content of innovative science, comparing the sites of intellectual change on methodological or social grounds, for example, the identification of communities, clusters, or groups of researchers, according to publication or citation frequency. We would prefer to see the profusion of cognitive detail peculiar to a particular site set forth, then placed in its social, cultural, and political contexts. More depth of analysis must precede breadth, as has been argued in a review of *Astronomy Transformed* (Chubin, 1978a; for other celebratory reviews of this book, see Crane, 1977; Sullivan and White, 1977; Gieryn and Merton, 1978).

7. In the Mullins et al. (1977) analysis of RT research, it is telling that research is labeled as belonging to the RT cluster beginning in *1967,* three years *prior* to the discovery of the enzyme. In a real sense the domain was already present as an anticipation prior to the discovery. The real question, though, is whether cocitation is a suitable method for discovering the confluence patterns which converge on the discovery process. What we demonstrated in Chapter 6 is how the anticipation period *is* mirrored somewhat in the citation structure of the domain (see Note 19).

8. Bhaskar forcefully underscores this realistic view in the following:

> Let us suppose that we could explain the emergence of organic life in terms of the physical and chemical elements out of which organic things were formed and perhaps even reproduce this process in the laboratory. Now would biologists lose their object of inquiry? Would living things cease to be real? Our apprehension of them unmasked as an illusion? No, for in as much as living things were capable of acting back on the materials out of which they were formed, biology would not be otiose. For a knowledge of biological structures and principles would still be necessary to account for any determinate state of the physical world. Whatever is capable of producing a physical effect is real and a proper object of scientific study [1975: 113].

9. The Central Dogma not only helped shape research strategy for the molecular biologist but it also symbolized tremendous confidence born of previous success. As the supply of surprises was depleted, however, the repetition of the research strategy seemed to some (Stent, 1969) to be a rather dull task. Dullness, alone, even for Stent, did not make him reject the Central Dogma; it simply became a shorthand notation for the end-point of progress. So, too, it would seem, the provirus hypothesis had much with which to contend. As Spiegelman (1978) told us,

> The real finding which would completely destroy the whole basis of molecular biology is not the reversal of RNA to DNA, but the reversal of proteins in nucleic acid. That would just completely shatter the whole field. That's what we meant by Central Dogma.

10. Such vocabularies are no doubt transmitted through the laboratory apprenticeship system, though certain researchers are better articulators (tacitly or otherwise) than others. This can be inferred from the success of their students to translate the evidential norms of a region into a vocabulary for participating in each of several problem domains throughout one's career. Hagstrom (1970) once referred to this capacity for intellectual migration as "skimming the milk" and moving on; we would propose as a new description of this capacity the analogy of "making various flavors of ice cream."

11. In another study of biomedical research organization (in reproductive endocrinology), we (Studer and Chubin, 1976) observed that historian-scientists often utilize the evidential norms of a problem domain to organize their narrative. Marc Klein, the endocrinologist-historian, writes,

> Once morphological exploration is complete, we have to turn to experimental investigation to clear up a problem. The simplest way is to remove an organ or parts of it, followed by extracting active products, first in crude and later in purified form. At that stage the exploration has already passed into the hands of chemists and physicists, who in the end specify the chemical formula and succeed in synthesizing the active principle [1963: 293].

Klein's theory of research is also Klein's historical chronology. An important historiographical question is whether other criteria or perspectives are possible for writing the history of science. Would, for instance, histories based on citation analysis reflect the evidential norms? If they would, why would they? If they would not reflect these norms—indeed we are skeptical that they do—what would they reflect?

12. Use of the parallel terms "cognitive structure" and "social structure" of science is revealing here with citation concentrations serving as the sole proxy for cognitive structure (e.g., Cole and Zuckerman, 1975; Cole et al., 1977a; Cole 1978).

13. On chance and luck in science, see Austin (1978) and Turner and Chubin (1979).

14. What was relevant to this discovery, we note, included tools found *outside* of the cognitive region of biology, namely, X-ray crystallography and concepts originating in physics. Thus, this example is exceptional for our purposes in that more than a discovery was made; a new discipline was founded (for a sociological analysis, see Mullins, 1972). Confluences beget problem domains, not institutionalized forms of science, according to our present conception of the theory.

15. Hence, a "linear" type of reductionism, while logically possible within biology, seems to be peripheral to the actual development of molecular biology (see Schaffner, 1974).

16. This is not to say that the participant scientists have identified the real world, just that they have modified their representations of it. Indeed, Barnes (1977) and Mulkay (1976) argue that scientists enjoy no privileged status vis-à-vis the apprehension of reality (also see Overington, 1979). To adopt this stance would place scientists on an "insider's pedestal" and preclude the debunking and comparing of their knowledge claims. To our mind, this has been the wont of sociologists of science. In the past few years, however, those committed to a sociology of knowledge or "cognitive" approach to science have endorsed the realistic epistemology (e.g., Barnes, 1974; Bloor, 1976); critics (e.g., Collins and Cox, 1977; Millstone, 1978; Meynell, 1977; Zenzen, 1978)—friendly and unfriendly alike—have responded in

kind. At the operational level, these epistemologies, again tending toward the poles of the realism-relativism dichotomy, translate into a continuum of skepticism concerning representations of scientific activity. Thus, some reject scientists' written descriptions of what they do (e.g., Gilbert, 1977; Edge, 1977; Knorr, 1977), while others reject scientists' oral accounts of what they do (Woolgar, 1976b) and are content only with *in situ* monitoring (in the laboratory) of the interaction processes by which scientists negotiate reality (Latour and Woolgar, 1979). For those of the latter ilk, science is "in the making," experiencing, or doing. Decreasing distance between subject and observer and between object and observer is almost a conversion experience (Goodfield, 1977). A glimpsing of the scientist's world from his or her perspective, even for a short time, is a needed anthropology—not understanding as an insider, but the empathic addition of that sample of reality to the systematically compiled observations of an outsider (see Bernstein, 1978). A rereading of Merton (1972) is bracing in this regard, for the methodology extolled in Latour and Woolgar (1979) is disturbing to anyone who has proceeded along the paths of triangulation. Alas, there is no way of avoiding epistemological relativism (Bhaskar, 1975; Elkana, 1978).

17. The prototype of center and periphery is Shils's (1972b) intellectual "metropolis" and "province." It is significant that subsequent uses of this metaphor at the approximate level (i.e., specialties) of analysis on which we have been operating have all yielded *status* interpretations of community structure (see Breiger, 1976; Mullins et al., 1977). Yet the hierarchization of the social dynamics relating central to peripheral scientists is superfluous (for theoretical critiques, see Mullins, 1975; Chubin, 1976; Chubin et al., 1977).

18. Still, the first place to discern confluence in science is within review articles. What is reviewed in such articles is generally a "line of inquiry"; what this entails is the specification of the progress that has been made. If one surveys the reviews in viral cell transformation, for example, tables much like those found in Chapter 1 are often an integral part of the survey. When such research is rehearsed, it narrates not only what has been discovered to date but it also presents the evidential criteria deemed sufficient for crediting an individual or team with having made an advance or some discovery. The retrospective aspects of the review thus points to the cognitive norms necessary for previous development and, by implication, suggests a similar thread of reasoning for the future. In surveying different problem domains the same research may be reviewed; a common point of relevance may thereby be established. But there is also a prospective, anticipatory aspect to review articles which brings together divergent lines of inquiry. In other words, review articles point to the reticulate nature of research within a biological domain; they mirror the researchers' comprehension of how reason must progress within it. What must be stressed here is that the technique for selecting sociologically interesting areas for analysis should not rest on judgments concerning social characteristics, especially since these characteristics are often isolated by methodological fiat. If one *knew* that social and intellectual characteristics were isomorphic, then one might draw upon social indicators (e.g., Anderson and Van Gelder, 1970). But that is precisely what *must be discovered and not assumed.*

19. This is not too unlike, as Mulkay remarked in his commentary on another version of this chapter, his "model of branching," which attempts to set forth the dynamics of scientific problems, definition, and negotiation (Mulkay, 1975). However, the model is essentially concerned with the process of social differentiation; it shares the virtues and vices of its many predecessors that we have discussed. Its orientation to scientific growth is similar to the neounilinearism found in the theories of Crane, Mullins, and Clark, that is, stages of growth predominate:

> Each stage is characterized by certain associated intellectual and social developments. During stage one participants are unlikely to have a clear conception of the research area to which they are contributing. It is only in the second stage, after a considerable degree of intellectual consensus has been achieved, that it becomes possible for participants or for outsiders to make reasonably clearcut decisions about which scientists actually contributed to the development of the field. Consequently, it is usually only possible to outline the growth of stage one retrospectively [Mulkay et al., 1975: 190].

Thus, the development of science is visualized as an unfolding and branching process, a view that has incorporated Kuhn's theory of paradigm development. But if the lines of research which make discoveries meaningful are taken into account, the adequacy of the branching model diminishes. The problem with which the sociologist must grapple is the confluence of lines of research onto new problems. The differentiation process, although undoubtedly at work, becomes subordinated to the more vexing issue of the confluence of scientific knowledge within domains of research. What the Kuhn and Mulkay models de-emphasize–the cumulative progress of science–becomes the crux of any attempt to explain the growth of science. Thus, the resemblance between branching and confluence is at best superficial. In the former, the cognitive is still an accessory to growth, not a cause. Nevertheless, the metaphorical reciprocity of converging versus branching out is an interesting coincidence.

20. We echo Edge and Mulkay's recommendation for future study, to wit, "as much attention must be given to those who respond to scientific innovations as to those who set these innovations in motion" (1976: 394). It was this aim that can be satisfied in part by "structural interviewing."

21. Some might argue that the boundaries which happen to separate biology, chemistry, and physics are historical accidents, and thus the grounds for asserting that these units display different styles of thought are fallacious. Historically accidental or not, we would respond, scientists are trained to think in a "disciplined" way about esoteric problems (Kuhn, 1963; Mitroff, 1974b); they develop disciplinary *Gestalten* which have been reified in the organization of university departments and in the bureaucratization of research patronage (e.g., Clark, 1973). The delineation of the object world into disciplines is a real and constraining specialization with which scientists must reckon.

22. Another example of this dialogue is renewed interest in scientific peer review–not only the issue of community autonomy in allocating society's resources for research but also the criteria by which the disposition of research proposals occurs. Contrary to analyses designed to show no bias in the review process (e.g., Cole et al., 1977b), the criteria issue can be constructively addressed in a dialectical policy analysis (Mitroff and Chubin, 1979).

23. Hargens (1978) recently termed this multidimensional approach "optimistic pluralism"; pluralistic it is, but the optimism may be groundless. A more tempered view, specifically relating "models of relevance" in sociology to policy, is found in Rule, "Accounts of how social arrangements could be 'better' do not necessarily provide grounds for reshaping the concrete interests and prerogatives of those who oppose such change" (1978: 96).

APPENDIX A Oncogenic Viruses by Year of Discovery[a]

	us (Tumor)	Host	Discoverers	Location	Journal	Support
	cken kemia	Chicken	Ellerman, V. Bang, O.	Kopenhagen	Centralbl. f. Bakt.	Kgl Fredericks Hospital (Bakteriologschen Lab.)
1911	Chicken Sarcoma	Chicken	Rous, P.	Lab. of the Rockefeller Inst. for Med. Res., N.Y.	Jour. A.M.A.	---
1911	Fowl Sarcoma	Chicken	Fujinami, A. Inamoto, K.	Japan	Gann	---
1912	Osteosarcoma in Fowl	Chicken	Rous, P.	Lab. of the Rockefeller Inst. for Med. Res., N.Y.	Jour. A.M.A.	---
1913	Angiosarcoma in Fowl	Chicken	Rous, P.	Lab. of the Rockefeller Inst. for Med. Res., N.Y.	J. Exp. Med.	---
1914	Myosarcoma of Ducks	Duck	Fujinami, K. Inamoto	Pathological Inst. of the Imperial Univ. in Kyoto, Japan	Z. f. Krebsforsch	---
1917	Human Wart Virus	---	Waelsch	---	Arch. f. Dermat u. Syph.	---
1919	Papillomata in Man	Man	Wile, U.J. Kinger, L.B.	Univ. Michigan Medical School	Jour. A.M.A.	---

(Appendix A continued)

Year	Virus (Tumor)	Host	Discoverers	Location	Journal	Support
1920	Bovine Papilloma	Cattle	Magalhaes, O.	---	Brasil-Medico	---
1932	Canine Oral Papilloma	Dog	Demonbreun, W.A. Goodpasteur, E.W.	Dept. Pathology Vanderbilt Med. School, Nashville, Tenn.	Am. J. Path	Grant from Pouch Fund
1932	Rabbit Fibroma	Rabbit	Shope, R.E.	Dept. Animal and Plant Pathology of the Rockefeller Inst. for Med. Res., Princeton, N.J.	J. Exp. Med.	---
1932	Papillomata of the Pharynx in Man	Man	Ullman, E.V.	---	Acta Oto-Laryng	---
1933	Rabbit Papilloma	Rabbit	Shope, R.E.	Dept. Animal and Plant Pathology of the Rockefeller Inst. for Med. Res., Princeton, N.J.	J. Exp. Med.	---
1933	Fowl Lymphoma	Chicken	Furth, J.	Dept. Path., Cornell Univ. Med. College, New York	J. Exp. Med.	Fund for the Study of Leukemia
1934	Frog Kidney Carcinoma	Frog	Balduin, L.	Lab. of Path., School of Med. Univ. Penn., Philadelphia, Penn.	Am J. Cancer	Grant from Mr. Wm. Donner and Int. Cancer Found. and Faculty Research Committee of Univ. Penn.
1935	Skin Cancer in Tritons	Triton	Champy, C Champy, M.	---	Bull. Assoc. France Etude Cancer	---

(Appendix A continued)

Year	Virus (Tumor)	Host	Discoverers	Location	Journal	Support
1936	Rabbit Oral Papilloma	Rabbit	Parsons, R.J. Kidd, J.G.	Lab. of the Rockefeller Inst. Med. Res., New York	Proc. Soc. Exp. Biol. Med.	---
1936	Mouse Mammary Carcinoma	Mouse	Bittner, J.J.	Jackson Memorial Lab. Bar Harbor, Maine	Science	---
1938	Frog Kidney Carcinoma	Frog	Lucke, B.	Lab. of Path., School of Med., Univ. Penn., Philadelphia	J. Exp. Med.	Int. Cancer Found. Nat. Research Council
1946	Pulmonary Adenomatosis of Sheep	Sheep	Dungal, N.	Dept. Path. Univ. Iceland Reykjavik, Iceland	Am J. Path.	---
1947	Lymphomatosis (and other forms of Leukosis)	Chicken	Burmester, B.R. Cottral, G.E.	U.S. Regional Poultry Research Lab., East Lansing, Michigan	Cancer Research	---
1950	Papilloma of Monkeys	Monkey	Lucke, B. Ratcliffe, H. Breedis, C.	Dept. Pathology Univ. Penn. School of Med., and Penrose Research Lab., Philadelphia Zoological Garden, Phil., Pa.	(Abst.) Fed. Proceedings	---
1951	Equine Cutaneous Carcinoma	Horse	Cook, R.H. Olson, C. Jr.	Dept. Animal Path. & Hygiene, Univ. Neb., Lincoln, Neb.	Am. J. Path.	National Cancer Inst. of the Nat. Inst. Health, Public Health Service, Bethesda, Maryland

(Appendix A continued)

Year	Virus (Tumor)	Host	Discoverers	Location	Journal	Support
1951	Mouse Leukemia (Lymphatic)	Mouse	Gross, L.	Cancer Research Unit Veterans Administra-tiona Hospital, Bronx, N.Y.	Proc. Soc. Exp. Biol & Med.	Veterans Admin.
1952	Sarcoma of the Fat Body in Frogs	Frog	Rose, S. M.	Dept. Zoology, Univ. Illinois, Urbana, Illinois	Ann. N.Y. Acad. Sci.	Amer. Cancer Soc. (Comm. Growth of the Nat. Res. Council)
1952	Cartilaginous Tumours caused by Lucke's Virus	Frog	Rose, S. M. Rose, F.	Dept. Zoology, Univ. Ill., Urbana, Illinois	Cancer Research	Amer. Cancer Society
1953	Mouse Parotid Tumor	Mouse	Gross, L.	Cancer Res. Unit, Veterans Adm. Hos-pital, Bronx, N. Y.	Proc. Soc. Exp. Biol & Med.	Damon Runyon Mem-orial Fund for Cancer Research
1953	Squirrel Fibroma	Grey Squirrel	Kilham, L. Herman, C.M. Fisher, E.R.	Federal Security Agency, Pub. Health Ser., NIH, Microbio-logical Inst., Nat. Inst. Arthritis & Metabolic Disease, Bethesda, Md., and Dept. Interior, Fish and Wildlife Service, Laurel, Md.	Proc. Soc. Exp. Biol. & Med.	---
1955	Deer Fibroma	White-tailed Deer	Shope, R. Mangold, R. Macnamara, L.G. Dumbell, K.R.	Rockefeller Inst; State of N.J. Dept. Conserv. and Economic Develop-ment, Division of Fish & Game, Trenton; Dept Bacteriology, The University, Liverpool	J. Exp. Med.	Nat. Inst. of Allergy and Infec-tious Diseases, U.S. Public Health Service

Year	Virus (Tumor)	Host	Discoverers	Location	Journal	Support
1956	Mouse Leukosis (Myeloid Forms)	Mouse	Graffi, A. Bielka, H. Fey, F.	Inst. f. Med. Biol. Deut Akad. Wissen-schaften Berlin	Acta Haemat	---
1956	Leukosis in Rats	Rat	Thurzo, V. Svec, F.	---	Cl. Onkol	---
1957	Mouse Leukosis	Mouse	Friend, C.	Sloan-Kettering Inst. for Cancer Res., Mem. Center for Cancer & Allied Diseases, N.Y.	Ann. N.Y. Acad. Sci.	---
1957	Mouse Leukosis	Mouse	Mazurenko, N.P. Nasornaia	---	Vopr. Onkol (Prob. Oncol.)	---
1957	Polyoma Virus (Mouse Parotid Tumor)	Mouse	Stewart, S.E. Eddy, B.E. Gochenour, A.M. Borgese, N.G. Grubbs, G.E.	Lab. of Biology, Nat. Cancer Inst. and Lab. of Viral Products, Div. Biol. Standards, Nat. Inst. Health, Public Service; U.S. Dept. H.E.W., Bethesda, Md.	Virology	---
1958	Mouse Leukosis	Mouse	Graffi, A.	---	Z. Ges. Inn. Med.	---
1959	Mouse Leukosis	Mouse	Schwartz, S.O. Schoolman, H.M.	Hematology Dept. Hektoen Inst. Med. Res., Cook Co. Hosp. Chicago, Ill.	Blood	---
1959	Mouse Leukosis	Mouse	Kaplan, H.S.	---	CIBA Fnd. Symp. Carcinogenesis, London	---
1959	Histiocytoma of Monkeys	Monkey	Andrewes, C.H.	---	Acta Int. Union Against Cancer	---

Year	Virus (Tumor)	Host	Discoverers	Location	Journal	Support
1960	Mouse Leukosis	Mouse	Moloney, J.B.	Lab. of Biol. Nat. Cancer Inst. Bethesda, Md. NIH, PHS, US Dept. HEW	J. Nat. Cancer Inst.	---
1960	Rat Leukosis	Rat	Moloney, J.B.	Lab. of Biol. Nat. Cancer Inst. Bethesda, Md. NIH, PHS, US Dept. HEW	Nat. Cancer Inst. Monog. 4	---
1960	SV 40 (Vacuolating Virus, SV 40)	Monkey but here cell culture	Sweet, B.H. Hilleman, M.R.	Division of Virus and Tissue Culture Research, Merck Inst. for Therapeutic Research, West Pt., Pa.	Proc. Soc. Exp. Biol. and Med.	---
1962	SV 40	Rhesus Monkey (Cultures)	Eddy, B.E. Borman, G.S. Grubbs, G.E. Young, R.D.	Div. Biol. Standards, Nat. Inst. Health, Bethesda, Md.	Virology	---
1962	Adenoviruses	Hamster	Huebner, R.J. Rowe, W. Land, W.	Lab. Infecticus Dis., Nat. Inst. Health, Bethesda, Md.	Proc. Nat. Acad. Sci.	U.S. Public Health Service, Cancer Control Unit
1962	SV 40	Hamster	Girard, A.J. Sweet, B.H. Slotnick, V.B. Hilleman, M.R.	Div. Virus and Tissue Culture Research, Merck Inst. for Therapeutic Research, West Pt., Pa.	Proc. Soc. Exp. Biol. and Med.	U.S. Public Health Service
1962	Human Adenovirus Type 12	Hamster	Trentin, J.J. Yabe, Y. Taylor, G.	Div. Exper. Biol., Baylor Univ. College Med., and Dept. Pediatrics, M.D. Anderson Hosp. Houston	Proc. Am. Assoc. Cancer Res.	---

Year	Virus (Tumor)	Host	Discoverers	Location	Journal	Support
1963	Cattle Leukosis	Cattle	Hoflund, S. Thorell, B. Winqwist, G.	---	Proc. Int. Symp. Comp. Leukemiares. Doc. III	---
1963	Canine Mastocytoma	Dog	Lombard, L.B. Moloney, J.B. Rickard, C. G.	Div. Biol. and Med. Res., Argonne Nat. Lab., Arbonne, Ill.	Ann N.Y. Acad. Sci.	U.S. Atomic Energy Commission and Public Health Service
1964	Cat Leukemia	Cat	Jarrett, W.F.H. Martin, W.B. Crishton, G.W. (Carnegie Res. Fellow), Dalton, R.G. Stewart, M.F.	Veterinary Hosp., Univ. Glasgow, and the Inst. of virol-ogy, Univ. Glasgow, Scotland)	Nature	British Empire Cancer Campaign
1966	Mouse Osteosarcoma	Mouse	Finkel, M.P. Birute, O.B. Jenkins, P.B.	Experimental Radiation Pathology, Argonne Nat. Lab., Argonne, Ill.	Science	USAEC

[a]Compiled from Gross (1970:1908-1966), Luria and Darnell (1968), Syverton (1960:1908-1957), and Zilber and Abelev (1968).

APPENDIX B Bacterial Species and Characters transformed and Their Major Researchers[a]

Year	Researcher	Species and Character	Year & Country of Birth	Year & Highest Degree	Institution of Highest Degree	Research Specialty
1928	Griffith, F.	Diplococcus pneumoniae synthesis of type specific capsular polysaccharide	Great Britain	---	---	---
1944	Avery, O.T. MacLeod, C.M. McCarty, M.	D. pneumoniae synthesis of type specific capsular polysaccharide	1877 Canada nat. --- 1911 U.S.	1904 MD --- 1937 MD	Columbia --- J. Hopkins	bacteriology --- med. bacter.
1945	Boivin, A. et. al.	Escherichia coli synthesis of type specific capsular polysaccharide	1895 France 1949 died	1931 DSc	Marseilles/ Strasbourg	chem; genetics
1946	McCarty, M. Avery, O.T.	D. pheumoniae synthesis of type specific capsular polysaccharide		see see	above above	
1947	MacLeod, C.M. Kraus, M.R.	D. pneumoniae Intermediate encapsulated types	--- ---	--- ---	--- ---	--- ---
1947	Weil, A.S. Binder, M.	Shigella paradysenteriae synthesis of type specific capsular polysaccharide	1900 Germany nat. ---	1932 MD ---	Munch ---	bacteriology ---
1949	Taylor, H.E.	D. pneumoniae intermediate encapsulated types	1913 Canada	1936 MD	Dalhousie	pathology

Year	Researcher	Species and Character	Year & Country of Birth	Year & Highest Degree	Institution of Highest Degree	Research Specialty
1949	Austrian, R. MacLeod, C.M.	D. pneumoniae specific protein antigens M protein	1916 U.S. ---	1941 MD ---	J. Hopkins ---	internal med; bact. genet. ---
1951	Hotchkiss, R.D.	D. pneumoniae - resistance to streptomycin	1911 U.S.	1935 PhD	Yale	biochem.
1951	Alexander, H.E. Leidy, G.	Hemophilus influenzae synthesis of type specific polysaccharides	--- ---	--- ---	--- ---	--- ---
1952	Austrian, R.	D. pneumoniae synthesis of type specific polysaccharides		see	above	
1953	Austrian, R.	D. pneumoniae filamentous type of growth		see	above	
1953	Alexander, H.E. Leidy, G.	H. influenzae resistance to streptomycin	--- ---	--- ---	--- ---	--- ---
1953	Austrian, R. Colowick, M.S.	D. pneumoniae systhesis of salicin fermentation enzyme	 ---	see ---	above ---	 ---
1953	Leidy, G. et. al.	H. influenzae mixed or binary encapsulation	---	---	---	---
1953	Alexander, H.E. Redman, W.	Neisseria meningitidis synthesis of type specific polysaccharide	---	---	---	---
1953	Klein, D.T. Klein, R.M.	Agrobacterium fumefaciens ability to induce crown-gall tumours in tomato	1928 U.S. ---	1961 PhD ---	Rutgers ---	micro bio; mol. bio. ---
1953	Klein, D.T. Klein, R.M.	A. radiobacter	 ---	see ---	above ---	 ---

Year	Researcher	Species and Character	Year & Country of Birth	Year & Highest Degree	Institution of Highest Degree	Research Specialty
1953	Klein, D.T. Klein, R.M.	A. Rubi	 ---	see ---	above ---	 ---
1954	Beiser, S.M. Hotchkiss, R.D.	D. pneumoniae abnormal capsular type	1923 U.S. ---	1951 PhD (bact.) ---	Columbia ---	microbio. ---
1954	Ephrussi-Taylor, H.E.	D. pneumoniae synthesis of lactic acid oxidase	1918 U.S.	1946 PhD (zool.)	Columbia	genetics microbio.
1954	Hotchkiss, R.D. Marmur, J.	D. pneumoniae synthesis of mannitol dehydrogenase	--- 1926 Poland (Canad. cit.)	--- 1951 PhD (bact. phys.)	--- Iowa St.	--- molec. bio. biochem.
1955, 1956	Balassa, R.	Rhizobium sp. ability to form nodules on alfafa	---	---	---	---
1955, 1956	Demerec, M. et. al.	Salmonella typhimurium ability to synthesize tryptophan; streptomycin resistance	1895 Yugoslavia nat.	1923 PhD (genet.)	Cornell	zoology genetics
1956	Leidy, G. et. al.	H. parainfluenzae resistance to streptomycin	---	---	---	---
1956	Leidy, G. et. al	H. suis resistance to streptomycin	---	---	---	---
1956	Schaeffer, P.	D. pneumoniae resistance to streptomycin	1905 U.S.	1936 PhD	Ohio St.	embryology
1957	Bracco, R.M. et. al.	Stretococcus viridans resistance to streptomycin	---	---	---	---

Year	Researcher	Species and Character	Year & Country of Birth	Year & Highest Degree	Institution of Highest Degree	Research Specialty
1957	Corey, R.R. Starr, M.P.	Xanthomonas phaseoli polysaccharide production	1926 U.S. 1917 U.S.	1955 PhD (micro) 1943 PhD (bact., biochem.)	CAL (Davis) Cornell	microbio. microbio.
	"	streptomycin resistance				
1957	Kanazir Subotic (referred to in Thomas)	Salmonella sp. ability to synthesize proline	--- ---	--- ---	--- ---	--- ---
1957	Drew, R.M.	D. pneumoniae resistance to amethopterin	1911 U.S.	1950 PhD (insect embryol.)	Radcliffe	bacteriology
1957	Goodgal, S.H. Herriott, R.M.	H. influenzae resistance to cathomycin	--- 1921 U.S.	--- 1950 PhD (bio.)	--- J. Hopkins	--- genet., biochem.
1957	Balassa, R.	Rhizobium sp. resistance to streptomycin	---	---	---	---
1957, 1958	Hotchkiss, R.D. Evans, A.H.	D. pneumoniae resistance to sulfanilamide	--- ---	--- ---	--- ---	--- ---
1957	Ephrussi-Taylor, H.E.	D. pheumoniae resistance to canavanine		see	above	
1958	Austrian, R.	D. pneumoniae mixed or binary encapsulation		see	above	
1958	Ephrussi-Taylor, H.E.	D. pneumoniae resistance to aminopterin		see	above	
1958	Pakula, R. et. al.	S. sbe resistance to streptomycin	---	---	---	---

(Appendix B continued)

Year	Researcher	Species and Character	Year & Country of Birth	Year & Highest Degree	Institution of Highest Degree	Research Specialty
1958	Pakula, R.	Stretococcus group H	---	---	---	---
1958	Spizizen, J.	Bacillus subtilus ability to synthesize indole, anthranilic acid, nicotinic acid	1917 Canada nat.	1942 PhD (bacteriol.)	Cal. Inst. Tech.	microbio. biochemistry
1958	Pakula, R.	S. viridans resistance to streptomycin	---	---	---	---
1959	Schaeffer, P. et. al.	B. subtilis sporulation		see	above	
1959	Spizizen, J.	B. subtilis synthesis of sucrase and B-galactosidase		see	above	
1959	Green, D.McD.	D. pneumoniae resistance to erythomycin	1930 U.S.	1958 PhD	Rochester	genetics
1959	Lerman, L.S. Tolmach, L.J.	D. pneumoniae resistance to optochin	1925 U.S.	1950 PhD (chemistry)	Cal. Inst. Tech.	molec. bio.
1959	Imshenetskii, A.A.	Staphlococcus aureus resistance to streptomycin	1905 Russia	1939 D. Bio. Sci.	Voronezh	microbio.
1960	Catlin, B.W.	Neisserin siccia	1917 U.S.	1947 PhD (micro)	Cal. (LA)	microbio.
1960	Kaiser, A.D. Hogness, R.D.	E. coli synthesis of two enzymes involved with galactose utilization	1927 U.S. 1925 U.S.	1954 PhD (bio) 1953 PhD (chem.)	Cal. Inst. Tech. Cal. Inst. Tech.	biochem. genet. biochem.

Year	Researcher	Species and Character	Year & Country of Birth	Year & Highest Degree	Institution of Highest Degree	Research Specialty
1960	Catlin, B.W.	N. meningitidis synthesis of type specific capsular polysaccharides		see	above	
1960	Sirotnak, F.M.	D. pneumoniae resistance to 8-azaguanine	1929 U.S.	1954 PhD (microbio.)	Maryland	microbiology genetics
1960	Marmur, J.	D. pneumoniae resistance to bryamycin		see	above	
1960	Balassa, R.	Rhizobium sp. enzyme necessary for synthesis of cysteing	---	---	---	---
1960	Lacks, S.	D. pneumonia synthesis of maltase	1934 U.S.	1960 PhD	Rockefeller	genetics; biochemistry
1961	Bryan, B.E.	D. pheumoniae resistance to streptomycin	---	---	---	---
1961	Ravin, A.W. Iyer, V.N.	D. pneumoniae resistance to erythomycin	1921 U.S.	1951 PhD (zool.)	Columbia	genetics

[a]Compiled from Ravin (1961), Foster (1970), Debus (1968), and American Men and Women of Science (1906-1972).

APPENDIX C

A Rationale and Algorithm for Structural Analysis

Relationships among journals, individuals, references, and citations can be analyzed in terms of their structural properties. But can one be used as a baseline to calibrate our understanding of another? Does it make sense to attempt to "control" for one relationship while studying others? What would be meant by "controlling for ideas" or "controlling for cocitations?" If disparate dimensions of science are not carefully analyzed in their own terms, the possibility of relating their respective contributions is nil. The approach of Chapters 5 and 6 probes what various dimensions of science may mean in terms of the development of a problem domain within biomedicine.

What our research was designed to elucidate is the manner in which the RT domain intertwines with other lines of research, various laboratory structures, and neighboring subject areas. Significantly, whereas Small's application of the cocitation technique is designed to isolate "hot areas" within science through citations–which it seems to do (Small, 1977; but see Sullivan et al., 1977b)–our strategy is to analyze only that literature which has been retrieved from indexing services on the subject of RT. Whereas Small's technique first isolates cocited documents which are subsequently subject analyzed, the present research begins with a "known" subject area, retrieves its article set, and then proceeds to analyze cocitation structures within this set. Obviously these two approaches to cocitation are complementary, but this is no guarantee that theories associated with them, or generated by them, will be compatible.

The very difficulty in capturing biological problem domains within a single conceptual framework (the difficulty of bibliographic taxonomy) in some sense mirrors the nature of biology itself. It would appear, however, that for some analyses, for example, coauthorship, once the sample of literature has been defined, a significant portion of the distribution *has* been captured (see Bradford, 1948; Donohue, 1973). We hasten to add that this statement can neither be demonstrated empirically nor falsified because the articles outside of the sample set that "belong" within the set will never be known. Some reassuring bibliometric evidence can be obtained, however, from the captured literature itself. As one studies the references contained within this literature, one readily surmises that the *authors* of articles that theoretically "should" have been captured are indeed represented within the article set. This appears to be the case, for instance, with the so-called in-house authors and the annual coauthorship networks in the RT domain.

A question, then, that speaks to the heart of our effort concerns the initial definition of the scientific area to be studied (Chapter 2). Why study aggregates of individuals, articles, institutions, and so on which have been initially defined in terms of subject matter? Our answer must be equally blunt: Research is conducted primarily to promote its subject matter and so any meaningful analysis of scientific growth must keep foremost in mind the cognitive content, the rationality, of the research domain. To invert this ordering and consider the cognitive as secondary, as essentially epiphenomena to social structure, is not simply a discredit to the scientists being studied, it is, as we have tried to demonstrate, a bad sociological theory of data.

An Algorithm for Network Analysis

Most of the analysis in Chapters 5 and 6 is couched in terms of a "network" of elements (see Bott, 1957; Nadel, 1957). The "generators" of the networks reduce to a relationship defined by the article as a research unit. For instance, coauthorship is a relationship sustained by individuals as defined by their appearance on the same article.

Less clear is the relationship established by the cocitation of articles. While the analysis carried out in Chapter 6 is based on a relationship defined over our basic article set, at the same time it *expands* the scope of this set. It includes those that are highly cited irrespective of their inclusion in the original set. Mindful of these defined relationships, we are able to expand and contract the analysis of different dimensions of the problem domain without defining relationships that forsake the mediating role of the basic article set. This affords much more intellectual control over the subject matter than if the basic generator of the networks changed (see Studer, 1977b: Avant-Propos).

The analysis we perform on the variously defined networks is relatively straightforward. The Pearson correlation analysis in Chapter 5 (see Mendenhall, 1971) makes use of a common technique in analyzing the coauthorship relation. We are concerned with uncovering similarities of citation profiles between individual scientists within a coauthorship network. However, citations are based upon an *article-to-article* relationship, whereas more than one author can be associated with each article. Thus, when an *author-to-author* citation network is constructed, the final distribution is not a simple sociometric matrix in which an individual is allowed to choose another individual; it is rather a matrix in which the *set of authors* of one article chooses another *set of authors* of another article.

Since the choice matrix is constructed *as if* individual authors were choosing other individual authors, one reference in an article can generate more than one choice. Each individual author of an article chooses each and every author on the reference list. The citations in an article are thus counted as the *product* of the number of coauthors on a referencing article multiplied by the number of coauthors on the cited article. For example, a referencing article with two authors and a cited article with five authors yield 10 citations, that is, a relationship among 10 individuals. After such a matrix is constructed, questions can be asked concerning the relationship of citation patterns to coauthorship structures.

Two individuals' profiles may well be identical because they were always cited in the same articles. Coauthorship, we could say, is the common factor which has constrained their individual citation profiles. This is precisely what we are trying to determine with this analysis: How much can two individuals be considered to be alike? Correlation in this case will be used to isolate coauthorship "identities": The higher the correlations, the more we infer that authors choose (reference) or are chosen (cited) as a unit.

In Chapter 5 and 6, we also use multidimensional scaling (see Alba and Gutmann, 1972; Green and Carmone, 1970; Green and Rao, 1972; McFarland and Brown, 1973) to summarize visually the relationships of coauthors and cocited articles within their respective network systems. Essential to this graphic technique is the translation of data matrices into a metric so that interpoint distances and geometric representations become possible. "Social distance" can be given a precise meaning within sociometric analysis when these techniques are used (see McFarland and Brown, 1973). In a triad, for instance, the assigned weights of a friendship relation can be directly and exhaustively interpreted in a two-dimensional triangular configuration. In general, if we are analyzing n individuals, their relationships can always be represented in an n-1 dimensional space. For the crux of the multidimentional scaling problem is to simplify the geometrical presentation by capturing as much information as possible in the fewest dimensions. The criterion for the goodness of fit which summarizes how well the reduced dimensions capture the information in a matrix is called "stress"—whose minimum value is zero (see Green and Carmone, 1970; Green and Rao, 1972). The stress value has been recorded on all of the scaled figures in Chapters 5 and 6; the stress levels are sufficiently low for two-dimensional representation of the network matrices. These figures present a *visual image* to which we can appeal in our technical discussion of RT research.

EIGENSTRUCTURE ANALYSIS

Once the graphic presentation of a network has been accomplished through multidimensional scaling, we continue our analysis by further decomposing the network structures. In essence, our tactic is to elaborate on the multidimensional scaling by taking into account several additional structural dimensions of the cocitation networks. We label the technique used "eigenstructure analysis" (see Cooley and Lohnes, 1971; Green, 1976) since it is based upon solution of the eigenvalues and eigenvectors (also called characteristic roots and vectors or latent roots and vectors) of a matrix. Because this method is the same as that employed in multidimensional scaling routines—and for that matter, in factor analysis and latent structure analysis as well—eigenstructure analysis provides us with a systematic approach to decomposing the visual network relationships presented in the scaled figures. To understand properly the reason why such analysis is needed and to suggest how it can be interpreted, we must review the underlying model upon which it is based. This will also aid understanding of the visual presentations yielded by the multideimensional scaling routines.

The cocitation networks which we study by means of eigenstructure analysis can all be represented by square symmetric matrices. More formally, an n x n matrix, $M = [M_{ij}]$ is symmetric if $M_{ij} = M_{ji}$, for all i, j, = 1, 2, . . . , n. The M_{ij} element is the number of times that article i and j are cited together (i.e., cocited). Because the networks can all be represented as real symmetric matrices, all of the eigenvalues are real numbers and all of the eigenvectors can be chosen to be real (for proof, see Bronson, 1969).

It is thus the structure of a symmetric, n x n, matrix that we must analyze; and because the only information we possess concerning this network is contained within the matrix, our analytical task is comparable to solving n homogeneous equations in n unknowns (see Boyce and DiPrima, 1969). A solution to this set of equations can be found by solving the following matrix equation for u: $Xu = \lambda u$, where X is the square symmetric matrix, u is an eigenvector, and λ (an eigenvalue) is a scalar such that λ sets the determinant of $(X - \lambda I)$ to zero (see Searle and Hausman, 1970). In short, we can derive *relative* solutions (Searle and Hausman, 1970) to homogeneous equations; there are infinitely many solutions to the above equation, but these all preserve the same internal proportions to one another. Thus, for any given eigenvalue, the elements in the solution vector will possess an invariant proportionality. In multidimensional scaling it is these solution vectors which are weighted by their respective eigenvalues to provide the criterion for locating points within an n-dimensional space. In our examples of multidimensional scaling of Chapters 5 and 6, we find that the two vectors associated with the largest eigenvalues capture very well the overall structure of these particular networks.

Because it is possible to find as many nonzero eigenvalues as there are linearly independent columns (or rows) in our symmetric matices (see

Searle and Hausman, 1970), the same number of dimensions could be scaled. The object, however, is to economize and use as few dimensions as possible; we want to be able to isolate *important* structures, not all features of a network. If we are attempting to locate such important structures of networks, we should not utilize the criterion that is established for principal-components or factor analysis, namely, explained variance. When one obtains the eigenstructure of a correlation matrix (i.e., principal-components analysis), the criterion for selecting the number of eigenvectors is relatively straightforward; each of the eigenvalues with their respective eigenvectors represents a variance-maximizing solution to the set of equations represented by a correlation matrix (see Cooley and Lohnes, 1971). In principal-components analysis, the amount of variance explained (R^2) by each of the eigenvector dimensions can be determined by dividing the corresponding eigenvalue by the sum of the eigenvalues. Variance can thus provide a criterion for choosing the number of dimensions needed for a meaningful decomposition of a correlation matrix.

Our network data (e.g., cocitations) comprise *neither* a correlation *nor* a covariance matrix (see Tinkler, 1972; Gould, 1967). Network matrices are structural matrices and the analysis that we conduct must therefore be interpreted in terms of the "structure-maximizing" properties of eigenvalues and eigenvectors; the vectors associated with the highest eigenvalues isolate the structurally most central features of a network system. But in a sense, a corelationship matrix is an empirically constructed "covariance" or "correlation" matrix (without subtracting the mean and dividing by the standard deviation to obtain unit variance and mean of zero); each element indicates how individual entities relate in a multidimensional space.

DATA REDUCTION AND NETWORK STRUCTURE

To elucidate further the nature of eigenstructure analysis, it is helpful to visualize how the coefficients on the various eigenvectors summarize information about a network structure. Pielou's description of what she terms "ordination," but what may perhaps more felicitously be called "data reduction," presents a clear picture of eigenstructure analysis:

> Ordination consists in plotting the n points in a space of fewer than s dimensions in such a way that none of the important features of the original s-dimensional pattern is lost. . . . Many possible methods of ordination have been devised. The most straightforward is to project the original s-space onto a space of fewer dimensions in such a way that the arrangement of the points suffers the least possible distortion. To take the simplest conceivable case, suppose we wished to project a swarm of points in the plane onto a line to obtain a linear ordination. *The distortion will be a minimum if the line is oriented so as to preserve as far as possible the spacing of the points* [1969: 250; italics added].

To translate this into network terms, if one could plot the dimensional space of our network data matrix, each eigenvalue and eigenvector represents the best line which could be drawn through the data to preserve the relative distances of each of the network units. The first eigenvector (associated with the highest eigenvalues) thus summarizes the best overall linear representation of the network. The greatest amount of information that can possibly be extracted with a one-dimensional transformation is obtained in the first eigenvector. The remaining eigenvectors (see Searle and Hausman, 1970, for methods of calculation) represent orthogonal (i.e., totally uncorrelated) solutions to the same set of equations.

Another approach to understanding eigenstructure analysis can be found in Tinkler's (1972) demonstration of the relationship of exponentiation of a sociometric matrix and eigenstructure analysis. The traditional means of determining clique structure within a dichotomous sociometric network (in which an individual either is or is not connected to another person) is to raise the matrix representation of the network to higher powers (see Festinger, 1949; Katz, 1953; Luce, 1950; Luce and Perry, 1949). The matrix powering method summarizes how accessible individuals are to one another in terms of the number of steps that must be taken to reach them. What is discovered, however, is that ordinarily the exponentiation eventually produces matrices in which the relative position of individuals—measured either on the main diagonal or as the sum of the column vectors of the exponentiated matrices—stabilizes. The relative position which is measured by this means is identical to the relations found within an eigenvector analysis. In fact, the exponentiation procedure is one method of arriving at the eigenvectors of a matrix (see Kendall, 1975).

An analytical question, however, concerns the weights given to the links within a network. Certainly simplicity may dictate that a Boolean or dichotomous matrix be analyzed; weighting the links may involve an unnecessary introduction of error. Whether to weight or not to weight must be decided by the questions one wants to pose concerning the network. If structure alone counts in the questions asked, then a dichotomous matrix is what one wants to analyze; if the strength of the linkage is important to the analysis, then weights should be utilized. But there is another important empirical consideration in using these two techniques, namely, what is the proportion of zero to nonzero cells in the network to be analyzed? For instance, in the case of the in-house cocitation analysis, the network is very dense in terms of connectivity, as almost every article is connected in some fashion to every other article. Reducing this matrix to a dichotomous one may produce a trivial analysis.

To utilize the information in the network without artificially truncating (e.g., every connection below five will be set to zero), the analysis demands that the strength of the linkage be used. Thus, in our analysis of cocitations, we use weighted matrices in the eigenstructure analysis because the intensity of cocitations is integral to understanding the importance of this network. We want to be able to discern not simply the structure but also the intensity or thickness of the linkages between highly cocited articles. It is, in sum, the analytical focus which determines to a large degree whether one uses dichotomous or weighted matrices.

THE PRESENTATION OF EIGENVECTORS

We have chosen to look at only the four vectors associated with the four largest eigenvalues. The criteria for choosing how many eigenvectors will be used in a network analysis is somewhat arbitrary: We cannot use, of course, the criterion of explained variance employed in principal-components factor analysis (see above). In general, however, the structures isolated by the eigenvectors associated with low eigenvalues represent network structures of decreasing interest; they represent articles, typically, that are less highly cited than those centrally clustered on the first four eigenvectors. But as Tinkler (1972) has stressed, in the analysis of network data we are not dealing with the same type of measurement error that must be taken into account in principal-components factor analysis. *All* of the eigenvectors isolate structural features of the network.

Note, too, that we have only attempted to interpret the relative positions of articles and keywords on the eigenvectors. The eigenvalues are recorded in tables (where appropriate), but the eigenvectors have neither been weighted (normed) in terms of their eigenvalue nor have the specific values explicitly entered into our discussion. There are several reasons for this: First, because we are only dealing with the first four eigenvectors, they all represent important structural features of our networks. Second, the eigenvalues are already implicitly present in the ordering of the four vectors we present. And third, given our descriptive interests in network analysis, interpretation of eigenvalues in terms of the rate of flow or the rate of growth is not particularly instructive (Tinkler, 1972: 31). What *is* flowing between two highly cocited articles, for instance, is problematic. There is, in other words, no need to confound the structural properties summarized by the eigenvectors by explicitly introducing into the analysis the specific eigenvalues associated with these vectors.

The eigenvectors are presented in orthonormal form. They are orthogonal (uncorrelated) to each other because all eigenvectors associated with distinct eigenvalues of symmetric real matrices are orthogonal (for proof, see Bronson, 1969). In addition, the vectors have been normed so that the sum of the squares of any vector equals one. This transformation does not, of course, affect the relative positions of elements on a vector.

What we are interested in isolating is the distribution of the structural influence of certain network nodes throughout the entire system. The principal eigenvector associated with the highest eigenvalue summarizes the most important central features of the network system. All of the values on this vector for our real symmetrical matrix (which contains only zeroes or positive values) will always be of the same sign. Subsequent vectors associated with lower eigenvalues will contain both positive and negative numbers. Because the solutions contained in all of the vectors are only relative solutions, however, the signs can all be reversed within a vector without altering relationships (see Tinkler, 1972).

The distributions on each eigenvector provide weights for every node within the networks which we analyze. It is, however, the most central nodes on each of the vectors that is of utmost interest; it is the high positive weights and the low negative weights (remember the signs could be changed) which describe the center of a particular system. The most central nodes are termed "clusters" throughout Chapters 5 and 6. They simply represent the local structural centers discerned by the eigen-structure analysis. The number to be included within a cluster is, of course, open to discussion. Our criterion will mainly be the ease of substantive interpretation of a set of articles defined by cocitations. The desirable size of a cluster is also a function of size of the network; it would not make sense to include every node in all of the clusters. A balance must be struck between simplicity and precision, between ease of interpre-tability and accuracy of interpretation.

Conclusion

Our fundamental interest in eigenstructure analysis is to facilitate our understanding of bibliometric relations within RT research. The methods which we have described in this appendix are simply ways of expressing systematically our insights into network structures. The methods, like the networks, are tools for understanding, not ends in themselves.

APPENDIX D

MOST HIGHLY CITED ($\geq$ 25) ARTICLES BY THE REVERSE

TRANSCRIPTASE ARTICLE SET[a]

1951 28 May
ID=1
CT=71
CC=343
WT=.0934

*Lowry, O.H., N.J. Rosebrough, N.J., A.L. Farr, and R.J. Randall
"Protein measurement with the Folin phenol reagent." J. Biol. Chem. 193:265-275, 1951.

Department of Pharmacology, Washington University School of Medicine, St. Louis.

Supported in part by a grant from the American Cancer Society on the recommendation of the Committee on Growth of the National Research Council.

1968 29 May
ID=2
CT=26
CC=246
WT=.0664

*Duesberg, P.H.
"Physical properties of Rous sarcoma virus RNA." Proc. N.A.S. 60:1511-1518, 1968.

Virus Laboratory, University of California, Berkeley.

This investigation was supported by U.S. Public Health Service research grant AI 01267 from the National Institute of Allergy and Infectious Diseases, and grants CA 04774, CA 05619, and training grant CA 05028 from the National Cancer Institute.

1969 16 Sept.
ID=3
CT=55
CC=447
WT=.1109

*Huebner, R.J. and G.J. Todaro
"Oncogenes of RNA tumor viruses as determinants of cancer." Proc. N.A.S. 64:1087-1094, 1969.

Viral Carcinogenesis Branch, National Cancer Institute, National Institutes of Health, Bethesda.

1970 24 March
ID=4
CT=30
CC=111
WT=.0332

*Baltimore, D., A.S. Huang, and M. Stampfer
"Ribonucleic acid synthesis of vesicular stomatitis virus, II. An RNA polymerase in the virion." Proc. N.A.S. 66(2):572-576, 1970.

Department of Biology, Massachusetts Institute of Technology.

Supported by USPHS grant AI-08388 and the American Cancer Society grant E-512. D.B. was supported by a Faculty Research Award from the American Cancer Society, and M.S. was supported by a predoctoral fellowship from the National Science Foundation.

1970 2 June
ID=5
CT=186
CC=1387
WT=.3845

Baltimore, D.
"Viral RNA-dependent DNA polymerase." Nature 226(June 27):1209-1211, 1970.

Department of Biology, Massachusetts Institute of Technology.

This work was supported by grants from the U.S. Public Health Service and the American Cancer Society and was carried out during the tenure of an American Society Faculty Research Award.

1970 15 June
ID=6
CT=194
CC=1414
WT=.3897

Temin, H.M. and S. Mizutani
"RNA-dependent DNA polymerase in virions of Rous sarcoma virus." Nature 226(June 27): 1211-1213, 1970.

McArdle Laboratory for Cancer Research, University of Wisconsin, Madison.

This work was supported by a U.S. public Health Service research grant from the National Cancer Institute. H.M.T. holds a research career development award from the National Cancer Institute.

1970 30 June
ID=7
CT=36
CC=368
WT=.1048

Green, M., M. Rokutanda, K. Fujinaga, R.K. Ray, H. Rokutanda, and C. Gurgo
"Mechanism of Carcinogenesis by RNA tumor viruses, I. An RNA-dependent DNA polymerase in murine sarcoma viruses." Proc. N.A.S. 67(Sept.):385-393, 1970.

Institute for Molecular Virology, Saint Louis University School of Medicine.

This investigation was supported by USPHS grant AI-01725 and research contract PH43-67-692 from the National Cancer Institute, Viral Carcinogenesis Branch, Etiology Area, National Institutes of Health, USPHS, Bethesda. M.G. Research Career Awardee (5-K6-AI-4739), National Institutes of Health, PHS.

1970 10 July
ID=8
CT=92
CC=829
WT=.2373

Spiegelman, S., A. Burny, M.R. Das, J. Keydar, J. Schlom, M. Travnicek, and K. Watson
"Characterization of the Products of RNA-directed DNA polymerases in oncogenic RNA viruses." Nature 227(August 8):563-567, 1970.

Institute of Cancer Reseach, Columbia University, and College of Physicians and Surgeons, New York.

The work was supported by a contract with the SVCP of the U.S. National Cancer Institute and an NCI grant.

1970 21 July
ID=9
CT=39
CC=502
WT=.1392

Rokutanda, M., H. Rokutanda, M. Green, K. Fujinaga, R.K. Ray, and C. Gurgo
"Formation of viral RNA-DNA hybrid molecules by the DNA polymerase of sarcoma-leukaemia viruses." Nature 227(Sept. 5):1026-1028, 1970.

Institute for Molecular Virology, St. Louis University School of Medicine.

This work was supported by a grant from the U.S. Public Health Service, a contract from the National Institute of Allergy and Infectious Diseases, Vaccine Development Branch, a contract from the National Cancer Institute, Viral Carcinogenesis Branch, Etiology Area and a research career award (M.G.) from the National Institutes of Health, USPHS.

1970 27 July
ID=10
CT=28
CC=325
WT=.0911

Spiegelman, S, A. Burny, M.R. Das, J. Keydar, J. Schlom, M. Travnicek, and K. Watson
"DNA-directed DNA polymerase activity in oncogenic RNA viruses." Nature 227(Sept. 5): 1029-1031, 1970.

Institute of Cancer Research, Columbia University, College of Physicians and Surgeons, New York.

The work was supported by a contract with the SVCP of the US National Cancer Institute and a NCI grant.

1970 14 Aug.
ID=11
CT=27
CC=333
WT=.0948

Mizutani, S. D. Boettiger, and H.M. Temin
"A DNA-dependent DNA polymerase and a DNA endonuclease in virions of Rous sarcoma virus." Nature 228(Oct. 31):424-427, 1970.

McArdle Laboratory, University of Wisconsin, Madison.

1970 16 Aug.
RV 5 Oct.
ID=12
CT=25
CC=285
WT=.0760

McDonnell, A-C. Garapin, W.E. Levinson, N. Quintrell, L. Fanshier, J.M. Bishop
"DNA polymerases of Rous sarcoma virus: delineation of two reactions with actinomycin." Nature 228(Oct. 31):433-435, 1970.

Department of Microbiology, University of California, San Francisco.

This work was supported by grants from the National Institutes of Health, the California Division of the American Cancer Society, and the Cancer Research Coordinating Committee of the University of California.

1970 24 Aug.
ID=13
CT=47
CC=473
WT=.1330

Spiegelman, S., A. Burny, M.R. Das, J. Keydar, J. Schlom, M. Trávníček, and K. Watson
"Synthetic DNA-RNA hybrids and RNA-RNA duplexes as templates for the polymerases of the oncogenic RNA viruses." Nature 228(Oct. 31):430-432, 1970.

Institute of Cancer Research, Columbia University, College of Physicians and Surgeons, New York.

The work was supported by a contract with the SVCP and a grant from the National Cancer Institute.

1970 18 Sept.
RV 23 Dec.
ID=14
CT=27
CC=220
WT=.0643

Moore, D.H., J. Charney, B. Kramarsky, E.Y. Lasfargues, N.H. Sarkar, M.J. Brennan, J.H. Burrows, S.M. Sirsat, J.C. Paymaster, and A.B. Vaidya
"Search for a human breast cancer virus." Nature 229(Feb. 26):611-615, 1970.

D.H.M., J.C., B.K., E.Y.L. and N.H.S., Institute for Medical Research, Camden, N.J., M.J.B. and J.H.B., Michigan Cancer Foundation, Detroit, and S.M.S., J.C.P. and A.B.V. Tata Memorial Centre, Parel, Bombay.

This work was supported by contracts and grants from the U.S. National Cancer Institute and the State of New Jersey.

1970 6 Oct.
ID=15
CT=37
CC=356
WT=.1001

Scolnick, E., E. Rands, S.A. Aaronson, and G.J. Todaro
"RNA-dependent DNA polymerase activity in five RNA viruses: divalent cation requirements." Proc. N.A.S. 67(Dec.):1789-1796, 1970.

Viral Leukemia and Lymphoma Branch, National Cancer Institute, E.R. Meloy Laboratories, Springfield, Va.

Supported by Contract PH-70-2047 from the National Cancer Institute.

1970 29 Oct.
ID=16
CT=40
CC=455
WT=.1177

Hanafusa, H., and T. Hanafusa
"Noninfectious RSV deficient in DNA polymerase." Virology 43:313-316, 1971.

Department of Viral Oncology, The Public Health Research Institute of the City of New York.

This investigation was supported by the U.S. Public Health Service Research Grant CA 08747 from the National Cancer Institute.

1970 6 Nov.
ID=17
CT=33
CC=373
WT=.1056

Schlom, D.H. Harter, A. Burny, and S. Spiegelman
"DNA polymerase activities in virions of visna virus, a causative agent of a 'slow' neurological disease." Proc. N.A.S. 68(Jan.):182-186, 1971.

Columbia University College of Physicians and Surgeons, New York.

The work was supported by a contract from the National Cancer Institute (with the SVCP, no. 70-2049) and National Cancer Institute grant CA-02332, also a grant from the National Institute of Neurological Diseases and Stroke (NS-06989) and a gift from the Miles Hodson Vernon Foundation, Inc.. D.H.H. is recipient of Career Research Development Award 1K3NS34,990 from the National Institute of Neurological Diseases and Stroke, USPHS.

1970 7 Nov.
ID=18
CT=29
CC=255
WT=.0717

Gurgo, C., R.K. ray, L. Thiry, M. Green
"Inhibitors of the RNA and DNA dependent polymerase activities of RNA tumour viruses." Nature New Biology 229(January 27):111-114, 1971.

Institute for Molecular Virology, St. Louis University School of Medicine, St. Louis.

This work was supported by a grant from the U.S. Public Health Service and a contract from the National Cancer Institute, U.S. National Institutes of Health.

1970 16 Nov.
ID=19
CT=66
CC=677
WT=.1868

Gallo, R.C., S.S. Yang, and R.C. Ting
"RNA dependent DNA polymerase of human acute leukaemic cells." Nature 228(Dec. 5): 927-929, 1970.

R.C.G., Section on Cellular Control Mechanisms, Human Tumor Cell Biology Branch, NCI-NIH, S.S.Y. and R.C.T., Bionetics Research Laboratories.

This work was supported by the U.S. National Cancer Institute and Bionetics Research Laboratories, Inc.

1971 4 Jan. Brockman, W.W., W.A. Carter, Li-H. Li, F. Reusser, F.R. Nichol
ID=20 CT=25 CC=261 WT=.0748
"Streptovaricins inhibit RNA dependent DNA polymerase present in an oncogenic RNA virus." Nature 230(March 26):249-250, 1971.

W.W.B. and W.A.C., Departments of Medicine and Microbiology, The Johns Hopkins University School of Medicine, Li-H.L., F.R., and F.R.N., The Upjohn Company, Kalamazoo, Mich.

W.A.C. was supported by a U.S. Public Health Service research career development award and research grant. Grants were also received from the Council for Tobacco Research and the American Cancer Society.

1971 5 Jan. Scolnick, E.M., S.A. Aaronson, G.J. Todaro, and W.P. Parks
ID=21 CT=33 CC=439 WT=.1217
"RNA dependent DNA polymerase activity in mammalian cells." Nature 229(January 29):318-321, 1971.

Viral Lymphoma and Leukemia Branch and Viral Carcinogenesis Branch, National Cancer Institute.

This work was supported in part by a contract from the National Cancer Institute.

1971 (1 Feb.)? Temin, H.M.
ID=22 CT=30 CC=229 WT=.0616
"The protovirus hypothesis: speculations on the significance of RNA-directed DNA synthesis for normal development and for carcinogenesis." J. Natl. Cancer. Inst. 46(3):III-VII, 1971.

McArdle Laboratory, University of Wisconsin, Madison.

Supported by Public Health Service research grant CA 071175 from the National Cancer Irstitute, and Research Career Development Award 10K 3-CA 8182 from the National Cancer Institute.

1971 17 Feb. Sutton, W.D.
ID=23 CT=30 CC=151 WT=.0378
"A crude nuclease preparation suitable for use in DNA reassociation experiments." Biochim. Biophys. Acta 240:522-531, 1971.

Medical Research Council Group on the Mammalian Genome. Department of Zoology, University of Edinburgh, Edinburgh (Great Britain).

This work was supported in part by a Postdoctoral Fellowship awarded by the New Zealand University Grants Committee, and in part by an M.R.C. Research Grant to Prof. P.M.B. Walker.

1971 19 Feb. Aaronson, S.A., W.P. Parks, E.M. Scolnick, and G.J. Todaro
ID=24 CT=35 CC=383 WT=.0950
"Antibody to the RNA-dependent DNA polymerase of mammalian C-type RNA tumor viruses." Proc. N.A.S. 68(May):920-924, 1971.

Viral Leukemia and Lymphoma Branch and Viral Carcinogenesis Branch, National Cancer Institute.

This work was supported in part by National Cancer Institute contract PH70-2047.

1971 16 April Schlom, J., S. Spiegelman, and D. Moore
ID=25 CT=44 CC=396 WT=.1039
"RNA-dependent DNA polymerase activity in virus-like particles isolated from human milk." Nature 231(May 14):97-100, 1971.

J.S. and S.S., Institute of Cancer Research, College of Physicians and Surgeons, Columbia University, and D.M., Institute for Medical Research, Camden, New Jersey.

This work was supported by contracts and grants from the U.S. National Cancer Institute and a grant from the State of New Jersey.

1971 26 April Baltimore, D. and D. Smoler
ID=26 CT=76 CC=706 WT=.1866
"Primer requirement and template specificity of the DNA polymerase of RNA tumor viruses." Proc. N.A.S. 68(July):1507-1511, 1971.

Department of Biology, Massachusetts Institute of Technology, Cambridge, Mass.

Supported by grants no. AI-08388 from the USPHS and grant no. E-512 from the American Cancer Society. D.B. is a Faculty Research Awardee of the American Cancer Society.

1971 30 April Ross, J., E.M. Scolnick, G.J. Todaro, and S.A. Aaronson
ID=27 CT=59 CC=472 WT=.1232
"Separation of murine cellular and murine leukaemia virus DNA polymerases." Nature New Biology 231(June 9):163-167, 1971.

Viral Leukemia and Lymphoma Branch, National Cancer Institute, National Institutes of Health.

This work was supported in part by a contract from the Special Virus Cancer Program of the US National Cancer Institute.

1971 3 May Theilen, G.H., D. Gould, M. Fowler, and D.L. Dungworth
RV 21 June
ID=28 CT=32 CC=278 WT=.0669
"C-type virus in tumor tissue of a woolly monkey (Lagothrix spp.) with fibrosarcoma." J. Nat. Canc. Inst. 47:881-885, 1971.

Departments of Clinical Sciences and Pathology, School of Veterinary Medicine, University of California, Davis.

This study was supported in part by Public Health Service Contract PH 70-2048 within the Special Virus Cancer Program of the National Cancer Institute and by grant CA 05457 from the National Cancer Institute.

1971 1 June Kacian, D.L., K.F. Watson, A. Burny and S. Spiegelman
ID=29 CT=79 CC=638 WT=.1716
"Purification of the DNA polymerase of avian myeloblastosis virus." Biochim. Biophys. Acta 246:365-383, 1971.

Institute of Cancer Research, College of Physicians and Surgeons, Columbia University.

This work was supported in part by the National Institutes of Health, National Cancer Institutes of Health, National Cancer Institute, Special Virus Cancer Program Contract 70-2049 Training Grant CA-05011, Research Grant CA-02332, and Postdoctoral Fellowship CA-38924.

1971 30 June
ID=30
CT=74
CC=701
WT=.1892

Goodman, N.C., and S. Spiegelman
"Distinguishing reverse transcriptase of an RNA tumor virus from other known DNA polymerases." Proc. N.A.S. 68(Sept.):2203-2206, 1971.

Institute of Cancer Research, College of Physicians and Surgeons, Columbia University.

This work was supported in part by the National Institutes of Health, National Cancer Institute, Special Virus Cancer Program Contract 70-2049, Training Grant CA-05011, Research Grant CA-02332, and Postdoctoral Fellowship CA-41173.

1971 19 July
ID=31
CT=27
CC=324
WT=.0850

Mölling, K., D.P. Bolognesi, H. Bauer, W. Büsen, H.W. Plassman, P. Hansen
"Association of viral reverse transcriptase with an enzyme degrading RNA moiety of RNA-DNA hybrids." Nature New Biology 234:240- , 1971.

Max Planck Institute für Virusforschung, Tübingen, Max Planck Institute für Biologie, Tübingen.

1971 19 Aug.
ID=32
CT=27
CC=292
WT=.0758

Verma, I.M., N.L. Meuth, E. Bromfeld, K.F. Manly, and D. Baltimore
"Covalently linked RNA-DNA molecule as initial product of RNA tumour virus DNA polymerase." Nature New Biology 233(Sept. 29):131-134, 1971.

Department of Biology, Massachusetts Institute of Technology.

This work was supported by a grant from the American Cancer Society and a contract from the Special Virus Cancer Program of the National Cancer Institute. I.M.V. was a fellow of the Jane Coffin Childs Memorial Fund for Medical Research, K.F.M. was a fellow of, and D.B. was a faculty research awardee of, the American Cancer Society.

1971 14 Sept.
ID=33
CT=50
CC=335
WT=.0781

Aaronson, S.A., G.J. Todaro, and E.M. Scolnick
"Induction of murine C-type viruses from clonal lines of virus-free BALB/3T3 cells." Science 174(Oct. 8):157-159, 1971.

Viral Leukemia and Lymphoma Branch, National Cancer Institute.

This work was supported in part by a contract from the Special Virus Cancer Program of the National Cancer Institute.

1971 21 Sept.
ID=34
CT=53
CC=353
WT=.0822

Lowy, D.R., W.P. Rowe, N. Teich, J.W. Hartley
"Murine leukemia virus: high-frequency activation in vitro by 5-iododeoxyuridine and 5-bromodeoxyuridine." Science 174(Oct. 8):155-156, 1971.

Laboratory of Viral Diseases, National Institute of Allergy and Infectious Diseases.

N.T. was a postdoctoral fellow of the American Association of University Women, holding the Margaret Comstock Snell Fellowship. Supported in part by the Etiology Area, the National Cancer Institute.

1971 30 Sept.
ID=35
CT=41
CC=433
WT=.1116

Hurwitz, J. and J.P. Leis
"RNA-dependent DNA polymerase activity of RNA tumor viruses, I. Directing influence of DNA in the reaction." Journal of Virology 9(Jan.):116-129, 1972.

Division of Biology, Department of Developmental Biology and Cancer, Albert Einstein College of Medicine, Bronx.

This study was conducted by Public Health Service contract 71-2251 within the Special Virus-Cancer Program of the Naitonal Cancer Institute, and by research grant GM-13344 from the National Institute of General Medical Sciences and American Cancer Society (P561-B). J.P.L. is a postdoctoral fellow of the Damon Runyon Cancer Foundation (DRF-659).

1971 12 Oct.
ID=36
CT=41
CC=371
WT=.0862

Parks, W.P., E.M. Scolnick, J. Ross, G.J. Todaro, and S.A. Aaronson
"Immunological relationships of reverse transcriptases from ribonucleic acid tumor viruses." Journal of Virology 9(Jan.):110-115, 1972.

Viral Carcinogenesis Branch and Viral Leukemia and Lymphoma Branch, National Cancer Institute.

This work was supported by a contract NCI 72-2006 from the Special Virus Cancer Program, National Cancer Institute, National Institutes of Health.

1971 26 Oct.
ID=37
CT=63
CC=495
WT=.1283

Schlom, J. and S. Spiegelman
"Simultaneous detection of reverse transcriptase and high molecular weight RNA unique to oncogenic RNA viruses." Science 174(Nov. 19):840-843, 1971.

Institute of Cancer Research, College of Physicians and Surgeons, Columbia University.

The work was supported by the National Cancer Institute special virus cancer program contract 70-2049 and research grant CA-02332.

1971 (1 Nov.)?
ID=38
CT=39
CC=391
WT=.1070

Gallo, R.C.
"Reverse transcriptase, the DNA polymerase of oncogenic RNA viruses." Nature 234(Nov. 26): 194-198, 1971.

National Cancer Institute

1971 12 Nov.
ID=40
CT=29
CC=246
WT=.0638

McAllister, R.M., M. Nicolson, M.B. Gardner, R.W. Rongey, S. Rasheed, P.S. Sarma, R.J. Huebner, M. Hatanaka, S. Oroszlan, R.V. Gilden, A. Kabigting, and L. Vernon
"C-type virus released from cultured human rhabdomyosarcoma cells." Nature New Biology 235(Jan. 5):3-6, 1972.

R.M.M. and M.N., Department of Pediatrics, University of Southern California School of Medicine, Children's Hospital of Los Angeles, M.B.G., R.W.R., and S.R., Department of Pathology, University of Southern California School of Medicine, P.S.S. AND R.J.H., Viral Carcinogenesis Branch, National Cancer Institute, NIH, M.H., S.O., and R.V.G., Flow Laboratories Incorporated, Maryland, A.K. and L.V., Microbiological Associates, Inc., Bethesda.

This work was supported by grants from the US Public Health Service within the Special Virus Cancer Program, National Cancer Institute, NIH, and a research grant from the National Cancer Institute.

1971 8 Nov. Yang, S.S., F.M. Herrera, R.G. Smith, M.S. Reitz, G. Lancini, R.C. Ting, and R.C. Gallo
RV 2 Mar. "Rifamycin antibiotics: inhibitors of Rauscher murine leukemia virus reverse transcriptase and of purified DNA polymerases from human normal and leukemic lymphoblasts." J. Natl. Cancer Inst. 49(July):7-25, 1972.
ID=39
CT=23
CC=149
WT=.0407

Bionetics Research Laboratories, Bethesda, Laboratory of Tumor Cell Biology, National Cancer Institute, R.C. Gallo, National Institutes of Health, Public Health Service, U.S. Department of Health, Education, and Welfare.

1971 16 Nov. Lai, M.M.C., and P.H. Duesberg
RV 11 Dec. "Adenylic acid-rich sequence in RNAs of Rous sarcoma virus and Rauscher mouse leukemia virus." Nature 235(Feb. 18):383-386, 1972.
ID=41
CT=35
CC=459
WT=.1153

Department of Molecular Biology and Virus Laboratory, University of California, Berkeley.

This investigation was supported by a grant from the National Cancer Institute, and a contract from the Special Virus-Cancer Program of the National Cancer Institute, NIH, of the US Public Health Service.

1971 26 Nov. Axel, R., J. Schlom, and S. Spiegelman
"Presence in human breast cancer of RNA homologous to mouse mammary tumour virus RNA." Nature 235(Jan. 7):32-36, 1972.
ID=42
CT=35
CC=375
WT=.0960

Institute of Cancer Research, College of Physicians and Surgeons, Columbia University.

This research was supported by the National Institutes of Health, National Cancer Institute, Special Virus Cancer Program contract and research grant.

1971 2 Dec. Scolnick, E.M., W.P. Parks, G.J. Todaro, and S.A. Aaronson
"Immunological characterization of primate C-type virus reverse transcriptases." Nature New Biology 235(Jan. 12):35-40, 1972.
ID=43
CT=45
CC=464
WT=.1079

Viral Leukemia and Lymphoma Branch and Viral Carcinogenesis Branch, National Cancer Institute, National Institutes of Health.

This work was supported in part by a contract from the Special Virus Cancer Program, National Cancer Institute.

1971 7 Dec. Hehlmann, R., D. Kufe, and S. Spiegelman
"RNA in human leukemic cells related to the RNA of a mouse leukemia virus." Proc. N.A.S. 69(Feb.):435-439, 1972.
ID=44
CT=39
CC=470
WT=.1170

Institute of Cancer Research, College of Physicians and Surgeons, Columbia University.

This research was supported by the National Institutes of Health, National Cancer Institute Special Virus Cancer Program Contract 70-2049 and Research Grant CA-02332.

1971 8 Dec. Kufe, D., R. Hehlmann, and S. Spiegelman
"Human sarcomas contain RNA related to the RNA of a mouse leukemia virus." Science 175 (Jan. 14):182-185, 1972.
ID=45
CT=30
CC=398
WT=.0998

Institute of Cancer Research, College of Physicians and Surgeons, Columbia University.

This study was conducted under contract 70-2049 within the Special Virus Cancer Program of NIH and NIH grant CA-02332.

1971 9 Dec. Ross, J., H. Aviv, E. Scolnick, P. Leder
"In vitro synthesis of DNA complementary to purified rabbit globin mRNA." Proc. N.A.S. 69(Jan.):264-268, 1972.
ID=46
CT=51
CC=297
WT=.0806

J.R. and E.S., Viral Leukemia Branch, National Cancer Institute, National Institutes of Health, H.A. and P.L., Laboratory of Molecular Genetics, National Institute of Child Health and Human Development.

1971 10 Dec. Fridlender, B., M. Fry, A. Bolden, and A. Weissbach
"A new synthetic RNA-dependent DNA polymerase from human tissue culture cells." Proc. N.A.S. 69(Feb.):452-455, 1972.
ID=47
CT=42
CC=396
WT=.1014

Roche Institute of Molecular Biology, Department of Cell Biology, Nutley, N.J.

1971 15 Dec. Schlom, J., S. Spiegelman, D.H. Moore
"Detection of high-molecular-weight RNA in particles from human milk." Science 175 (Feb. 4):542-544, 1972.
ID=48
CT=31
CC=274
WT=.0700

J.S. and S.S., Institute of Cancer Research, College of Physicians and Surgions, Columbia University, D.H.M. Institute for Medical Research, Camden, N.J.

This study was conducted under contract 70-2049 within the special virus cancer program of the National Cancer Institute, and grant CA-02332.

1971 17 Dec. Kacian, D.L., S. Spiegelman, A. Bank, M. Terada, S.Metafora, L. Dow, and P.A. Marks
"In vitro synthesis of DNA components of human genes for globins." Nature New Biology 235(Feb. 9):167-169, 1972.
ID=49
CT=36
CC=198
WT=.0484

D.L.K. and S.S., Institute of Cancer Research, Columbia University and Francis Delafield Hospital, A.B., M.T., S.M., L.D., P.A.M., Department of Medicine, College of Physicians and Surgeons, Columbia University, and the Medical Service, Presbyterian Hospital, N.Y.

This study was supported in part by the NIH Special Virus Cancer Program and by the National Science Foundation. A.B. is a recipient of a Faculty Research award from the American Cancer Society.

1971 29 Dec. Robert, M.S., R.G. Smith, R.C. Gallo, P.S. Sarin, and J.W. Abrell
RV '72 23 Mar. "Viral and cellular DNA polymerase: comparison of activities with synthetic and natural RNA templates." Science 176(May 19):798-800, 1972.
ID=50
CT=41
CC=448
WT=.1106

M.S.R., R.G.S., AND R.C.G., Laboratory of tumor cell biology, National Cancer Institute, P.S.S., and J.W.A. Bionetics Research Laboratories, Bethesda.

Supported in part by the Leukemia Society of America. M.S.R. is a fellow of the Leukemia Society of America.

1972 10 Jan.
ID=51
CT=37
CC=277
WT=.0758

Ting, R.C., S.S. Yang, and R.C. Gallo
"Reverse transcriptase, RNA tumour virus transformation and derivatives of rifamycin SV." Nature New Biology 236(April 12):163-166, 1972.

R.C.T. and S.S.Y., Bionetics Research Laboratories, Bethesda, R.C.G., Laboratory of Tumor Cell Biology, National Cancer Institute.

This work was supported by contracts from the Chemotherapy Area and Special Virus Cancer Program of the National Cancer Institute.

1972 26 Jan.
ID=52
CT=28
CC=393
WT=.0992

Green, M. and M. Cartas
"The genome of RNA tumor viruses contains polyadenylic acid sequences." Proc. N.A.S. 69(April):791-794, 1972.

Institute for Molecular Virology, Saint Louis University School of Medicine.

This study was conducted under Contract no. PH43-67-692 within the Special Virus Cancer Program of the National Cancer Institute, NIH, USPHS, and by USPHS Grant AI-01725.

1972 31 Jan.
ID=53
CT=27
CC=292
WT=.0740

Faras, A.J., J.M. Taylor, J.P. McDonnell, W.E. Levinson, and J.M. Bishop
"Purification and characterization of the deoxyribonucleic acid polymerase associated with Rous sarcoma virus." Biochemistry 11(12):2334-2342, 1972.

Department of Microbiology, University of California, San Francisco.

This investigation was supported by U.S. Public Health Service Grants AI 08864, CA 12380, CA 12705, AI 06862, and AI 00299 and Contract 71-2147 within the Special Virus-Cancer Program of the National Cancer Institute, NIH, PHS.

1972 14 Feb.
ID=54
CT=32
CC=443
WT=.1092

Gillespie, D., S. Marshall, R.C. Gallo
"RNA of RNA tumour viruses contains poly A." Nature New Biology 236(April 26):227-231, 1972.

D.G. and S.M., Laboratory of Molecular Aging, Gerontology Research Center, NICHD, NIH, and Baltimore City Hospitals, R.C.G., Laboratory of Tumor Cell Biology, National Cancer Institute.

1972 27 Mar.
ID=55
CT=31
CC=353
WT=.0888

Kang, C-Y. and H.M. Temin
"Endogenous RNA-directed DNA polymerase activity in uninfected chicken embryos." Proc. N.A.S. 69(June):1550-1554, 1972.

McArdle Laboratory for Cancer Research, University of Wisconsin, Madison.

This investigation was supported by Public Health Service Research Grant CA-07175 from the National Cancer Institute and grant VC-7 from the American Cancer Society. C.-Y. K. was supported by Training Grant T01-CA-5002 from the Naitonal Cancer Institute. H.M.T. holds Research Career Development Award 10K3-CA-8182 from the National Cancer Institute.

1972 (1 Apr.)?
ID=56
CT=34
CC=257
WT=.0638

Todaro, G.J. and R.J. Huebner
"The viral oncogene hypothesis: new evidence." Proc. N.A.S. 69(April):1009-1015, 1972.

Viral Leukemia and Lymphoma Branch, and Viral Carcinogenesis Branch, National Cancer Institute.

1972 24 Apr.
ID=57
CT=31
CC=402
WT=.1011

Hehlmann, R., D. Kufe, and S. Spiegelman
"Viral-related RNA in Hodgkins' disease and other human lymphomas." Proc. N.A.S. 69(July):1727-1731, 1972.

Institute of Cancer Research, College of Physicians and Surgeons, Columbia University.

This research was supported by the National Institutes of Health, National Cancer Institute, Special Virus Cancer Program Contract 70-2049 and Research Grant CA-02332.

1972 18 May
ID=58
CT=32
CC=366
WT=.0891

Gulati, S.C., R. Axel, and S. Spiegelman
"Detection of RNA-instructed DNA polymerase and high molecular weight RNA in malignant tissue." Proc. N.A.S. 69(Aug.):2020-2024, 1972.

Institute of Cancer Research, College of Physicians and Surgeons, Columbia University.

This research was supported by the National Institutes of Health, National Cancer Institute, Special Virus Cancer Program Contract 70-2049 and by Research Grant CA-02332.

1972 (1 June)?
ID=59
CT=34
CC=321
WT=.0774

Temin, H.M. and D. Baltimore
"RNA-directed DNA synthesis and RNA tumor viruses." Advan. Virus Res. 17:129-186, 1972.

H.M.T., McArdle Laboratory, University of Wisconsin, Madison, D.B., Department of Biology, Massachusetts Institute of Technology.

H.M.T. supported by Public Health Service Research Grant CA-07175 and Research Career Development Award 10K3-CA-8182 from the Natioal Cancer Institute, D.B. supported by Grant E-512 and a Faculty Research Award from the American Cancer Society and a contract from The Special Virus Cancer Program of the National Cancer Institute.

1972 5 June
RV 24 July
ID=60
CT=33
CC=317
WT=.0735

Scolnick, E.M., W.P. Parks, G.J. Todaro
"Reverse Transcriptase of Primate viruses as immunological markers." Science 177(Sept. 22):1119-1121, 1972.

Viral Leukemia and Lymphoma Branch and Viral Carcinogenesis Branch, National Cancer Institute.

Supported in part by a contract to Meloy Labs., Springfield, Va., from the Special Virus Cancer Program, National Cancer Institute, National Institutes of Health.

1972 8 June RV 3 Aug. ID=61 CT=56 CC=550 WT=.1359	Sarngadharan, M.G., P.S. Sarin, and M.S. Reitz "Reverse transcriptase activity of human acute leukaemic cells: purification of the enzyme, response to AMV 70S RNA, and characterization of the DNA product." Nature New Biology 240(Nov. 15):87-72, 1972. M.G.S., P.S.S., and M.S.R., Department of Molecular Biology, Bionetics Research Laboratories, Bethesda, R.C.G., Laboratory of Tumor Cell Biology, National Cancer Institute, NIH.
1972 8 June RV 27 July ID=62 CT=50 CC=439 WT=.1095	Baxt, W., R. Hehlmann, and S. Spiegelman "Human leukaemic cells contain reverse transcriptase associated with a high molecular weight virus- related RNA." Nature New Biol 240(Nov. 15):72- , 1972. Institute of Cancer Research and Department of Human Genetics and Development, College of Physicians and Surgeons, Columbia University. Research supported in part by NIH and NCI grants.
1972 21 Aug. ID=63 CT=26 CC=284 WT=.0659	Axel, R., S.C. Gulati, S. Spiegelman "Particles containing RNA-instructed DNA polymerase and virus-related RNA in human breast cancer." Proc. N.A.S. 69(Nov.):3133-3137, 1972. Institute of Cancer Research and Department of Human Genetics and Development, College of Physicians and Surgeons, Columbia University. Research supported in part by NIH, National Cancer Institute, Special Virus Cancer Program, contract 70-2049, Research Grant CA 02332.
1972 (1 Oct.)? ID=64 CT=33 CC=378 WT=.0935	Smith, R.G., and R.C. Gallo "DNA-dependent DNA polymerases I and II from normal human-blood lymphocytes." Proc. N.A.S. 69(Oct.):2879-2884, 1972. Laboratory of Tumor Cell Biology, National Cancer Institute.
1972 7 Nov. ID=65 CT=39 CC=353 WT=.0849	Grandgenett, D.P., G.F. Gerard, and M. Green "A sigle subunit from avian myeloblastosis virus with both RNA-directed DNA polymerase and ribonuclease H activity." Proc. N.A.S. 70(Jan.):230-234, 1973. Institute for Molecular Virology, St. Louis University School of Medicine. This work was supported by Contract PH43-67-692 within the Special Virus-Cancer Program of the NCI, NIH, PHS. M.G. is a Research Career Awardee of the National Institutes of Health (5K6-AI-4739), and D.P.G. is a postdoctoral fellow of the American Cancer Society.
1973 16 Mar. ID=66 CT=28 CC=248 WT=.0577	Abrell, J.W., and R. Gallo "Purification, characterization, and comparison of the DNA polymerases from two primate RNA tumor viruses. J. Virology 12:431-439, 1973. Laboratory of Tumor Cell Biology, National Cancer Institute. This work was supported by contracts from PHS, NCI, NIH-71-2025.

---

[a]The total number of citations received (CT), the total number of co-citations (CC), and the weight received by the article on the first eigenvector (WT) (see Table 6.2) are recorded for each bibliographic entry in this table. Below the bibliographic information, the attributed location of the authors and funding information are given as they are found within the respective articles. The articles have been ordered according to submission dates, which are recorded to the left of the article. Question marks signify that the information recorded was determined with difficulty. In some cases we have also obtained revision dates (RV).

APPENDIX E

MOST HIGHLY CITED (≥ 10) ARTICLES BY THE REVERSE TRANSCRIPTASE

ARTICLE SET IN THE PREDISCOVERY PERIOD [a]

1936
ID=1
CT=11
CC=34
WT=.0659

Bittner, J.J.
"Some possible effects of nursing on the mammary gland tumor incidence in mice." Science 84:162, 1936.

Jackson Memorial Laboratory, Bar Harbor, Maine.

1951 28 May
ID=2
CT=71
CC=82
WT=.1341

Lowry, O.H., N.J. Rosebrough, A.L. Farr, and R.J. Randall
"Protein measurement with the folin phenol reagent." J. Biol. Chem. 193:265-275.

The Department of Pharmacology, Washington University School of Medicine, St. Louis.

Supported in part by a grant from the American Cancer Society on the recommendation of the Committee on Growth of the National Research Council.

1958 11 Feb.
ID=3
CT=10
CC=42
WT=.1093

Bernhard, W.
"Electron microscopy of tumor cells and tumor viruses: a review." Cancer Res. 18: 491-509, 1958.

Institut de Recherches sur le Cancer, Villejuif, Seine, France.

1959 10 Sept.
ID=4
CT=14
CC=67
WT=.1812

Bernhard, W.
"The detection and study of tumor viruses with the electron microscope." Cancer Res. 20:712-727, 1960.

Institut de Recherches sur le Cancer, Villejuif, Seine, France.

This work was aided by Grant C-4602 from the National Cancer Institute, National Institutes of Health, Public Health Service; and by financial aid from the Mutuelle Générale de l'Education Nationale.

1960 5 Dec.
ID=5
CT=13
CC=30
WT=.0717

Martin, R.G., and B.N. Ames
"A method for determining the sedimentation behavior of enzymes: application to protein mixtures." Journal of Biol. Chem. 236(May):1372-1379, 1961.

National Institute of Arthritis and Metabolic Diseases, Naitonal Institutes of Health.

This work was begun during service as an officer in the United States Public Health Service under the Commissioned Officers: Student Training and Extern Program (CO-STEP).

1960 8 Dec,
ID=6
CT=12
CC=27
WT=.0534

Hall, B.D., and S. Spiegelman
"Sequence complementarity of T2-DNA and T2-specific RNA." Proc. N.A.S. 47(Feb. 15): 137-146, 1961.

Departments of Chemistry and Microbiology, University of Illinois

This investigation was aided by grants in aid from the U.S. Public Health Service, National Science Founcation, and the Office of Naval Research.

1961 14 Aug.
ID=7
CT=14
CC=21
WT=.0451

Aposhian, H.V., and A. Kornberg
"Enzymatic synthesis of deoxyribonucleic acid." Journal of Biol. Chem. 237(Feb.): 519-525, 1962.

The Department of Biochemistry, Stanford University School of Medicine, Palo Alto, Calif.

This work was aided by grants from the United States Public Health Service.

1962 27 Feb.
ID=8
CT=10
CC=24
WT=.0600

Rauscher, F.J.
"A virus-induced disease of mice characterized by erythrocytopoiesis and lymphoid leukemia." J. Natl. Cancer Inst. 29(Sept.):515-532, 1962.

Laboratory of Viral Oncology, National Cancer Institute, Bethesda.

1963 11 April
ID=9
CT=12
CC=58
WT=.1620

Temin, H.M.
"The effects of actinomycin D on growth of Rous sarcoma virus in vitro." Virology 20:577-582, 1963.

McArdle Memorial Laboratory, Univerisy of Wisconsin, Madison.

This investigation was supported by a PHS grant, C-5250, from the National Cancer Institute, United States Public Health Service.

1963 9 Dec.
ID=10
CT=12
CC=42
WT=.1195

Bader, J.P.
"The role of deoxyribonucleic acid in the synthesis of Rous sarcoma virus." Virology 22:462-468, 1964.

Macromolecular Chemistry Section, Laboratory of Viral Oncology, National Cancer Institute.

Preliminary work on this problem was done at the California Institute of Technology during the tenure of a Postdoctoral Fellowship from the National Cancer Institute.

1964 31 March
ID=11
CT=23
CC=90
WT=.2466

Temin, H.M.
"Nature of the provirus of Rous sarcoma." Nat. Canc. Inst. Mono. 17:557-570, 1964.

McArdle Laboratory, University of Wisconsin, Madison.

This investigation was supported by grants C-5250 and CA-07175 from the National Cancer Institute, National Institutes of Health, Public Health Service.

1964 13 April
ID=12
CT=18
CC=83
WT=.2217

Temin, H.M.
"The participation of DNA in Rous sarcoma virus production." Virology 23:486-494, 1964.

McArdle Memorial Laboratory, University of Wisconsin, Madison.

This investigation was supported by a PHS grant, C-5250, from the National Cancer Institute, Public Health Service.

1964 17 June
ID=13
CT=12
CC=55
WT=.1683

Temin, H.M.
"Homology between RNA from Rous sarcoma virus and DNA from Rous sarcoma virus-infected cells." Proc. N.A.S. 52:323-329, 1964.

McArdle Memorial Laboratory, University of Wisconsin, Madison.

This investigation was supported by U.S. Public Health Service grant CA-07175 from the National Cancer Institute.

1964 15 Oct.
RV 9 Nov.
ID=14
CT=19
CC=32
WT=.0767

Studier, F.W.
"Sedimentation studies of the size and shape of DNA." J. Mol. Biol. 11:373-390, 1965.

Department of Biochemistry, Stanford University School of Medicine, Palo Alto, Calif.

This work was done while the author was a Postdoctoral Fellow of the National Science Foundation and was supported in part by research grants from the National Institutes of Health, United States Public Health Service.

1965 1 March
ID=15
CT=13
CC=40
WT=.0907

Hartley, J.W., W.P. Rowe, W.I. Capps, and R.J. Huebner
"Complement fixation and tissue culture assays for mouse leukemia viruses." Proc. N.A.S. 53:931-938, 1965.

Laboratory of Infectious Diseases, National Institutes of Health, Bethesda.

This research supported by NCI Field Studies.

1965 5 April
ID=16
CT=11
CC=20
WT=.0460

Ando, T.
"A nuclease specific for heat-denatured DNA isolated from a product of Aspergillus oryzae." Biochim. Biophys. Acta 114:158-168, 1966.

Laboratory of Microbiology, Institute of Physical and Chemical Research, Bunkyo-ku, Tokyo, Japan.

1965 13 May
ID=17
CT=12
CC=76
WT=.2111

Robinson, W.S., A. Pitkanen, and H. Rubin
"The nucleic acid of the Bryan strain of Rous sarcoma virus: purification of the virus and isolation of the nucleic acid." Proc. N.A.S. 54:137-144.

Virus Laboratory, University of California, Berkeley.

This investigation was supported by research grants CA 04774 and CA 05619 and by USPHS fellowship 1 F2 CA 23487-01 from the National Cancer Institute, National Institutes of Health, U.S. Public Health Service.

1965 22 Nov.
ID=18
CT=13
CC=44
WT=.1191

Duesberg, P.H., and W.S. Robinson
"Nucleic acid and proteins isolated from the Rauscher mouse leukemia virus (MLV)." Proc. N.A.S. 55:219-227, 1966.

Department of Molecular Biology and Virus Laboratory, University of California, Berkeley.

This investigation was supported in part by a U.S. Public Health Service research grant AI 01267 from the National Institute of Allergy and Infectious Diseases, research grants CA 04774 and CA 05619 from the National Cancer Institute, NIH, USPHS, and a grant from the Rockefeller Foundation.

1966 24 Feb.
ID=19
CT=12
CC=43
WT=.0892

Hartley, J.W., and W.P. Rowe
"Production of altered cell foci in tissue culture by defective Moloney sarcoma virus particles." Proc. N.A.S. 55:780-786, 1966.

National Institute of Allergy and Infectious Diseases, National Institutes of Health, Bethesda.

1966 27 June
ID=20
CT=17
CC=56
WT=.0983

Duc-Nguyen, H., E.N. Rosenblum, and R.F. Zeigel
"Persistent infection of a rat kidney cell line with Rauscher murine leukemia virus." Jour. of Bacteriology 92:1133-1140, 1966.

National Institutes of Health, National Cancer Institute, Bethesda.

1966 29 Aug.
ID=21
CT=13
CC=49
WT=.1113

Huebner, R.J., J.W. Hartley, W.P. Rowe, W.T. Lane, and W.I. Capps
"Rescue of the defective genome of Moloney sarcoma virus from a noninfectious hamster tumor and the production of pseudotype sarcoma viruses with various murine leukemia viruses." Proc. N.A.S. 56:1164-1169, 1966.

U.S. Public Health Service, National Institutes of Health, National Institute of Allergy and Infectious Diseases, Laboratory of Infectious Diseases, Bethesda.

This work was partially supported by the Etiology Area, National Cancer Institute, NIH.

1967 (1 Sept.)? Robinson, W.S., H.L. Robinson, and P.H. Duesberg
"Tumor virus RNA's." Proc. N.A.S. 58:825-834, 1967.
ID=22
CT=14
CC=72
WT=.1780

Department of Molecular Biology and Virus Laboratory, University of California, Berkeley.

This investigation was supported in part by U.S. Public Health Service research grants CA 08557, CA 04774, and CA 05619, and training grant CA 5028 from the National Cancer Institute, U.S. Public Health Service; H.R. is a National Science Foundation postdoctoral fellow.

1968 18 March
AC 20 May
ID=23
CT=12
CC=58
WT=.1726

Payne, L.N., and R.C. Chubb
"Studies on the nature and genetic control of an antigen in normal chick embryos which reacts in the COFAL test." J. Gen. Virol. 3:379-391, 1968.

Houghton Poultry Research Station, Houghton, Huntington, Great Britain.

1968 29 May
ID=24
CT=26
CC=117
WT=.3051

Duesberg, P.H.
"Physical properties of Rous sarcoma virus RNA." Proc. N.A.S. 60:1511-1518, 1968.

Virus Laboratory, University of California, Berkeley.

This investigation was supported by U.S. Public Health Service research grant AI 01267 from the National Institute of Allergy and Infectious Diseases, and grants CA 04774, CA 05619, and training rant CA 05028 from the National Cancer Institute.

1968 7 June
AC 23 July
ID=25
CT=10
CC=25
WT=.0443

Aaronson, S.A. and G.J. Todaro
"Development of 3T3-like lines from Balb/c mouse embryo cultures: transformation susceptibility to SV40." J. Cell Physiol. 72:141-148, 1968.

Viral Carcinogenesis Branch, National Cancer Institute, National Institutes of Health, Bethesda.

This work was supported in part by Contract PH 43-65-641 from the National Cancer Institute.

1968 (1 Aug.)?
ID=26
CT=22
CC=39
WT=.1016

Britten, R.J., and D.E. Kohne
"Repeated sequences in DNA." Science 161(9 Aug.):529-540, 1968.

Department of Terrestrial Magnetism of the Carnegie Institution of Washington, Washington, D.C.

1968 20 Sept.
ID=27
CT=12
CC=26
WT=.0401

Shatkin, A.J., and J.D. Sipe
"RNA polymerase activity in purified reoviruses." Proc. N.A.S. 61:1462-1469, 1968.

Laboratory of Biology of Viruses, National Institute of Allergy and Infectious Diseases National Institutes of Health, Bethesda.

1968 26 Sept.
ID=28
CT=13
CC=76
WT=.2253

Erikson, R.L.
"Studies on the RNA from avian myeloblastosis virus." Virology 37:124-131, 1969.

Department of Pathology, University of Colorado Medical Center, Denver

This work was supported by grants from the American Cancer Society (E-389a) and the National Institute of Allergy and Infectious Diseases (AI-06844).

1968 30 Sept.
ID=29
CT=10
CC=76
WT=.1505

Duesberg, P.H., and R.D. Cardiff
"Structural relationships between the RNA of mammary tumor virus and those of other RNA tumor viruses." Virology 36:696-700, 1968.

P.H.D., Virus Laboratory, University of California, Berkeley, R.D.C., Cancer Research Genetics Laboratory, University of California, Berkeley.

This investigation was supported by Public Health Service research grant AI 01267 from the National Institute of Allergy and Infectious Disseases, Us. Public Health Service; and grants CA 04774, CA 05619, F3-CA-34, 561-02, and training grant CA 05028 from the National Cancer Institute, U.S. Public Health Service.

1968 30 Sept.
ID=30
CT=13
CC=60
WT=.1592

Gregoriades, A., and L.J. Old
"Isolation and some characteristics of a group-specific antigen of the murine leukemia viruses." Virology 37:189-202, 1969.

Division of Immunology, Sloan-Kettering Institute for Cancer Research, and Sloan-Kettering Division, Cornell University Graduate School of Medical Sciences, Cornell University Medical College, New York.

This work was supported by National Cancer Institute Grant CA 08747 and a grant from the John A. Hartford Foundation, Inc.

1968 6 Nov.
ID=31
CT=20
CC=22
WT=.0391

Jovin, T.M., P.T. Englund, and L.L. Bertsch
"Enzymatic synthesis of deoxyribonucleic acid." Jour. of Biol. Chem. 214(June 10): 3996-3008, 1969.

Department of Biochemistry, Stanford University School of Medicine.

This study was supported in part by grants from the National Institutes of Health (United States Public Health Service), the National Science Foundation, and the National Aeronautics and Space Administration. T.M.J., National Science Foundation Postdoctoral Fellow, P.T.E., National Institutes of Health Postdoctoral Fellow.

1968 14 Nov.
ID=32
CT=11
CC=36
WT=.0742

Hartley, J.W., W.P. Rowe, W.I. Capps, and R.J. Huebner
"Isolation of naturally occurring viruses of the murine leukemia virus group in tissue culture." Jour. of Virology 3(Feb.):126-132, 1969.

Laboratory of Viral Diseases, National Institute of Allergy and Infectious Diseases, Bethesda.

This investigation was supported by the Etiology Area of the National Cancer Institute.

1969 25 Feb.
ID=33
CT=10
CC=24
WT=.0568

Toyoshima, K., and P.K. Vogt
"Enhancement and inhibition of avian sarcoma viruses by polycations and polyanions." Virology 38:414-426, 1969.

Department of Microbiology, University of Washington, School of Medicine, Seattle.

Supported by the U.S. Public Health Service Research Grant No. CA 10569, from the National Cancer Institute.

1969 10 April
ID=34
CT=12
CC=46
WT=.1074

Klement, V., W.P. Rowe, J.W. Hartley, and W.E. Pugh
"Mixed culture cytopathogenicity: a new test for growth of murine leukemia viruses in tissue culture." Proc. N.A.S. 63:753-758, 1969.

Laboratory of Viral Diseases, National Institute of Allergy and Infectious Diseases, National Institutes of Health, Bethesda.

1969 30 April
ID=35
CT=15
CC=40
WT=.0700

Moore, D.H., N.H. Sarkar, C.E. Kelly, N. Pillsbury, and J. Charney
"Type B particles in human milk." Texas Reports on Biology and Medicine 27(Winter): 1027-1039, 1969.

Institute for Medical Research, Camden, N.J.

Supported in part by Contract No. Ph-43-68-1000 and Grant No. 08740 from the National Cancer Institute, National Institutes of Health, and by a Grant from the Lillia Babbitt Hyde Foundation.

1969 17 June
ID=36
CT=15
CC=10
WT=.0123

Burgess, R.R.
"A new method for the large scale purification of Escherichia coli deoxyribonucleic acid-dependent ribonucleic acid polymerase." Jour. of Biol. Chem. 244(Nov. 25):6160-6167, 1969.

The Biological Laboratory, Harvard University, Cambridge, Mass.

The work was supported by grants from the National Institutes of Health, and the National Science Foundation. National Science Foundation Predoctoral Fellow, Helen Haw Whitney Postdoctoral Fellow.

1969 19 June
ID=37
CT=14
CC=72
WT=.1989

Bader, J.P., and T.L. Steck
"Analysis of the ribonucleic acid of murine leukemia virus." Jour. of Virology 4(Oct.): 454-459, 1969.

Chemistry Branch, National Cancer Institute, Bethesda.

1969 14 July
ID=38
CT=18
CC=36
WT=.0921

Aaronson, S.A., J.W. Hartley, and G.J. Todaro
"Mourse leukemia virus: "spontaneous" release by mouse embryo cells after longterm in vitro cultivation." Proc. N.A.S. 64:87-94, 1969.

National Institutes of Health, Bethesda. S.A.A. and G.J.T., Viral Carcinogenesis Branch, Natioanl Cancer Institute. J.W.H., Laboratory of Viral Oncology, National Institute of Allergy and Infectious Diseases.

This work was supported in part by National Cancer Institute Contract PH43-65-641.

1969 15 July
ID=39
CT=12
CC=31
WT=.0598

Jainchill, J.L., S.A. Aaronson, and G.J. Todaro
"Murine sarcoma and leukemia viruses: assay using clonal lines of contact-inhibited mouse cells." Jour. of Virology 4(Nov.):549-553, 1969.

Viral Carcinogenesis Branch, National Cancer Institute, Bethesda.

This investigation was supported by Public Health Service contract no. PH-43-65-641.

1969 15 Sept.
ID=40
CT=12
CC=38
WT=.0748

Feller, W.F., and H.C. Chopra
"Studies of human milk in relation to the possible viral etiology of breast cancer." Cancer 24:1250-1254, 1969.

W.F.F., Georgetown University School of Medicine, Washington, D.C., and H.C.C., The John L. Smith Memorial for Cancer Research, Charles Pfizer and Company, Inc., Maywood, N.J.

Supported by Public Health Service Contracts PH 43-65-53 and 43-67-1176.

1969 16 Sept.
ID=41
CT=10
CC=16
WT=.0200

Skehel, J.J., and W.K. Joklik
"Studies on the in vitro transcription of reovirus RNA catalyzed by reovirus cores." Virology 39:822-831, 1969.

Department of Microbiology and Immunology, Duke University Medical Center, Durham, N.C.

This work was supported by Grant No. GB-8077 from the National Science Foundation, Grant No. AT-(40-1)-3857 from the United States Atomic Energy Commission, and Grant No. AI-08909-01 from the United States Public Health Service.

1969 16 Sept.
ID=42
CT=55
CC=153
WT=.3450

Huebner, R.J., and G.J. Todaro
"Oncogenes of RNA tumor viruses as determinants of cancer." Proc. N.A.S. 64:1087-1094, 1969.

Viral Carcinogenesis Branch, National Cancer Institute, National Institutes of Health, Bethesda.

1969 24 Oct.
ID=43
CT=10
CC=16
WT=.0288

Diggelmann, H., and C. Weissmann
"Rifampicin inhibits focus formation in chick fibroblasts infected with Rous sarcoma virus." Nature 224(Dec. 27):1277-1279, 1969.

Institut für Molekularbiologie der Universität Zürich, Switzerland.

The investigation was supported by grants from the Schweizerische Nationalfonds and the Jane Coffin Childs Fund.

1969 18 Dec.
RV '70 27 Feb.
ID=44
CT=12
CC=25
WT=.0476

Hausen, P., and H. Stein
"Ribonuclease H: an enzyme degrading the RNA moiety of DNA-RNA hybrids." Eur. J. Biochem. 14(2):278-283, 1970.

Max-Planck-Institut für Biologie, Abteilung Beermann, Tübingen.

Supported by the Duetsche Forschungsgemeinschaft.

1970 19 Jan.
ID=45
CT=14
CC=54
WT=.1308

Geering, G., T. Aoki, and L.J. Old
"Shared viral antigen of mammalian leukaemic viruses." Nature 226(April 18):265-266, 1970.

Sloan-Kettering Institute for Cancer Research, New York.

The work is supported in part by an NCI grant and a grant from the John A. Hartford Foundation, Inc.

1970 11 Feb.
AC 2 April
ID=46
CT=20
CC=45
WT=.0869

Chopra, H.C., and M.M. Mason
"A new virus in a spontaneous mammary tumor of a rhesus monkey." Cancer Research 30(Aug.): 2081-2086, 1970.

John L. Smith Memorial for Cancer Research, Charles Pfizer and Co., Inc., Maywood, N.J. (H.C.C. and Mason Research Institute, Worcester, Mass. (M.M.M.).

Supported by Breast Cancer Task Force Contract PH 43-67-1176, NIH.

1970 26 Feb.
ID=47
CT=10
CC=64
WT=.1924

Baluda, M.A., and D.P. Nayak
"DNA complementary to viral RNA in leukemic cells induced by avian myeloblastosis virus." Proc. N.A.S. 66(June):329-336, 1970.

Department of Medical Microbiology and Immunology, University of California School of Medicine, Los Angeles.

This investigation was supported by U.S. Public Health Service research grant CA-10197 from the National Cancer Institute and by the California Institute for Cancer Research. M.A.B. recipient of American Cancer Society award (PRA-34) for faculty position support, D.P.N. recipient of a senior Dernham Fellowship, American Cancer Society, California division.

1970 24 March
ID=48
CT=30
CC=36
WT=.0572

Baltimore, D., A.S. Huang, and M. Stampfer
"Ribonucleic acid synthesis of vesicular stomatitis virus, II. an RNA polymerase in the virion." Proc. N.A.S. 66(June):572-576, 1970.

Department of Biology, Massachusetts Institute of Technology.

Supported by USPHS grant AI-08388 and the American Cancer Society grant E-512. D.B. was supported by a Faculty Research Award from the American Cancer Society, and M.S. was supported by a predoctoral fellowship from the National Science Foundation.

1970 30 March
ID=49
CT=11
CC=70
WT=.1962

Duesberg, P.H., G.S. Martin, and P.K. Vogt
"Glycoprotein components of avian and murine RNA tumor viruses." Virology 41:631-646, 1970.

Virus Laboratory and Department of Molecular Biology, University of California, Berkeley, Department of Microbiology, University of Washington, Seattle, Washington.

This investigation was supported by U.S. Public Health Service research grants CA 11426, CA 05619, and CA 10569 from the National Cancer Institute, and by a grant from the Jane Coffin Childs Memorial Fund for Medical Research.

1970 7 April
AC 22 May
ID=50
CT=10
CC=28
WT=.0584

Jensen, E.M., I. Zelljadt, H.C. Chopra, and M.M. Mason
"Isolation and propagation of a virus from a spontaneous mammary carcinoma of a rhesus monkey." Cancer Research 30(Sept.):2388-2393, 1970.

The John L. Smith Memorial for Cancer Research, Pfizer, Inc., Maywood, N.J. (E.M.M., I.Z., H.C.C.), and Mason Research Institute, Worcester, Mass (M.M.M.).

This study was conducted under USPHS contracts PH 43-66-98 (NIH 70-2080) and PH 43-67-1176 within the Special Virus-Leukemia Program of the National Cancer Institute, Bethesda.

1970 14 April
ID=51
CT=10
CC=44
WT=.1073

Aaronson, S.A., and W.P. Rowe
"Nonproducer clones of murine Sarcoma virus transformed BALB/3T3 cells." Virology 42: 9-19, 1970.

Viral Carcinogenesis Branch, National Cancer Institute, and Laboratory of Viral Diseases, National Institute of Allergy and Infectious Diseases, Bethesda.

This work was supported in part by National Cancer Institute Contract No. PH43-66-641.

1970 16 April
ID=52
CT=15
CC=51
WT=.1226

Bassin, R.H., N. Tuttle, and P.J. Fischinger
"Isolation of murine sarcoma virus-transformed mouse cells which are negative for leukemia virus from agar suspension cultures." Int. J. Cancer 6:95-107, 1970.

Viral Leukemia and Lymphoma Branch, National Cancer Institute, Bethesda.

These studies were initiated while one of us (R.H.B.) was working at the Imperial Cancer Research Fund, London, and were supported in part by US Public Health Service Fellowship 2-F2-CA-31, 749-02.

1970 27 May
ID=53
CT=13
CC=56
WT=.1546

Bishop, J.M., W.E. Levinson, N. Quintrell, D. Sullivan, L. Fanshier, and J. Jackson
"The low molecular weight RNAs of Rous sarcoma virus: I. The 4 S RNA." Virology 42:182-195, 1970.

Department of Microbiology, University of California School of Medicine, San Francisco, Calif.

The work was supported by USPHS grants CA 10223 and AI 06862, USPHS training grant AI00299, and grants from the Cancer Coordinating Committee of the University of California and the California Division of the American Cancer Society.

1970 (1 June)?
ID=54
CT=10
CC=24
WT=.0668

Green, M.
"Oncogenic Viruses." Ann. Rev. Biochem. 39:701-756, 1970.

Institute for Molecular Virology, St. Louis University School of Medicine, St. Louis.

Work cited in this review by the author was supported by Public Health Service grant AI-01725, contract PH43-64-928 from the National Institute of Allergy and Infectious Diseases, and contract PH43-67-692 from the National Cancer Institute. Research Career Awardee of the National Institutes of Health (5-K6-AI-4739).

---

[a]The total number of citations received (CT), the total number of co-citations (CC) and the weight received by the article on the first eigenvector (WT) (see Table 6.4) are recorded for each bibliographic entry in this table. Below the bibliographic information, the attributed location of the authors and the funding information are given as they are found within the respective articles. The articles have been ordered according to submission dates, which are recorded to the left of the article. Question marks signify that the information recorded was determined with difficulty. In some cases we have also obtained revision dates (RV).

REFERENCES

Aaronson, Stuart A., Janet W. Hartley, and George J. Todaro

1969 "Mouse leukemia virus: 'Spontaneous' release by mouse embryo cells after long-term in vitro cultivation." *Proceedings of the National Academy of Sciences* 64: 87-94.

Ahlström, C. G. and C. H. Andrewes

1938 "Fibroma virus infection in tarred rabbits." *Journal of Pathology and Bacteriology* 47: 65-86.

Alba, Richard D. and Myron P. Gutmann

1972 "SOCK: A sociometric analysis system." *Behavioral Science* 17: 326.

Allen, Garland

1975 *Life Science in the Twentieth Century.* New York: Wiley.

Allison, P. D. and J. A. Stewart

1974 "Productivity differences among scientists: Evidence for accumulative advantage." *American Sociological Review* 39: 596-606.

American Men and Women of Science

1906- 1972 The Physical and Biological Sciences. 1st-12th Editions. New York: Cattell Press/Bowker.

1976 The Physical and Biological Sciences. 13th Edition. New York: Cattell Press/Bowker.

Amos, Harold

1977 "Basic science and public policy." *Yale Journal of Biology and Medicine* 50: 261-264.

Anderson, Sydney and Richard G. Van Gelder

1970 "The history and status of the literature of mammalogy." *BioScience* 20: 949-957.

Anonymous

1970a "New enzyme found in leukemia patients." *Chemical and Engineering News* 48: 46-49.

1970b "Reverse transcriptases: Roundabouts and swings from our cell biology correspondent." *Nature* 228 (December 26): 1255.

1971 "Happy birthday, reverse transcriptase?" *Nature (New Biology)* 231 (June 9): 161.

1972 "Germ weapon center to be converted for cancer work." *Wall Street Journal,* June 26: 14.

1973 "Reverse transcriptase in acute leukemia." *Lancet* ii (September 8): 542-544.

Arber, Agnes
1954 *The Mind and the Eye: A Study of the Biologist's Standpoint.* Cambridge, MA: Cambridge University Press.

Arnold, David O.
1970 "Dimensional sampling: An approach for studying a small number of cases." *American Sociologist* 5: 147-150.

Astbury, W. T.
1952 "Adventures in molecular biology." *Harvey Lectures,* Series 46 (1950-1951): 3-44.

Atlanta Constitution
1978 "Cancer-virus link proof near." September 22.

Austin, James H.
1978 *Chase, Chance, and Creativity. The Lucky Art of Novelty.* New York: Columbia University Press.

Avery, O. T., C. M. MacLeod, and M. McCarty
1944 "Induction of transformation by a desoxyribonucleic acid fraction isolated from pneumococcus type III." *Journal of Experimental Medicine* 79: 137-157.

Bader, John P.
1967 "Metabolic requirements in Rous sarcoma virus replication." Pp. 697-708 in J. S. Colter and W. Paranchych (eds.), *The Molecular Biology of Viruses.* New York: Academic Press.
1978 Personal interview (May 10).

Baker, Carl G., Louis M. Carrese, and Frank Rauscher
1968 "The Special Virus-Leukemia Program of the National Cancer Institute—scientific aspects and program logic." Pp. 259-278 in R. N. Fiennes (ed.), *Some Recent Developments in Comparative Medicine.* Symposia of the Zoological Society of London 17. London: Academic Press.

Baltimore, David
1970 "Viral RNA-dependent DNA polymerase." *Nature* 226 (June 27): 1209-1211.
1971 "Expression of animal virus genomes." *Bacteriological Reviews* 35: 235-241.
1975 "Tumor viruses: 1974." *Cold Springs Harbor Symposium on Quantitative Biology* 28: 1187-1200.
1976a "The strategy of RNA viruses." *Harvey Lectures,* Series 46 (1974-1975): 57-74.
1967b "Viruses, polymerases, and cancer." *Science* 192 (May 14): 632-636.
1977 Personal communication (January 31).
1978 Personal interview (March 20).

Baltimore, David, A. S. Huang, and M. Stampfer
1970 "Ribonucleic acid synthesis of vesicular stomatitis virus. II. An RNA polymerase in the virion." *Proceedings of the National Academy of Sciences* 66: 572-576.

Baluda, M. and P. Markham
1971 "Nucleotide composition of RNA hybridizing to homologous DNA from cells transformed by avian tumor viruses." *Nature (New Biology)* 231: 90-91.

Baluda, M. and D. P. Nayak
1970 "DNA complementary to viral RNA in leukemic cells induced by avian myeloblastosis virus." *Proceedings of the National Academy of Sciences* 66: 329-336.

Barber, Bernard
1952 *Science and the Social Order.* New York: Macmillan.
1961 "Resistance by scientists to scientific discovery." *Science* 134 (August 25): 596-602.

Barnes, Barry
1972 "On the reception of scientific beliefs." Pp. 269-291 in S. B. Barnes (ed.), *Sociology of Science.* Hammondsworth, England: Penguin Books.
1974 *Scientific Knowledge and Sociological Theory.* London: Routledge and Kegan Paul.
1977 *Interests and the Growth of Knowledge.* London: Routledge Direct Editions.

Baxt, W., R. Hehlmann, and S. Spiegelman
1972 "Human leukaemic cells contain reverse transcriptase associated with a high molecular weight virus-related RNA." *Nature (New Biology)* (November 15): 72-75.

Bayne-Jones, S., R. G. Harrison, C. C. Little, J. Northrop, and J. B. Murphy
1938 "Fundamental cancer research: Report of a committee appointed by the Surgeon General." *Public Health Reports 53: 2121-2130.*

Beadle, G. W.
1963 *Genetics and Modern Biology.* Philadelphia: American Philosophical Society.

Bearden, J., W. Atwood, P. Freitag, C. Hendricks, B. Mintz, and M. Schwartz
1975 "The nature and extent of bank centrality in corporate networks." Presented at the Annual Meeting of the American Sociological Association, San Francisco (August).

Ben-David, Joseph
1960 "Roles and innovations in medicine." *American Journal of Sociology* 65: 557-568.
1963 "Scientific growth: A sociological view." *Minerva* 2: 455-476.
1971 *The Scientist's Role in Society.* Englewood Cliffs, NJ: Prentice-Hall.

Ben-David, Joseph and Randall Collins
1966 "Social factors in the origins of a new science: The case for psychology." *American Sociological Review* 31: 451-465.

Ben-David, Joseph and A. Zloczower
1962 "Universities and academic systems in modern societies." *European Journal of Sociology* 31: 45-85.

Bendix, Reinhard
1975 "Science and the purposes of knowledge." *Social Research* 332-359.

Bernal, J. D.
1939 "Structures of protein." *Nature* 143: 663-667.

Bernhard, W.
1958 "Electron microscopy of tumor cells and tumor viruses." *Cancer Research* 18: 491-509.
1960 "The detection and study of tumor viruses with the electron microscope." *Cancer Research* 20: 712-727.

Bernstein, Jeremy
1978 *Experiencing Science*. New York: Basic Books.

Berry, G. P. and H. M. Dedrick
1936 "A method for changing the virus of rabbit fibroma (Shope) into that of infectious myxomatosis (Sanarelli)." *Journal of Bacteriology* 31: 50-51.

Bhaskar, R.
1975 *A Realist Theory of Science*. Leeds, England: Leeds Books.

Bittner, John J.
1936 "Some possible effects of nursing on the mammary gland tumor incidence in mice." *Science* 84: 162.

Bloor, David
1976 *Knowledge and Social Imagery*. London: Routledge and Kegan Paul.

Blume, S. S.
1974 *Toward a Political Sociology of Science*. New York: Macmillan.
1977 "Sociology of sciences and sociologies of science." Pp. 1-20 in S. S. Blume (ed.), *Perspectives in the Sociology of Science*. New York: Wiley.

Boehme, Gernot
1975 "The social function of cognitive structures: A concept of the scientific community within a theory of action." Pp. 205-225 in K. D. Knorr, H. Strasser, and H. G. Zilian (eds.), *Determinants and Controls of Scientific Development*. Dordrecht, Holland: D. Reidel.
1977 "Models for the development of science." Pp. 319-351 in Ina Spiegel-Roesing and Derek de Solla Price (eds.), *Science, Technology and Society: A Cross-Disciplinary Perspective*. Beverly Hills, CA: Sage.

Boehme, Gernot, W. van den Daele, and W. Krohn
1973 "Die Finalisierung der Wissenschaft." *Zeitschrift fuer Soziologie* 2: 128-144.

Bollum, F. J. and V. R. Potter
1958 "Incorporation of thymidine into deoxyribonucleic acid by enzymes from rat tissues." *Journal of Biological Chemistry* 233: 478-482.

Borsa, J. and A. F. Graham
1968 "Reovirus: RNA polymerase activity in purified virions." *Biochemical Research Communications* 33: 895-901.

Bott, Elizabeth
1957 *Family and Social Network*. London: Tavistock.

Bourdieu, P.
1975 "The specificity of the scientific field and the social conditions of the progress of reason." *Social Science Information* 14: 19-47.

Boveri, Theodor
1929 *The Origin of Malignant Tumors*. Trans. by Marcella Boveri from 1902 German edition. Baltimore: Williams and Wilkins.

Boyce, William E. and Richard C. DiPrima
1969 *Elementary Differential Equations and Boundary Value Problems*. New York: Wiley.

Bradford, Samuel Clement
1948 *Documentation.* London: Crosby Lockwood.
Breiger, R. L.
1976 "Career attributes and network structure: A blockmodel study of a biomedical research specialty." *American Sociological Review* 41: 117-135.
Brittain, J. M. and M. B. Line
1973 "Sources of citations and references for analysis purposes: A comparative assessment." *Journal of Documentation* 29: 72-80.
Bronson, Richard
1969 *Matrix Methods.* New York: Academic Press.
Brush, S. G.
1974 "Should the history of science be rated X?" *Science* 183 (March 22): 1164-1172.
Bud, R. F.
1978 "Strategy in American cancer research after World War II: A case study." *Social Studies of Science* 8 (November): 425-459.
Burnet, F. M.
1968 "A modern basis for pathology." *Lancet* (June 29): 1383-1387.
Butel, J. S., S. S. Tevethia, and J. L. Melnick
1972 "Oncogenicity and cell transformation by papovavirus SV40: The role of the viral genome." *Advances in Cancer Research* 15: 1-55.

Cairns, J., G. S. Stent, and J. D. Watson (eds.)
1966 *Phage and the Origins of Molecular Biology.* Cold Spring Harbor, NY: Cold Spring Harbor Laboratory.
Carlson, E. A.
1966 *The Gene: A Critical History.* Philadelphia: W. B. Saunders.
Carrese, Louis
1978 Personal interview (February 24).
Carrese, Louis M. and Carl G. Baker
1967 "The convergence technique: A method for the planning and programming of research efforts." *Management Science* 13: 420-438.
Chargaff, Erwin
1947 "On the nucleoproteins and nucleic acids of micro-organisms." *Cold Spring Harbor Symposium on Quantitative Biology* 12: 28-34.
1955 "Isolation and composition of the deoxypentose nucleic acids and of the corresponding nucleoproteins." Pp. 307-371 in E. Chargaff and J. N. Davidson (eds.), *The Nucleic Acids,* Vol. 1. New York: Academic Press.
Chubin, Daryl E.
1975 "The journal as a primary data source in the sociology of science: With some observations from sociology." *Social Science Information* 14: 157-168.
1976 "The conceptualization of scientific specialties." *Sociological Quarterly* 17: 448-476.
1978a "Review of Edge and Mulkay's *Astronomy Transformed.*" *Technology and Culture* 19: 580-583.

1978b *Intellectual Mobility, Mentorship, and Confluence in Biomedical Problem Domains: The Case of Reverse Transcriptase.* Final Technical Report on Grant No. SOC77-11593 to the National Science Foundation (November).

Chubin, Daryl E., P. T. Carroll, and K. E. Studer
1977 "Underpinnings and overselling: A comment upon two blockmodel studies of cocitation clusters." (Unpublished)

Chubin, Daryl E. and S. Moitra
1975 "Content analysis of references: Adjunct or alternative to citation counting?" *Social Studies of Science* 5: 423-441.

Chubin, D. E. and K. E. Studer
1978 "The politics of cancer." *Theory and Society* 6 (July): 55-74.
1979 "Knowledge and structures of scientific growth: Measurement of a cancer problem domain." *Scientometrics* 1 (January): 171-193.

Clark, Terry N.
1972 "The stages of scientific institutionalization." *International Social Science Journal* 24: 658-671.
1973 *Prophets and Patrons.* Cambridge, MA: Harvard University Press.

Cole, Jonathan R. and Stephen Cole
1972 "The Ortega hypothesis." *Science* 178 (October 27): 368-375.
1973 *Social Stratification in Science.* Chicago: University of Chicago Press.

Cole, Jonathan R. and H. A. Zuckerman
1975 "The emergence of a scientific specialty: The self-exemplifying case of the sociology of science." Pp. 139-174 in Lewis A. Coser (ed.), *The Idea of Social Structure: Papers in Honor of Robert K. Merton.* New York: Harcourt Brace Jovanovich.

Cole, R. K. and J. Furth
1941 "Experimental studies on the genetics of spontaneous leukemia in mice." *Cancer Research* 1: 957-965.

Cole, Stephen
1978 "Scientific reward systems: A comparative analysis." *Research in Sociology of Knowledge, Sciences, and Art* 1: 167-190.

Cole, Stephen, Jonathan R. Cole, and Lorraine Dietrich
1977a "Measuring the cognitive state of scientific disciplines." Pp. 209-251 in Y. Elkana et al. (eds.), *Toward a Metric of Science.* New York: Wiley.

Cole, Stephen, L. Rubin, and J. R. Cole
1977b "Peer review and the support of science." *Scientific American* 237: 34-41.

Collins, H. M.
1974 "The TEA set: Tacit knowledge and scientific networks." *Science Studies* 4: 165-186.

Collins, Harry and Graham Cox
1977 "Relativity revisited: Mrs. Keech—A suitable case for special treatment?" *Social Studies of Science* 7: 372-380.

Comroe, Julius H.
1978 "The road from research to new diagnosis and therapy." *Science* 200 (May 26): 931-937.

Comroe, Julius H. and Robert D. Dripps

1976 "Scientific basis for the support of biomedical science." *Science* 192 (April 9): 105-111.

Cooley, William W. and Paul R. Lohnes

1971 *Multivariate Data Analysis.* New York: Wiley.

Cooper, G. M. and Howard M. Temin

1974 "Infectious Rous sarcoma virus and reticul oendotheliosis virus DNAs." *Journal of Virology* 14: 1132-1141.

Corner, George W.

1964 *A History of the Rockefeller Institute, 1902-1953: Origins and Growth.* New York: Rockefeller Institute Press.

Cotgrove, S. and S. Box

1970 *Science, Industry, and Society: Studies in the Sociology of Science.* London: Allen & Unwin.

Crane, Diana

1965 "Scientists at major and minor universities: A study of productivity and recognition." *American Sociological Review* 30: 699-714.

1967 "The gatekeepers of science: Some factors affecting the selection of articles for scientific journals." *American Sociologist* 2: 195-201.

1971 "Transnational networks in basic science." *International Organization* 25: 585-601.

1972 *Invisible Colleges.* Chicago: University of Chicago Press.

1977 "Review of Edge and Mulkay's *Astronomy Transformed.*" *Newsletter of the Society for Social Studies of Science* 2: 27-29.

Crick, Francis H. C.

1958 "On protein synthesis." *Symposium of the Society of Experimental Biology* 12: 138-163.

1970 "Central dogma of molecular biology." *Nature* 227 (August 8): 561-563.

Crowley, C. J. and D. E. Chubin

1976 "The occupational structure of science: A log-linear analysis of the inter-sectoral mobility of American sociologists." *Sociological Quarterly* 17: 197-217.

Culliton, Barbara J.

1971 "Reverse transcription: One year later." *Science* 172 (May 28): 926-928.

1973 "Biomedical research (II): Will the 'wars' ever get started?" *Science* 181 (September 7): 921-925.

1974 "Virus cancer program: Review panel stands by criticism." *Science* (April 12): 143-145.

1976 "Kennedy hearings: Year-long probe of biomedical research begins." *Science* 193 (July 2): 32-35.

1977 "Arthur Canfield Upton: New direction of the NCI." *Science* 197 (August 19): 737-739.

Davidson, J. N. and E. Chargaff

1955 "Introduction." Pp. 1-8 in E. Chargaff and J. N. Davidson (eds.), *The Nucleic Acids,* Vol. 1. New York: Academic Press.

Dawson, M. H.

1930 "The transformation of pneumococcal types. II. The interconvertibility of type specific S pneumococci." *Journal of Experimental Medicine* 51: 123-147.

de Kervasdoue, Jean and Francois Billon

1978 "Development of research and external influences: The case of cancer and respiratory diseases." *Social Science Information* 17: 735-774.

Day, M. S.

1974 "Computer-based retrieval services at the National Library of Medicine." *Federation Proceedings* 33: 1717-1718.

Debus, A. G. (ed.)

1968 *World Who's Who in Science*. Chicago: Marquis.

Donohue, Joseph C.

1973 *Understanding Scientific Literatures: A Bibliometric Approach*. Cambridge: MIT Press.

Doppelt, Gerald

1978 "Kuhn's epistemological relativism: An interpretation and defense." *Inquiry* 21: 33-86.

Dulbecco, Renato

1966 "The plaque technique and the development of quantitative animal virology." Pp. 287-291 in J. Cairns, G. S. Stent, and J. D. Watson (eds.), *Phage and the Origins of Molecular Biology*. Cold Spring Harbor, NY: Cold Spring Harbor Laboratory of Quantitative Biology.

1967 "The induction of cancer by viruses." *Scientific American* (April): 28-37.

1973 "Cell transformation by viruses and the role of viruses in cancer." *Journal of General Microbiology* 79: 7-17.

1974 "Oncongenic viruses: The last twelve years." *Cold Spring Harbor Symposium on Quantitative Biology* 39: 1-7.

1976 "From the molecular biology of oncogenic DNA viruses to cancer." *Science* 192 (April 30): 437-440.

Duncan, O. D.

1959 "Human ecology and population studies." In P. Hauser and O. D. Duncan (eds.), *The Study of Population*. Chicago: University of Chicago Press.

Duran-Reynals, F.

1940-1941 "Production of degenerative inflammatory or neoplastic effects in the new born rabbit by the Shope fibroma virus." *Yale Journal of Biology and Medicine* 13: 99-110.

Eckhart, Walter

1972 "Oncogenic viruses." *Annual Review of Biochemistry* 41: 503-516.

1975 "The 1975 Nobel prize for physiology or medicine." *Science* 190 (November 14): 650; 712; 714.

Edge, D. O.

1977 "Why I am not a co-citationist." *Newsletter of the Society for Social Studies of Science* 2: 13-19.

Edge, D. O. and M. J. Mulkay

1976 *Astronomy Transformed: The Emergence of Radio Astronomy in Britain*. New York: Wiley.

Edsall, John T.

1962 "Proteins as macromolecules: An essay on the development of the macromolecule concept and some of its vicissitudes." *Archives of Biochemistry and Biophysics,* Supplement 1: 12-20.

Elkana, Yehuda

1978 "Two-tier thinking: Philosophical realism and historical relativism." *Social Studies of Science* 8: 309-326.

Ellermann, V. and O. Bang

1908 "Experimentelle Leukaemie bei Huhnern." *Zentralblatt fuer Bakteriologie,* I Abt. Originale 46: 595-609.

Enders, John F., F. C. Robbins, and T. H. Weller

1964 "The cultivation of the poliomyelitis viruses in tissue culture." Pp. 448-467 in *Nobel Lectures in Physiology or Medicine, 1942-1962.* New York: Elsevier.

Endicott, Kenneth M.

1969 "Trends in the support of cancer research in the United States." *Canadian Cancer Conference* 8: 1-8.

Ezrahi, Y.

1971 "The political resources of American science." *Science Studies* 1: 117-133.

Festinger, Leon

1949 "The analysis of sociograms using matrix albegra." *Human Relations* 2: 153-158.

Fisher, C. S.

1966 "The death of of a mathematical theory: A study in the sociology of knowledge." *Archive for History of Exact Sciences* 3: 137-159.

1967 "The last invariant theorists." *European Journal of Sociology* 8: 216-244.

Foster, A.

1970 *A History of Medical Bacteriology and Immunology.* London: Heineman.

Franklin, R. M. and David Baltimore

1962 "Patterns of macromolecular synthesis in normal and virus-infected mammalian cells." *Cold Spring Harbor Symposium on Quantitative Biology* 27: 175-198.

Friedkin, N. E.

1978 "University social structure and social networks among scientists." *American Journal of Sociology* 83: 1444-1465.

Fruton, Joseph S.

1966 "The Rockefeller Institute for Medical Research: An essay review." *Journal of the History of Medicine* 21: 71-77.

Furth, Jacob

1959 "A meeting of ways in cancer research: Thoughts on the evolution and nature of neoplasms." *Cancer Research* 19: 241-258.

1976 "The making and missing of discoveries: An autobiographical essay." *Cancer Research* 36: 871-880.

Gallo, Robert C.

1972 "RNA-dependent DNA polymerase in viruses and cells: Views on the current state." *Blood* 39: 117-137.

1974 "On the origin of human acute myeloblastic leukemia: Virus-'hot spot' hypothesis." Pp. 227-236 in Rolf Neth, Robert Gallo, Sol Spiegelman, and Frederick Stohlman, Jr. (eds.), *Modern Trends in Human Leukemia: Biological, Biochemical, and Virological.* London: Grune and Stratton.

Gallo, Robert C. and Sol Spiegelman

1974 "Reverse transcriptase in acute leukaemia." *Lancet* (June 1): 1117-1118.

Gallo, Robert C. and R. C. Ting

1972 "Cancer viruses." *CRC Critical Reviews in Clinical Laboratory Sciences* (December): 403-449.

Gardner, John

1966 "The government, the universities, and biomedical research." *Science* 153 (September 30): 1602-1604.

Garfield, Eugene

1972 "Citation analysis as a tool in journal evaluation." *Science* 178 (November 3): 471-479.

1974 "Journal citation studies. XV. Cancer journals and articles." *Current Contents* (October 16): 5.

1977 *Essays of an Information Scientist.* Volume 1, 1962-1973; Volume 2, 1974-1976. Philadelphia: ISI Press.

Garfield, Eugene, Morton V. Malin, and Henry Small

1977 "Citation data as science indicators." Pp. 179-207 in Y. Elkana et al. (eds.), *Toward a Metric of Science.* New York: Wiley.

Garvey, W. D. and K. Tomita

1972 "Continuity of productivity by scientists in the years 1968-71." *Science Studies* 2: 379-383.

Gaston, Jerry

1973 *Originality and Competition in Science.* Chicago: University of Chicago Press.

1978 *The Reward System in British and American Science.* New York: Wiley.

Geiduschek, E. P., T. Nakamoto, and S. B. Weiss

1961 "The enzymatic synthesis of RNA: Complementaty interaction with DNA." *Proceedings of the National Academy of Sciences* 47: 1405-1415.

Gieryn, Thomas F,

1978 "Problem retention and problem change." Pp. 96-115 in Jerry Gaston (ed.), *The Sociology of Science.* San Francisco: Jossey-Bass.

Gieryn, Thomas F. and R. K. Merton

1978 "The sociological study of scientific specialties." *Social Studies of Science* 8 (May): 257-261.

Gilbert, G. N.

1977 "Referencing as persuasion." *Social Studies of Science* 7 (February): 113-122.

1978 "Measuring the growth of science: A review of indicators of scientific growth." *Scientometrics* 1: 9-34.

Gilbert, G. N. and S. W. Woolgar

1974 "The quantitative study of science: An examination of the literature." *Science Studies* 4: 279-294.

Gilden, Raymond V.

1978 Personal interview (February 9).

Gillespie, David and Robert C. Gallo

1975 "RNA processing and RNA tumor virus origin and evolution." *Science* 188 (May 23): 802-811.

Glass, Bentley

1955 "A survey of biological abstracting, Part I." *AIBS Bulletin* 5 (January): 20-24.

1965 "A century of biochemical genetics." *Proceedings of the American Philosophical Society* 109: 227-236.

1974 "The long neglect of genetic discoveries and the criterion of prematurity." *Journal of the History of Biology* 7 (Spring): 101-110.

Goodfield, June

1977 "Humanity in science: A perspective and a plea." *Science* 198 (November 11): 580-585.

Gordon, G. and S. Marquis

1966 "Freedom, visibility of consequences and scientific innovation." *American Journal of Sociology* 72 (September): 195-202.

Gould, P. R.

1967 "On the geographical interpretation of eigenvalues." *Transactions, Institute of British Geographers,* No. 42 (December): 53-86.

Goulder, A. W.

1976 *The Dialectic of Ideology and Technology.* New York: Seabury Press.

Granovetter, Mark

1973 "The strength of weak ties." *American Journal of Sociology* 78: 1360-1380.

1976 "Network sampling: Some first steps." *American Journal of Sociology* 81: 1287-1303.

Green, Maurice

1978 Personal interview (March 15).

Green, Maurice and Gary F. Gerard

1974 "RNA-directed DNA polymerase–properties and functions in oncogenic RNA viruses and cells." *Progress in Nucleic Acid Research and Molecular Biology* 14: 187-334.

Green, Paul E.

1976 *Mathematical Tools for Applied Multivariate Analysis.* New York: Academic Press.

Green, P. E. and F. J. Carmone

1970 *Multidimensional Scaling.* New York: Allyn and Bacon.

Green, P. E. and V. R. Rao

1972 *Applied Multidimensional Scaling.* New York: Holt, Rinehart & Winston.

Greenberg, Daniel S.

1967 *The Politics of Pure Science.* New York: New American Library.

1975 "Cancer: Now, the bad news." Washington *Post* (January 19).

Greene, J. C.
1971 "The Kuhnian paradigm and the Darwinian revolution in natural history." Pp. 3-25 in D.H.D. Roller (ed.), *Perspectives in the History of Science and Technology.* Norman: University of Oklahoma Press.

Griffith, B. C., M. C. Drott, and H. G. Small
1977 "On the use of citations in studying scientific achievements and communication." *Newsletter of the Society for Social Studies of Science* 2 (Summer): 9-13.

Griffith, B. C. and N. C. Mullins
1972 "Coherent social groups in scientific change." *Science* 177 (September 15): 959-964.

Griffith, B. C., H. E. Small, J. A. Stonehill, and S. Dey
1974 "The structure of scientific literatures II: Toward a macro- and microstructure for science." *Science Studies* 4: 339-365.

Griffith, F.
1928 "The significance of pneumococcal types." *Journal of Hygiene* 27: 113-159.

Gross, L.
1970 *Oncogenic Viruses.* Oxford, England: Pergamon.

Gustafson, T.
1975 "The controversy over peer review." *Science* 190 (December 12): 1060-1066.

Haberer, Joseph
1969 *Politics and the Community of Science.* New York: Litton.

Hackett, Edward J.
1979 *Social and Cultural Influences on Contemporary Biomedical Science: A Case Study of Friend Virus Research.* Cornell University: Unpublished doctoral dissertation.

Hagstrom, Warren O.
1965 *The Scientific Community.* New York: Basic Books.
1970 "Factors related to the use of different modes of publishing research in four scientific fields." Pp. 85-124 in Carnot E. Nelson and D. K. Pollock (eds.), *Communication Among Scientists and Engineers.* Lexington, MA: Lexington Books.
1974 "Competition in science." *American Sociological Review* 39 (February): 1-18.

Hamblin, R. L., R. B. Jacobsen, and J.L.L. Miller
1973 *A Mathematical Theory of Social Change.* New York: Wiley.

Hargens, Lowell L.
1969 "Patterns of mobility of new Ph.D.s among American academic institutions." *Sociology of Education* 42 (Winter): 18-37.
1975 *Patterns of Scientific Research: A Comparative Analysis of Research in Three Scientific Fields.* Washington, DC: American Sociological Association.
1978 "Theory and method in the sociology of science." Pp. 121-139 in J. Gaston (ed.), *Sociology of Science.* San Francisco: Jossey-Bass.

Harmon, L. R.
1965 *Profiles of Ph.D.s in the Sciences: Summary Report on the Follow-Up Doctorate Cohorts, 1935-60.* Washington, DC: National Academy of Sciences–National Research Council, Publication 1293.

Hayes, W.
1966 "The discovery of pneumococcal type transformation: An appreciation." *Journal of Hygiene* 64: 177-184.

Henle, Werner, Gertrude Henle, and Evelyn T. Lennette
1979 "The Epstein-Barr virus." *Scientific American* 241 (July): 48-59.

Hershey, A. D. and M. Chase
1952 "Independent functions of viral protein and nucleic acid in growth of bacteriophage." *Journal of General Physiology* 36: 39-56.

Hess, Eugene L.
1970 "Origins of molecular biology." *Science* 168 (May 8): 664-669.

Heumann, K. F. (ed.)
1974 "Biomedical literature and information services" (Special topic issue with ten articles on information services in biomedicine). *Federation Proceedings* 33 (June): 1693-1723.

Hill, M. and J. Hillova
1972 "Virus recovery in chicken cells tested with Rous sarcoma cell DNA." *Nature (New Biology)* 237: 35-39.
1974 "RNA and DNA forms of the genetic material of C-type viruses and the integrated state of the DNA form in the cellular chromosome." *Biochimica et Biophysica Acta* 355: 7-48.

Hixson, Joseph
1976 *The Patchwork Mouse.* Garden City, NJ: Anchor Doubleday.

Holton, Gerald
1961 "On the recent past of physics." *American Journal of Physics* 29 (December): 805-810.
1962 "Models for understanding the growth and excellence of scientific research." In S. R. Graubard and G. Holton (eds.), *Excellence and Leadership in a Democracy.* New York: Columbia University Press.

Holton, Gerald and Robert S. Morison (eds.)
1978 "Limits of scientific inquiry." Thematic issue. *Daedalus* 107 (Spring).

Horsfall, F. L., Jr.
1960 "The expanding body of scientific knowledge: Implications for medical education and medical care." Presented at the Teaching Institute, Association of American Medical Colleges, Hollywood Beach, Florida.

Hotchkiss, R. E.
1965 "Oswald T. Avery." *Genetics* 31 (January): 1-10.

Huang, A. S., David Baltimore, and M. A. Bratt
1971 "Ribonucleic acid polymerase in virions of Newcastle disease virus: Comparison with vesicular stomatitis virus polymerase." *Journal of Virology* 7: 389-394.

Huebner, Robert J.
1977 "Immune protection against spontaneous and induced cancers in mice and rats based on endogenous virogene and sarcogene specific immunity: A strategy for protection against cancer in man." VI International Conference on Cancer, Perugia, Italy (July).

1978 Private communication (January 4).

Huebner, Robert J. and George J. Todaro

1969 "Oncogenes of RNA tumor viruses as determinants of cancer." *Proceedings of the National Academy of Sciences* 64: 1087-1094.

Huebner, Robert J., George J. Todaro, Padman Sarma, Janet W. Hartley, Aaron E. Freeman, Robert L. Peters, Carrie E. Whitmire, Hans Meier, and Raymond V. Gilden

1970 " 'Switched off' vertically transmitted C-type RNA tumor viruses as determinants of spontaneous and induced cancer: A new hypothesis of viral carcinogenesis." *International Symposiums of the Centre National de la Recherche Scientifique* 183: 33-57.

Hufbauer, Karl

1978 "The role of inter-specialty migrants in scientific innovation: The case of research on the stellar-energy problem, 1919-1938." Presented at the Third Annual Meeting of the Society for Social Studies of Science, Bloomington, Indiana (November 4-6).

Hull, David

1974 *Philosophy of Biological Science*. Englewood Cliffs, NJ: Prentice-Hall.

Ihde, A. J.

1969 "An inquiry into the origins of hybrid sciences: Astrophysics and biochemistry." *Journal of Chemical Education* 46 (April): 193-196.

Jacob, François and Jacques Monod

1961 "Genetic regulatory mechanisms in the synthesis of proteins." *Journal of Molecular Biology* 3: 318-356.

Johnston, Ron

1976 "Contextual knowledge: A model for the overthrow of the internal/external dichotomy in science." *Australian and New Zealand Journal of Sociology* 12 (October): 193-203.

Jones, K. S. and C. J. van Rybergen

1976 "Information retrieval test collections." *Journal of Documentation* 32 (March): 59-75.

Kalberer, John T., Jr.

1975 "Impact of the National Cancer Act on grant support." *Cancer Research* 35: 473-481.

Kang, C.-Y. and Howard M. Temin

1972 "Endogenous RNA-directed DNA polymerase activity in uninfected chicken embryos." *Proceedings of the National Academy of Sciences* 69: 5050-5054

1973 "Early DNA-RNA complex from endogenous RNA-directed DNA polymerase activity of uninfected chicken embryos." *Nature (New Biology)* 242: 206-208.

Kaplan, Abraham

1964 *The Conduct of Inquiry: Methodology for Behavioral Science*. San Francisco: Chandler.

Kaplan, N.

1965 "The norms of citation behavior: Prolegomena to the footnote." *American Documentation* 16: 179-184.

Kates, J. R. and B. R. McAuslan
1967 "Poxvirus DNA-dependent RNA polymerase." *Proceedings of the National Academy of Sciences* 58: 1134-1141.

Katz, Leo
1953 "A new status index derived from sociometric analysis." *Psychometrika* 18: 39-43.

Kendall, M. G.
1957 *A Course in Multivariate Analysis.* London: Charles Griffin.

Kennedy, T. J., Jr., R. Lamont-Havers, and J. F. Sherman
1972 "Factors contributing to current distress in the academic community." *Science* 175 (February 11): 599-607.

King, M. D.
1971 "Reason, tradition and the progressiveness of science." *History and Theory* 10: 3-32.

Klein, Marc
1963 "Trends in the methodology of endocrinological techniques." Pp. 289-302 in P. Eckstein and F. Knowles (eds.), *Techniques in Endocrine Research.* New York: Academic Press.

Knorr, Karin D.
1977 "Producing and reproducing knowledge: Descriptive or constructive?" *Social Science Information* 16: 669-696.

Kolata, G. B.
1977 "Animal viruses: Probes of cell function." *Science* 196 (April 22): 417-418.

Kornberg, Arthur
1959 "Enzymatic synthesis of deoxyribonucleic acid." Pp. 83-112 in *The Harvey Lectures,* 1957-1958, Series LIII. New York: Academic Press.
1961 *Enzymatic Synthesis of DNA.* New York: Wiley.

Kornberg, Arthur, I. R. Lehman, and E. S. Simms
1956 "Polydeoxyribonucleotide synthesis by enzymes from Escherichia coli." *Federation Proceedings* 15: 291-292.

Krohn, R. G.
1977 "Scientific ideology and scientific process: The natural history of a conceptual shift." Pp. 69-99 in E. Mendelsohn, P. Weingart, and R. Whitley (eds.), *The Social Production of Scientific Knowledge.* Sociology of the Sciences, Vol. 1. Boston: D. Reidel.

Kuhn, Thomas S.
1962 *The Structure of Scientific Revolutions.* Chicago: University of Chicago Press.
1963 "The essential tension: Tradition and innovation in scientific research." In C. W. Taylor and F. Barron (eds.), *Scientific Creativity, Its Recognition and Development.* New York: Wiley.
1970 *The Structure of Scientific Revolutions.* Chicago: University of Chicago Press.
1974 "Second thoughts on paradigms." Pp. 459-482 in F. Suppe (ed.), *The Structure of Scientific Theories.* Urbana: University of Illinois Press.

1977 "Preface." Pp. ix-xiii in T. S. Kuhn, *The Essential Tension. Selected Studies in Scientific Tradition and Change.* Chicago: University of Chicago Press.

Lakatos, Imre

1970 "Falsification and the methodology of scientific research programmes." Pp. 91-196 in I. Lakatos and A. Musgrave (eds.), *Criticism and the Growth of Knowledge.* Cambridge, MA: Cambridge University Press.

1971 "History of science and its rational reconstructions." Pp. 91-136 in Roger C. Buck and R. S. Cohen (eds.), *Boston Studies in the Philosophy of Science,* Vol. 8. Dordrecht, Holland: Reidel.

Lancaster, F. W.

1968 *Evaluation of the MEDLARS Demand Search Service.* Washington, DC: National Library of Medicine, U.S. Department of Health, Education and Welfare.

Latour, Bruno and Steve Woolgar

1979 *Laboratory Life: The Social Construction of Scientific Facts.* Beverly Hills, CA: Sage.

Laudan, Larry

1977 *Progress and Its Problems.* Berkeley: University of California Press.

Law, J.

1973 "The development of specialties in science: The case of X-ray protein crystallography." *Science Studies* 3: 275-303.

Lazarsfeld, P. F. and N. W. Henry

1968 *Latent Structure Analysis.* Boston: Houghton Mifflin.

Lederberg, Joshua

1972 "Reply to H. V. Wyatt." *Nature* 239 (September 22): 234.

Lemaine, Gerard, Roy MacLeod, Michael Mulkay, and Peter Weingart

1976 "Problems in the emergence of new disciplines." Pp. 1-23 in Lemaine et al. (eds.), *Perspectives on the Emergence of Scientific Disciplines.* The Hague, Holland: Mouton.

Levene, P. A. and L. W. Bass

1931 *Nucleic Acids.* New York: Chemical Catalog Company.

Little, C. C.

1941 "A review of progress in the study of the genetics of spontaneous tumor incidence." *Journal of the National Cancer Institute* 1 (June): 727-736.

Longo, Lawrence D.

1973 "Some problems facing biomedical research." *Federation Proceedings* 32: 2078-2085.

Lowenstein, Douglas

1979 "Despite soaring research budgets, killer diseases persist." Atlanta *Journal-Constitution* (April 8): 13-A.

Lowry, O. H., N. J. Rosebrough, A. L. Farr, and R. J. Randall

1951 "Protein measurement with the Folin phenol reagent." *Journal of Biological Chemistry* 193: 265-275.

Lowy, D. R., W. P. Rowe, N. Teich, and J. W. Hartley

1971 "Murine leukemia virus: High frequency activation *in vitro* by 5-iododeoxyuridine and 5-bromodeoxyuridine." *Science* 174: 155-156.

Luce, R. Duncan

1950 "Connectivity and generalized cliques in sociometric group structure." *Psychometrika* 15: 169-190.

Luce, R. Duncan and Albert D. Perry

1949 "A method of matrix analysis of group structure." *Psychometrika* 14: 95-116.

Luhmann, N.

1968 "Selbstseuerung der Wissenschaft." *Jahrbuch fuer Sozialwissenschaft* 19: 147-170.

Luria, S. E. and J. A. Darnell, Jr.

1968 *General Virology.* New York: Wiley.

Luria, S. E., J. E. Darnell, Jr., David Baltimore, and Allan Campbell

1978 *General Virology.* New York: Wiley.

Lwoff, Andre

1953 "Lysogeny." *Bacteriological Reviews* 17: 269-337.

1962 *Biological Order.* Cambridge: MIT Press.

1966 "The prophage and I." Pp. 88-99 in J. Cairns, G. S. Stent, and J. D. Watson (eds.), *Phage and the Origins of Molecular Biology.* Cold Spring Harbor, NY: Cold Spring Harbor Laboratory.

1972 "Interaction among virus, cell, and organism." Pp. 174-185 in *Nobel Lectures in Physiology or Medicine,* 1963-1970. New York: Elsevier.

Lyons, Gene M.

1969 *The Uneasy Partnership: Social Science and the Federal Government in the Twentieth Century.* New York: Russell Sage Foundation.

MacLeod, Roy

1977 "Changing perspectives in the social history of science." Pp. 149-195 in I. Spiegel-Roesing and D. de S. Price (eds.), *Science, Technology, and Society: A Cross-Disciplinary Perspective.* Beverly Hills, CA: Sage.

Maisin, J.

1949 *Cancer, Tome II.* Paris: Casterman Tournai.

Mannheim, Karl

1936 *Ideology and Utopia.* New York: Harcourt Brace Jovanovich.

Margalith, Miriam, Helen Thornton, Roman Narconis, Henry Pinkerton, and Maurice Green

1975 "Studies on virus induction by 5-bromodeoxyuridine in nonproducer murine sarcoma virus-transformed 3T3 cells." *Virology* 65: 27-39.

Marshino, O.

1944 "Administration of the National Cancer Institute Act, August 5, 1937 to June 30, 1943." *Journal of the National Cancer Institute* 4: 429-443.

Martins, H.

1972 "The Kuhnian 'revolution' and its implications for sociology." Pp. 13-58 in T. J. Nossiter (ed.), *Imagination and Precision in the Social Sciences.* London: Faber and Faber.

Marx, J. L.

1977 "Persistent infections: The role of viruses." *Science* 196 (April 8): 151-152.

1978a "RNA tumor viruses: Getting a handle on transformation." *Science* 199 (January 13): 161-164.

1978b "Function of the *src* gene product." *Science* 201 (August 15): 702.

Maugh, Thomas H.

1974a "Chemical carcinogenesis: A long-neglected field blossoms." *Science* 183 (March 8): 940-944.

1974b "RNA viruses: The age of innocence ends." *Science* (March 22): 1181-1185.

McAllister, Robert M.

1973 "Viruses in human carcinogenesis." *Progress in Medical Virology* 16: 48-85.

McFarland, David D. and Daniel J. Brown

1973 "Social distance as a metric: A systematic introduction to smallest space analysis." Pp. 213-253 in Edward O. Laumann, *Bonds of Pluralism: The Form and Substance of Urban Social Networks.* New York: Wiley-Interscience.

McGinnis, Robert

1972 *Federal Funding and Graduate Education in Bioscience.* Report prepared for the Office of Scientific Personnel, National Research Council (February).

Meadows, A. J. and J. G. O'Connor

1971 "Bibliographical statistics as a guide to growth points in science." *Science Studies* 1 (January): 95-98.

Medvedev, Zhores A.

1969 *The Rise and Fall of T. D. Lysenko.* New York: Anchor Doubleday.

Menard, H. W.

1971 *Science: Growth and Change.* Cambridge, MA: Harvard University Press.

Mendelsohn, Everett

1969 "Commentary." *Journal of the History of Biology* 2: 135-140.

1977 "The social construction of scientific knowledge." Pp. 3-26 in E. Mendelsohn, P. Weingart, and R. Whitley (eds.), *The Social Production of Scientific Knowledge.* Sociology of the Sciences, Volume I. Boston: Reidel.

Mendelsohn, Everett, Dorothy Nelkin, and Peter Weingart

1979 "The social assessment of science (Bielefeld, 26-28 May 1978)." *Social Studies of Science* 9: 125-133.

Mendenhall, William

1971 *Introduction to Probability and Statistics.* Belmont, CA: Duxbury Press.

Merton, Robert K.

1942 "Science and technology in a democratic order." *Journal of Legal and Political Sociology* 1: 115-126.

1949 *Social Theory and Social Structure.* New York: Macmillan.

1957 "Priorities in scientific discovery: A chapter in the sociology of science." *American Sociological Review* 22: 635-659.

1961 "Singletons and multiples in scientific discovery: A chapter in the sociology of science." *Proceedings of the American Philosophical Society* 105 (October 13): 470-486.

1965 "The ambivalence of scientists." Pp. 112-132 in N. Kaplan (ed.), *Science and Society.* Skokie, IL: Rand McNally.

1968 "The Matthew effect in science." *Science* 159 (January 5): 56-63.

1972 "Insiders and outsiders: A chapter in the sociology of knowledge." *American Journal of Sociology* 77 (July): 9-47.

1977 "The sociology of science: An episodic memoir." Pp. 3-141 in R. K. Merton and J. Gaston (eds.), *The Sociology of Science in Europe*. Carbondale: Southern Illinois University Press.

Meynell, Hugo

1977 "On the limits of the sociology of knowledge." *Social Studies of Science* 7 (November): 489-500.

Miller, James A.

1970 "Carcinogenesis by chemicals: An overview." *Cancer Research* 30 (March): 559-576.

Millstone, Erik

1978 "A framework for the sociology of knowledge." *Social Studies of Science* 8: 111-125.

Mitroff, I. I.

1974a "Norms and counter-norms in a select group of the Apollo moon scientists: A case study of the ambivalence of scientists." *American Sociological Review* 39 (August): 579-595.

1974b *The Subjective Side of Science: A Philosophical Enquiry into the Psychology of the Apollo Moon Scientists.* New York: Elsevier.

Mitroff, I. I. and D. E. Chubin

1979 "Peer review at NSF: A dialectical policy analysis." *Social Studies of Science* 9 (May): 199-232.

Monaghan, Jean

1974 "Flow Labs–Leading producer of biological products." *Investment Dealers Digest 40 (March 5): 19-20.*

Moore, D. H., J. Charney, B. Kramarsky, E. Y. Lasfargues, M. J. Brennan, J. H. Burrows, S. M. Sirsat, J. C. Paymaster, and A. B. Vaidya

1970 "Search for a human breast cancer cirus." *Nature* 229 (February 26): 611-615.

Moravcsik, M. J.

1973 "Measures of scientific growth." *Research Policy* 2: 266-275.

Moravcsik, M. J. and P. Murugesan

1975 "Some results on the function and quality of citations." *Science Studies* 5: 86-92.

Morison, Robert S.

1969 "Science and social attitudes." *Science* 165 (July 11): 150-165.

Mulkay, M. J.

1969 "Some aspects of cultural growth in the natural sciences." *Social Research* 36 (Spring): 22-52.

1972 *Social Process of Innovation.* New York: Macmillan.

1974a "Methodology in the sociology of science: Some reflections on the study of radio astronomy." *Social Science Information* 13: 107-119.

1974b "Conceptual displacement and migration in science: A prefatory paper." *Science Studies* 4: 205-234.

1975 "Three Models of scientific development." *Sociological Review* 23: 509-538.

1976 "Norms and ideology in science." *Social Science Information* 15: 637-656.

1978 "Consensus in science." *Social Science Information* 17: 107-122.

Mulkay, M. J. and D. O. Edge

1973 "Cognitive, technical and social factors in the growth of radio astronomy." *Social Science Information* 12: 25-61.

Mulkay, M. J., G. N. Gilbert, and S. Woolgar

1975 "Problem areas and research networks in science." *Sociology* 9: 187-203.

Mullins, Nicholas C.

1968 "The distribution of social and cultural properties in informal communication networks among biological scientists." *American Sociological Review* 33: 786-797.

1972 "The development of a scientific specialty: The phage group and the origins of molecular biology." *Minerva* 10 (January): 52-82.

1973 *Theories and Theory Groups in Contemporary American Sociology.* New York: Harper and Row.

1975 "A sociological theory of normal and revolutionary science." In K. D. Knorr et al. (eds.), *Determinants and Controls of Scientific Development.* Boston: Reidel.

Mullins, N. C., L. L. Hargens, P. K. Hecht, and E. L. Kick

1977 "The group structure of cocitation clusters: a comparative study." *American Sociological Review* 42 (August): 552-562.

Munyon, W., E. Paoletti, and J. T. Grace, Jr.

1967 "RNA polymerase activity in purified infectious vaccinia virus." *Proceedings of the National Academy of Sciences* 58: 2280-2287.

Nadel, S. F.

1957 *Theory of Social Structure.* London: Cohen and West.

Narin, F.

1976 *Evaluative Bibliometrics, Final Report to NSF.* Cherry Hill, N.J: Computer Horizons.

Neiman, P. E.

1972 "Rous sarcoma virus nucleotide sequences in cellular DNA: Measurement by RNA-DNA hybridization." *Science* 178: 750-753.

Nelkin, Dorothy

1975a "Changing images of science: New Pressures on old stereotypes." *Newsletter 14 of the Program on Public Conceptions of Science,* Harvard University: 21-31.

1975b "The political impact of technical expertise." *Social Studies of Science* 5 (February): 35-54.

1978 "Threats and promises: Negotiating the control of research." *Daedalus* 107 (Spring): 191-209

Northrup, J. H.

1962 "Infectious macromolecules." *Archives of Biochemistry and Biophysics,* Supplement 1: 7-11.

O'Connor, T. E.

1973 "Reverse transcriptase–progress, problems and prospects." Pp. 1165-1181 in R. M. Dutcher and L. Chieco-Bianchi (eds.), *International Symposium of Comparative Leukemia Research* 39. Basel, Switzerland: Karger.

Olby, Robert

1970 "Francis Crick, DNA, and the central dogma." *Daedalus* 99: 938-987.

1972 "Avery in retrospect." *Nature* 239 (September 29): 295-296.

1974a "The origins of molecular genetics." *Journal of the History of Biology* 7 (Spring): 93-100.

1974b *The Path to the Double Helix*. New York: Macmillan.

Orlans, Harold

1971 "Social science research policies in the United States." *Minerva* 9: 7-31.

1975 "Neutrality and advocacy in policy research." *Policy Sciences* 6: 107-119.

Overington, Michael A.

1979 "Doing what comes rationally: Some developments in metatheory." *American Sociologist* 14 (February): 2-12.

Park, Robert E.

1928 "Human migration and the marginal man." *American Journal of Sociology* 33: 881-892.

Parks, W. P., R. V. Gilden, A. F. Bykovsky, G. G. Miller, V. M. Zhadanov, V. D. Soloviev, and E. M. Scolnick

1973 "Mason-Pfizer virus characterization: A similar virus in a human amniotic cell line." *Journal of Virology* 12: 1540-1547.

Pelz, Donald C. and Frank M. Andrews

1976 *Scientists in Organizations: Productive Climates for Research and Development*. Ann Arbor: University of Michigan.

Peterson, James C. and Gerald E. Markle

1979 "Politics and science in the Laetrile controversy." *Social Studies of Science* 9 (May): 139-166.

Phillips, D. L.

1974 "Epistemology and the sociology of knowledge: The contributions of Mannheim, Mills, and Merton." *Theory and Society* 1: 59-88.

Pielou, R. V.

1969 *An Introduction to Mathematical Ecology*. New York: Wiley-Interscience.

Pigman, Ward

1973 "Government support of biomedical research." *Federation Proceedings* 32: 1731-1734.

Pirsig, Robert M.

1974 *Zen and the Art of Motorcycle Maintenance*. New York: Bantam Books.

Polanyi, Michael

1966 *The Tacit Dimension*. New York: Anchor Doubleday.

Popper, Karl R.

1973 "The rationality of scientific revolutions." Pp. 72-101 in R. Harre (ed.), *Problems of Scientific Revolution: Progress and Obstacles to Progress in the Sciences*. Oxford, England: Clarendon Press.

Potter, Van Rensselaer
1964 "Biochemical perspectives in cancer research." *Cancer Research* 24: 1085-1098.

Price, Derek de Solla
1963 *Little Science, Big Science.* New York: Columbia University Press.
1965 "Networks of scientific papers." *Science* 149 (July 30): 510-515.
1969 "Measuring the size of science." *Proceedings of the Israel Academy of Sciences and Humanities* 4: 98-111.
1970 "Citation measures of hard science, soft science, technology and non-science." Pp. 3-22 in Carnot Nelson and D. Pollock (eds.), *Communication Among Scientists and Engineers.* Lexington, MA: D. C. Heath.
1975 *Science Since Babylon.* New Haven, CT: Yale University Press.

Pyenson, Lewis
1977 " 'Who the guys were': Prosopography in the history of science." *History of Science* 15: 155-188.

Rauscher, Frank J.
1974 "Budget and the National Cancer Program." *Science* 184 (May 24): 871-875.
1975 "Research and the National Cancer Program." *Science* 189 (July 11): 115-119.
1978 Personal interview (21 March).

Ravetz, J. R.
1971 *Scientific Knowledge and Its Social Problems.* Oxford, England: Oxford University Press.

Ravin, A. W.
1961 "The genetics of transformation." *Advances in Genetics* 10: 61-163.

Reif, Arnold E.
1958 "International cancer congress." *Science* 128 (December 12): 1512-1522.

Rettig, Richard A.
1977 *Cancer Crusade: The Story of the National Cancer Act of 1971.* Princeton, NJ: Princeton University Press.
1978 "Testimony before the Subcommittee on Nutrition, Committee on Agriculture, Nutrition, and Forestry, U.S. Senate." (June 12) (Mimeo).

Richter, Maurice N., Jr.
1972 *Science as a Cultural Process.* Cambridge, MA: Schenkman.

Rokutanda, M., H. Rokutanda, M. Green, K. Fujinaga, R. K. Ray, and C. Gurgo.
1970 "Formation of viral RNA-DNA hybrid molecules by the DNA polymerase of sarcoma-leukemia Viruses." *Nature* 227 (September 5): 1026-1028.

Rose, Steven
1967 "The S curve considered." *Technology and Society* 4: 33-39.

Ross, J., E. M. Scolnick, G. J. Todaro, and S. A. Aaronson
1971 "Separation of murine cellular and murine leukaemia virus DNA polymerases." *Nature (New Biology)* 231 (June 9): 163-167.

Rous, Peyton
1911a "A sarcoma of the fowl transmissible by an agent separable from the tumor cells." *Journal of Experimental Medicine* 13: 397-411.

1911b "Transmission of a malignant new growth by means of a cell-free filtrate." *Journal of American Medical Association* 56 (January 21): 198.
1959 "Surmise and fact on the nature of cancer." *Nature* 183: 1357-1361.

Rous, P. and J. W. Beard
1934-1935 "Carcinomatous changes in virus-induced papillomas of the skin of the rabbit." *Proceedings of the Society of Experimental Biology and Medicine* 32: 578-580.

Rule, J. B.
1978 "Models of relevance: The social effects of sociology." *American Journal of Sociology* 84 (July): 78-98.

Ruse, M. E.
1970 "The revolution in biology." *Theoria* 36: 1-22.
1971a "Two biological revolutions." *Dialectica* 25: 17-28.
1971b "Reduction, replacement, and molecular biology." *Dialectica* 25: 39-72.
1973 *The Philosophy of Biology.* London: Hutchinson.

Ryder, N. B.
1965 "The cohort as a concept in the study of social change." *American Sociological Review* 30 (December): 843-861.

Salomon, J.-J.
1972 "The mating of knowledge and power." *Impact of Science on Society* 22 (January-June): 123-132.

Sambrook, Joe
1972 "Transformation by polyoma virus and simian virus 40." *Advances in Cancer Research* 16: 141-180.

Sawyer, R. A.
1963 *Experimental Spectroscopy.* New York: Dover.

Schaffner, Kenneth F.
1969 "Theories and explanations in biology." *Journal of the History of Biology* 2: 19-32.
1974 "The peripherality of reductionism in the development of molecular biology." *Journal of the History of Biology* 7: 111-139.
1976 "The Watson-Crick model and reductionism." Pp. 101-127 in R. S. Cohen and M. W. Wartofsky (eds.), *Boston Studies in the Philosophy of Science,* Vol. 27. Boston: D. Reidel.

Scheffler, I.
1967 *Science and Subjectivity.* Indianpolis: Bobbs-Merrill.

Schlom, Jeffrey
1978 Personal interview (February 28).

Schon, D. A.
1963 *Displacement of Concepts.* London: Tavistock.

Science Citation Index
1965-1977 *Source Index* and *Citation Index.* Philadelphia: Institute for Scientific Information.

Searle, S. R. and W. H. Hausman
1970 *Matrix Algebra for Busii.ess and Economics.* New York: Wiley-Intersience.

Shapere, Dudley
1966 "Meaning and scientific change." Pp. 41-85 in R. G. Colodny (ed.), *Mind and Cosmos: Essays in Contemporary Science and Philosophy.* Pittsburgh: University of Pittsburgh Press.

1969a "Biology and the unity of science." *Journal of the History of Biology* 2: 3-18.

1969b "Notes toward a post-positivistic interpretation of science." Pp. 115-160 in P. Achinstein and S. F. Barker (eds.), *Legacy of Logical Positivism.* Baltimore: Johns Hopkins Press.

1974 "Scientific theories and their domains." Pp. 518-565 in F. Suppe (ed.), *Structure of Scientific Theories.* Urbana: University of Illinois Press.

Shatkin, A. J. and J. D. Sipe

1968 "RNA polymerase activity in purified reoviruses." *Proceedings of the National Academy of Sciences* 61: 1462-1463.

Shils, Edward

1961 "Centre and periphery." Pp. 117-130 in *Logic of Personal Knowledge: Essays Presented to Michael Polanyi on His Seventieth Birthday, 11th March 1961.* London: Routledge and Kegan Paul.

1972a "Anti-science: Observations on the recent 'crisis' of science." Pp. 33-49 in *CIBA Foundation Symposium, Civilization and Science in Conflict or Collaboration?* Amsterdam: Associated Scientific Publishers.

1972b "Metropolis and province in the intellectual community." Pp. 355-371 in Edward Shils, *Intellectuals and the Powers and Other Essays.* Chicago: University of Chicago Press.

Shimkin, Michael B.

1974 "History of cancer research: A starter reading list and guide." *Cancer Research* 34 (June): 1519-1520.

Shockley, William

1957 "On the statistics of individual variations of productivity in research laboratories." *Proceedings of the IRE* (January): 279-290.

Shope, Richard E.

1932 "A filtrable virus causing a tumor-like condition in rabbits and its relationship to virus myxomatosum." *Journal of Experimental Medicine* 56: 803-822.

1933 "Infectious papillomatosis of rabbits." *Journal of Experimental Medicine* 58: 607-623.

1937 "Immunization of rabbits to infectious papillomatosis." *Journal of Experimental Medicine* 65: 219-231.

1966 "Evolutionary episodes in the concept of viral oncogenesis." *Perspectives on Biological Medicine* 9 (Winter): 258-274.

Shoyab, M., M. A. Baluda, and R. Evans

1974 "Acquisition of new DNA sequences after infection of chicken cells with avian myeloblastosis virus." *Journal of Virology* 13: 331-339.

Slye, M.

1931 "The relation of heredity to the occurrence of spontaneous leukemia, pseudo-leukemia, lymphosarcoma and allied diseases in mice (preliminary report)." *American Journal of Cancer* 15: 1361-1368.

Small, Henry G.

1973 "Co-citation in the scientific literature: A new measure of the relationship between two documents." *Journal of the American Society for Informational Sciences* 24: 265-269.

1974 "Multiple citation patterns in scientific literature: The circle and hill models." *Information Storage and Retrieval* 10: 393-402.

1977 "A co-citation model of a scientific specialty: A longitudinal study of Collagen research." *Social Studies of Science* 7 (May): 139-166.

Small, Henry and B. C. Griffith

1974 "The structure of scientific literatures I: Identifying and graphing specialties." *Science Studies* 4: 17-40.

1978 "The mapping of science." Presented at the Third Annual Meeting, Society for Social Studies of Science, Bloomington, Indiana (3-5 November).

Smart, J.J.C.

1963 *Philosophy and Scientific Realism.* London: Routledge and Kegan Paul.

Smith, R. Jeffrey

1979 "NCI bioassays yield a trail of blunders." *Science* 204 (June 22): 1287-1292.

Spiegel-Roesing, Ina

1977 "The study of science, technology, and society (SSTS): Recent trends and future challenges." Pp. 7-42 in I. Spiegel-Roesing and D. de S. Price (eds.), *Science, Technology, and Society: A Cross-Disciplinary Perspective.* Beverly Hills, CA: Sage.

Spiegel-Roesing, Ina and D. de S. Price (eds.)

1977 *Science, Technology and Society: A Cross-Disciplinary Perspective.* Beverly Hills, CA: Sage.

Spiegelman, Sol

1978 Personal interview (March 21).

Spiegelman, S., A. Burny, M. R. Das, J. Keydar, J. Schlom, M. Travnicek, and K. Watson

1970 "Characterization of the products of RNA-Directed DNA polymerases in oncogenic RNA viruses." *Nature* 227 (August 8): 563-567.

Stent, Gunther S.

1967 "Induction and repression of enzyme synthesis." Pp. 152-161 in G. C. Quarton, T. Melnechuk, and F. O. Schmitt (eds.), *Neurosciences.* New York: Rockefeller University Press.

1969 *The Coming of the Golden Age.* Garden City, NY: Natural History Press.

1972 "Prematurity and uniqueness in scientific discovery." *Scientific American* 227 (December): 84-93.

Storer, Norman W.

1966 *The Social System of Science.* New York: Holt, Rinehart & Winston.

1967 "The hard sciences and the soft." *Bulletin of the Medical Library Association* 55 (January): 75-84.

1974 "Science as nonautonomous: Book review of *Toward a Political Sociology of Science.*" *Science* 185 (July 12): 137.

Strickland, S.

1972 *Politics, Science, and Dread Disease.* Cambridge, MA: Harvard University Press.

Studer, Kenneth E.

1977a "Interpreting scientific growth: A comment on Derek Price's 'Science since Babylon.' " *History of Science* 15: 44-51.

1977b *Growth and Specialization in Contemporary Biomedicine: The Case of Reverse Transcriptase.* Cornell University: Unpublished doctoral dissertation.

Studer, Kenneth E. and Daryl E. Chubin

1976 "The heroic age of reproductive endocrinology: Its development and structure." *Proceedings of the First Annual Meeting, Society for Social Studies of Science.* Ithaca, NY: Cornell University (November 4-6).

1977 "Ethics and the unintended consequences of social research: A perspective from the sociology of science." *Policy Sciences* 8: 111-124.

Sullivan, D. F.

1975 "Competition in bio-medical science: Extent, structure, and consequences." *Sociology of Education* 48 (Spring): 223-241.

Sullivan, D. F. and D. H. Whyte

1977 "Review of Edge of Mulkay's *Astronomy Transformed.*" *Newsletter of the Society for Social Studies of Science* 2 (Fall): 25-27.

Sullivan, D., D. H. Whyte, and E. J. Barboni

1977a "The state of a science: Indicators in the specialty of weak interactions." *Social Studies of Science* 7 (May): 167-200.

1977b "Co-citation analyses of science: An evaluation." *Social Studies of Science* 7 (May): 223-240.

Syverton, Jerome T.

1960 "Present status of studies on tumor producing viruses." *National Cancer Monograph* 4: 345-353.

Tagliacozzo, Renata

1977 "Self-citations in scientific literature." *Journal of Documentation* 33 (December): 251-265.

Teich, Mikulas

1975 "A single path to the double helix?" *History of Science* 13: 264-283.

Temin, Howard M.

1963 "The effects of actinomycin D on growth of Rous sarcoma virus *in vitro.*" *Virology* 20: 577-582.

1964a "Homology between RNA from Rous sarcoma virus and DNA from Rous sarcoma virus-infected cells." *Proceedings of the National Academy of Sciences* 52: 323-329.

1964b "Nature of the provirus of Rous sarcoma." *National Cancer Institute Monograph* 17: 557-570.

1967 "Studies on carcinogenesis by avian sarcoma viruses." Pp. 709-715 in J. S. Colter and W. Paranchych (eds.), *The Molecular Biology of Viruses.* New York: Academic Press.

1970a "Formation and activation of the provirus of RNA sarcoma viruses." Pp. 233-249 in R. D. Barry and B.W.J. Mahy (eds.), *The Biology of Large RNA Viruses.* New York: Academic Press.

1970b "Malignant transformation of cells by viruses." *Perspectives in Biology and Medicine* 13 (Autumn): 11-26.

1971 "The protovirus hypothesis: Speculations on the significance of RNA-directed DNA synthesis for normal development and for carcinogenesis." *Journal of the National Cancer Institute* 46: iii-vii.

1972 "RNA-directed DNA synthesis." *Scientific American* 226: 25-33.

1974 "On the origin of RNA tumor viruses." *Annual Review of Genetics* 8: 155-177.

1976 "The DNA provirus hypothesis: The establishment and implications of RNA-directed DNA synthesis." *Science* 192 (June 11): 1075-1080.

1978 Personal interview (March 16).

Temin, Howard M. and David Baltimore

1972 "RNA-directed DNA synthesis and RNA tumor viruses." *Advances in Virus Research* 17: 129-186.

Temin, Howard M. and Satoshi Mizutani

1970 "RNA-dependent DNA polymerase in virions of Rous sarcoma virus." *Nature* 226 (June 27): 1211-1213.

Thackray, Arnold

1977 "Measurement in the historiography of science." Pp. 11-30 in Y. Elkana et al. (eds.), *Toward a Metric of Science.* New York: Wiley.

Thomas, Lewis

1977 "Biomedical science and human health: The long-range prospect." Pp. 163-171 in *Discoveries and Interpretations: Studies in Contemporary Scholarship,* Vol. 1, *Daedalus* (Summer).

Tinkler, K. J.

1972 "The physical interpretation of eigenfunctions of dichotomous matrices." *Transactions, Institute of British Geographers* 55 (March): 17-46.

Todaro, George

1978 Personal interview (February 23).

Todaro, G. J., R. E. Benveniste, R. Callahan, M. M. Lieber, and C. J. Sherr

1975 "Endogenous primate and feline type C viruses." *Cold Spring Harbor Symposium on Quantitative Biology* 29: 1159-1168.

Todaro, George J. and Robert J. Huebner

1972 "The viral oncogene hypothesis: New evidence." *Proceedings of the National Academy of Sciences* 69: 1009-1015.

Toulmin, Stephen

1972 "The historical background to the anti-science movement." Pp. 23-32 in *CIBA Foundation Symposium, Civilization and Science in Conflict or Collaboration?* Amsterdam: Associated Scientific Publishers.

1977 "From form to function: Philosophy and history of science in the 1950s and now." Pp. 143-162 in *Discoveries and Interpretations: Studies in Contemporary Scholarship,* Vol. 1. *Daedalus* (Summer).

Turner, S. P. and D. E. Chubin

1976 "Another appraisal of Ortega, the Coles, and science policy: The Ecclesiastes hypothesis." *Social Science Information* 15: 657-662.

1979 "Chance and eminence in science: Ecclesiastes II." *Social Science Information* 18: 437-449.

U.S. National Institutes of Health (NIH)

1975 *NIH Almanac, 1975.* Washington, DC: Government Printing Office (DHEW Publication, NIH 75-5).

U.S. National Library of Medicine

1974 *Medical Subject Headings Tree Structures.* U.S. Department of Commerce: National Technical Information Service.

U.S. Senate

1971a *Conquest of Cancer Act, 1971.* Hearings before the Subcommittee on Health of the Committee on Labor and Public Welfare, U.S. Senate, Ninety-Second Congress. Washington, DC: U.S. Government Printing Office.

1971b *National Program for the Conquest of Cancer.* Report of the National Panel of Consultants on the Conquest of Cancer, prepared for the Committee on Labor and Public Welfare, U.S. Senate. Washington, DC: Government Printing Office.

1972 *National Heart, Blood Vessel, Lung, and Blood Act of 1972.* Hearing before the Subcommittee on Health of the Committee on Labor and Public Welfare, U.S. Senate, Ninety-Second Congress. Washington, DC: Government Printing Office.

van den Daele, W., W. Krohn, and P. Weingart

1977 "The political direction of scientific development." Pp. 219-242 in E. Mendelsohn et al. (eds.), *The Social Production of Scientific Knowledge.* Sociology of the Sciences, Vol. 1. Boston: D. Reidel.

Varmus, H. E., S. Heasley, and J. M. Bishop

1974 "Use of DNA-DNA annealing to detect new virus-specific DNA sequences in chicken embryo fibroblasts after infection by avian sarcoma virus." *Journal of Virology* 14: 895-903.

Virgo, J. A.

1970 "An evaluation of *Index Medicus* and *MEDLARS.*" *Journal of the American Society for Information Science* 21: 254-270.

Waddington, C. H.

1969 "Some European contributions to the prehistory of molecular biology." *Nature* 221 (January 15): 318-321.

Wade, Nicholas

1976 "Cancer Institute: Expert charges neglect of carcinogenesis studies." *Science* 192 (May 7): 529-531.

Wagner, Robert P.

1968 "Genetics–A century after Mendel." *Graduate Journal* 8: 179-197.

Waksman, S. A.

1969 "Microbiology as a field of science and application." *American Scientist* 57 (Autumn): 364-371.

Watson, James D.

1965 *Molecular Biology of the Gene.* Menlo Park, CA: Benjamin/Cummings.

1968 *The Double Helix.* New York: Atheneum.

1970 *Molecular Biology of the Gene.* Menlo Park, CA: Benjamin/Cummings.

1976 *Molecular Biology of the Gene.* Menlo Park, CA: Benjamin/Cummings.

Watson, James D. and Francis H. C. Crick

1953 "Genetical implications of the structure of deoxyribonucleic acid." *Nature* 171: 964-967.

Webb, E. J., D. T. Campbell, R. D. Schwartz, and L. Sechrest

1966 *Unobtrusive Measures: Nonreactive Research in the Social Sciences.* Skokie, IL: Rand-McNally.

Weinberg, Alvin M.

1961 "Impact of large-scale science on the United States." *Science* 134 (July 21): 161-164.

1965 "The coming age of biomedical science." *Minerva* 4: 3-14.

1967 *Reflections on Big Science.* Cambridge: MIT Press.

Weingart, Peter

1977 "Science policy and the development of science." Pp. 51-70 in S. S. Blume (ed.), *Perspectives in the Sociology of Science.* New York: Wiley.

Weinstock, M.
1971 "Citation indexes." Pp. 16-40 in *Encyclopedia of Library and Information Science.* New York: Marcel Dekker, Inc.

Weiss, S. B.
1960 "Enzymatic incorporation of ribonucleotide triphosphates into the inter-polynucleotide linkages of ribonucleic acid." *Proceedings of the National Academy of Sciences* 46: 1020-1030.

Whitley, R. D.
1972 "Black boxism and the sociology of science: A discussion of the major developments in the field." Pp. 61-92 in P. Halmos (ed.), *Sociology of Science. Sociological Review Mongraph* 18 (September).
1974 "Cognitive and social institutionalization of scientific specialties and research areas." Pp. 69-95 in R. D. Whitley (ed.), *Social Processes of Scientific Development.* London: Routledge and Kegan Paul.
1977 "The sociology of scientific work and the history of scientific developments." Pp. 21-50 in S. S. Blume (ed.), *Perspectives in the Sociology of Science.* New York: Wiley.

Williams, A. O., G. M. Carter, A. J. Harmon, E. B. Keeler, W. G. Manning, Jr., C. R. Neu, M. L. Pearce, and R. A. Rettig.
1976 *Policy Analysis for Federal Biomedical Research.* Prepared for the President's Biomedical Research Panel. Santa Monica, CA: Rand Corporation.

Williams, G.
1960 *Virus Hunters.* London: Hutchinson.

Winch, Peter
1958 *The Idea of a Social Science and Its Relation to Philosophy.* London: Routledge and Kegan Paul.

Wood, W. B.
1961 *From Miasmas to Molecules.* New York: Columbia University Press.

Woolgar, S. W.
1976a "The identification and definition of scientific collectivities." Pp. 233-245 in Gerard Lamaine et al. (eds.), *Perspectives on the Emergence of Scientific Disciplines.* The Hague, Holland: Mouton.
1976b "Writing an intellectual history of scientific development: The use of discovery accounts." *Social Studies of Science* 6: 395-422.

Wu, A. M. and R. C. Gallo
1974 "Life cycle of RNA oncogenic viruses." Pp. 148-156 in Rolf Neth, Robert Gallo, Sol Spiegelman, and Frederick Stohlman, Jr. (ed.), *Modern Trends in Human Leukemia: Biological, Biochemical, and Virological.* London: Grune and Stratton.

Wyatt, H. V.
1972 "When does information become knowledge?" *Nature* 235 (January 14): 86-89.
1975 "Knowledge and prematurity: The journey from transformation to DNA." *Perspectives in Biology and Medicine* 18: 149-156.

Zenzen, Michael J.
1978 "Sociology of knowledge as theory of rationality." Presented at the Third Annual Meeting of the Society for Social Studies of Science, Bloomington, Indiana (November 4-6).

Zhadnov, V. M. and T. I. Tikchonenko
1974 "Viruses as a factor of evolution: Exchange of genetic information in the biosphere." *Advances in Virus Research* 19: 361-394.

Zilber, L. A. and G. I. Abelev
1968 *The Virology and Immunology of Cancer.* Trans. from Russian by Ruth Schachter. New York: Pergamon.

Ziman, John
1968 *Public Knowledge: An Essay Concerning the Social Dimension of Science.* New York: Cambridge University Press.

Zubrod, C. G., S. Schepartz, L. M. Carrese, and C. G. Baker
1966 "The chemotherapy program of the National Cancer Institute: History, analysis, and plans." *Cancer Chemotherapy Reports* 50: 348-540.

Zuckerman, Harriet A.
1968 "Patterns of name ordering among authors of scientific papers: A study of social symbolism and its ambiguity." *American Journal of Sociology* 74: 276-291.
1972 "Interviewing an ultra-elite." *Public Opinion Quarterly* 36 (Summer): 159-175.
1977 *Scientific Elite: Nobel Laureates in the United States.* New York: Macmillan.

Zuckerman, Harriet and Robert K. Merton
1972 "Age, aging, and age structure in science." In M. W. Riley, M. Johnson, and A. Foner (eds.), *A Sociology of Age Stratification,* Vol. 3. New York: Russell Sage Foundation.

ABOUT THE AUTHORS

Kenneth E. Studer is Assistant Professor of Sociology and Anthropology at Virginia Commonwealth University and is also an Advisory Editor of *Sociological Quarterly*. He is the coauthor of "Reflections on Alvin M. Weinberg: A Case Study on the Social Foundations of Science Policy" published in *Research Policy* (1975) and "Ethics and the Unintended Consequences of Social Research: A Perspective from the Sociology of Science" published in *Policy Research* (1976). Mr. Studer is currently pursuing further research in network analysis and studies of the social structure of hypertension.

Daryl E. Chubin is Associate Professor in the Department of Social Sciences at the Georgia Institute of Technology. His current interests center on ethical and value dimensions of research, interdisciplinary problem solving, and theory-method relations in science studies. He is completing a book on these and other themes. Dr. Chubin serves as an associate editor of *Scientometrics, Social Studies of Science,* and *The American Sociologist*, and as a member of the Council of the Society for Social Studies of Science.